MW00950725

PANCE AND PANRE QUESTION BOOK
SECOND EDITION

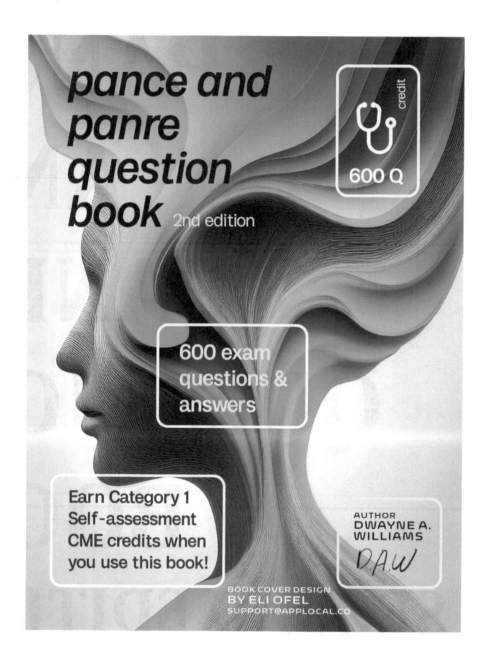

Copyright © 2024 Dwayne A. Williams
All rights reserved
ISBN: 9798333293565
Imprint: Independently published

Printed by Kindle direct publishing platform

Book cover design: Eli Ofel: support@applocal.co

Earn 20 AAPA-approved Self-Assessment CME credit when using this book!!

Go to www.pancepreppearls.com to download the forms to claim your credit for using this book.

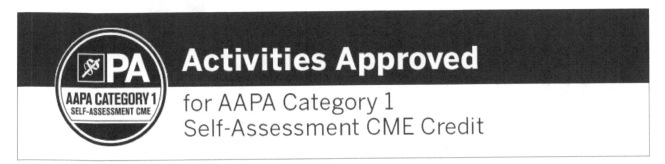

Want to earn even more AAPA-approved Self-Assessment CME credits???
PANCE PREP APP AVAILABLE ON IPHONE PLATFORMS!
EARN 20 CATEGORY 1 SELF-ASSESSMENT CME CREDITS
Go to Panceprepapp.io for more information

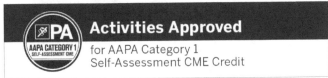

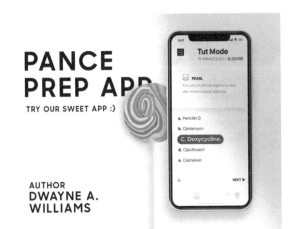

Over 15,000 clinically based practice examination questions specifically formulated to enhance clinical skills and improve performance on examinations, such as the PANCE, PANRE, OSCES, USMLE, end of rotation examinations and comprehensive medical examinations.

Download the PancePrep app from the App store now!

Go to **www.panceprepapp.io** to download the forms to claim your credit for using this app.

Get the book that started it all! Pance Prep Pearls 10th anniversary collector's edition!

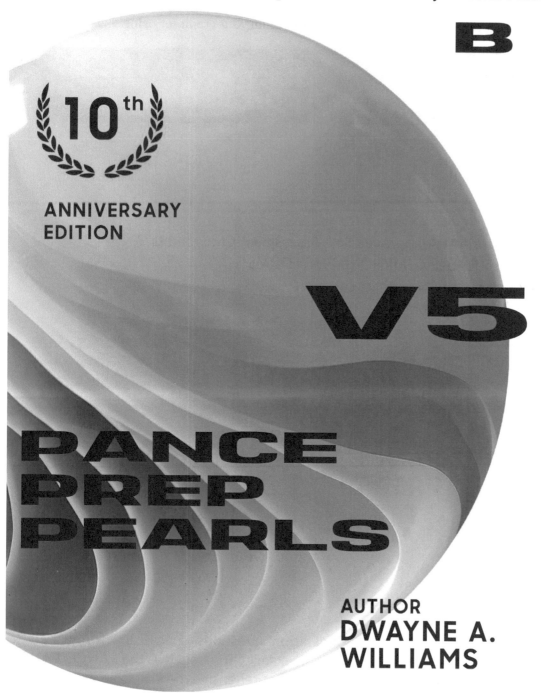

B

10th ANNIVERSARY EDITION

V5

PANCE PREP PEARLS

AUTHOR
DWAYNE A. WILLIAMS

TABLE OF CONTENTS

1. A 59-year-old female presents to the emergency department with headache, sweating, palpitations, and chest pain for 1 hour. She was recently notified her husband of 30 years died unexpectedly. An ECG is positive for ST segment elevation in the anterior precordial leads. Troponin level is 0.9 ng/mL (0-0.4). Urine catecholamines are negative. Coronary angiography reveals widely patent coronary vessels. Echocardiograph reveals severe anterior-apical akinesis and compensatory inferior-posterior hyperkinesis. Which of the following is the most likely diagnosis?
a. Atherosclerotic heart disease
b. Variant (Prinzmetal) angina
c. Takotsubo cardiomyopathy
d. Pheochromocytoma
e. Restrictive cardiomyopathy

2. A 32-year-old male presents to the clinic because he has been unable to go out with his friends and girlfriend. He has a fear of experiencing panic symptoms, fainting, or consequent embarrassment in conditions outside of his home where he does not feel "safe", such as taking buses or subways, being where large crowds gather, or being in unfamiliar places. When he has gone out, he experienced dry mouth, heart palpitations, and leg weakness. He has to have his cellphone fully charged, sits close next to exits or doors, takes an anti-nauseant before going out, and carries a paper bag in case of hyperventilation. Which of the following is the most effective treatment of choice?
a. Psychodynamic therapy and Buspirone
b. Interpersonal therapy and Lorazepam
c. Dialectical behavioral therapy and Sertraline
d. Cognitive behavioral therapy and Escitalopram
e. Exposure and response prevention and Clomipramine

3. A 36-year-old male presents to the clinic with intermittent bilateral flank pain and episodic hematuria. His brother died suddenly at age 45 years from a Subarachnoid hemorrhage. Vital signs reveal a blood pressure of 150/92 mmHg. Physical examination is notable for palpable nontender bilateral flank masses with no costovertebral angle tenderness. Urinalysis is positive for 2+ protein and 40 RBCs/hpf without pyuria or nitrates. Which of the following is the most appropriate next step in the evaluation of this patient?
a. 24-hour urine metanephrines
b. Radionuclide renal scan
c. Renal biopsy
d. Renal ultrasound
e. Cystoscopy

4. Which of the following cranial nerves is responsible for keeping the eyelids open?
a. II
b. III
c. IV
d. VI
e. VII

5. A 9-year-old male presents with bleeding from the right nare. Direct pressure is applied for 15 minutes after application of Oxymetazoline nasal spray. On nasal speculum examination, active bleeding is noted, and the site is visualized. Which of the following is the most appropriate next step in the management of this patient?
a. Foley catheter placement
b. Anterior nasal packing with a nasal tampon
c. Posterior nasal packing
d. Irrigation with normal saline
e. Cauterization

6. A 22-year-old woman is being evaluated in the clinic for irregular menses for the last 12 months. On examination, her BMI is 33 kg/m^2. Facial acne and velvety, hyperpigmented plaques are noted on the skin of the axillae and posterior neck. A transvaginal ultrasound is performed (see photo). Which of the following would most likely be seen on physical examination of this patient?

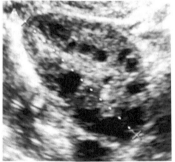

a. Cervical motion tenderness
b. Diffusely enlarged (globular), soft, mobile tender uterus
c. Discrete, firm, nontender, asymmetric mobile enlarged masses in the pelvis
d. Excessive growth of terminal hair in the periareolar, face, and linea alba regions
e. Adnexal tenderness

Photo credit:
Anne Mousse, CC0, via Wikimedia Commons

7. Which of the following is the most common sign of Pulmonary embolism?
a. Accentuated pulmonic component of the second heart sound
b. Tachycardia
c. Calf or thigh swelling
d. Tachypnea
e. Rales

8. A 20-year-old male was ejected off of his motorcycle and received two units of packed red cells. 60 minutes later, he develops chills, 9/10 flank pain, and oozing of blood from his intravenous sites. There is pink-red urine noted in the urinary catheter bag. Vitals reveal temperature 103°F (39.44°C), blood pressure 132/74 mmHg, pulse 118 bpm, respiratory rate 20 breaths/min, and SaO2: 99% on room air. The transfusion is discontinued. Which of the following is the most likely etiology of his reaction?
a. IgA deficiency
b. Donor blood products contaminated by bacteria or bacterial byproducts
c. ABO incompatibility
d. Reaction to cytokines stored in the transfused blood
e. Activation of recipient's neutrophils by antigens & anti-leukocyte antibodies in the transfused donor product

9. A 10-year-old boy presents to the urgent care clinic for a 3-day history of right eyelid swelling, ocular pain, and blurred vision. He has a 10-day history of nasal discharge, nasal obstruction, and cough. Vitals are significant for a temperature 101°F (38.3°C). Right eyelid swelling and erythema & pain with eye movement without proptosis or ocular discharge are noted. There is no vision deficit. Which of the following is the most likely etiology of his presentation?
a. Severe bacterial infection of the conjunctiva
b. Infection posterior to the orbital septum
c. Infection anterior to the orbital septum
d. Thrombus within the cavernous sinus
e. Mucormycosis fungal infection involving the orbit

10. A 22-year-old male presents to the dermatology clinic for follow-up of treatment for Acne vulgaris. He has been consistently using topical Tretinoin, topical Benzoyl peroxide, and oral Minocycline with minimal improvement of his Acne. On examination, there are multiple deep-seated, inflamed, and tender erythematous nodules >1 cm and pitting of the face, shoulders, and chest. Which of the following is the most appropriate next step in the management?
a. Add topical Clindamycin
b. Switch to oral Doxycycline
c. Switch to oral Isotretinoin
d. Add oral Cephalexin
e. Add topical Erythromycin

11. A 16-year-old male is complaining of eye redness. There is copious amounts of purulent thick yellow ocular discharge at the lid margins and in the corners of the eye which reappears within minutes of wiping the lids. Gram stain of the discharge reveals polymorphonuclear cells & Gram-negative diplococci. Which of the following is the recommended treatment?
a. Bacitracin ophthalmic ointment
b. Erythromycin ophthalmic ointment
c. Single dose of IM Ceftriaxone, topical Ofloxacin, oral Doxycycline
d. Topical Ofloxacin ophthalmic solution
e. Single dose of intramuscular (IM) Penicillin G

12. A 40-year-old female presents to the emergency department for colicky abdominal pain, nausea, and nonbloody, bilious vomiting for 48 hours. She has not passed any flatus or bowel movements during this time. She also endorses decreased appetite. She has a past surgical history of cesarean section. On physical examination, high-pitched tinkling bowel sounds are auscultated. An abdominal radiograph is performed (see photo).

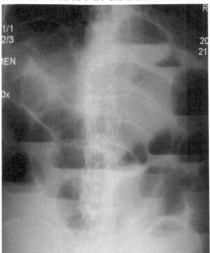

Which of the following is the most likely etiology of her presentation?
a. Hypokalemia
b. Prior abdominal surgery
c. Chronic constipation
d. Abdominal hernia
e. GI malignancy

Photo credit:
James Heilman, MD, CC BY-SA 3.0 <https://creativecommons.org/licenses/by-sa/3.0>, via Wikimedia Commons

13. A 17-year-old male presents to the emergency department complaining of fatigue, polyuria, increased thirst, and abdominal pain. Physical examination is notable for deep continuous breathing and abdominal tenderness. A basic metabolic panel reveals:
Na+: 139 mEq/L (135-145)
Cl-: 100 mEq/L (96-106)
K+: 3.0 mEq/L (3.5-5)
HCO3-: 19 mEq/L (22-26)
Glucose: 409 mg/dL (70-110).
Which of the following is the most appropriate next step in management?
a. Insulin, IV 0.9% sodium chloride, and IV potassium
b. IV Insulin, IV potassium, and IV D5 0.9% sodium chloride
c. IV 0.9% sodium chloride
d. IV Insulin and IV 0.9% sodium chloride
e. IV Potassium and IV 0.9% sodium chloride

14. A 58-year-old male is brought to the emergency department for confusion, diarrhea, and cough. He recently returned from vacation in an old hotel where other people experienced similar symptoms. On examination, he is confused. Moist mucous membranes, normal skin turgor, and localized crackles are noted on chest auscultation. Initial labs are positive for transaminitis, serum sodium of 127 mEq/L (135-45), and serum osmolality 260 mOsm/kg (275-295). Chest radiographs reveal scattered patchy infiltrates. In addition to Azithromycin, Which of the following is the first line management for this patient?
a. Fluid restriction
b. IV 3% sodium chloride
c. IV 0.9% sodium chloride
d. Dextrose 5% in water
e. Salt tablets

15. A 12-year-old male presents to the clinic with a 4-day history of low-grade fever, chills, headache, and myalgias. He recently returned home from a camping trip in Tennessee. Physical examination is notable for a nonpruritic maculopapular rash on the arms and wrists without nuchal rigidity. Initial labs are remarkable for a serum sodium of 128 mEq/L (135-145), platelet count 30,000 platelets/mcL (150,000-450,000) and elevated transaminases. Which of the following is the most likely causative organism of his presentation?
a. Ehrlichia chaffeensis
b. Borrelia burgdorferi
c. Neisseria meningitidis
d. West Nile virus
e. Rickettsia rickettsii

16. A 29-year-old male presents to the urgent care clinic with fatigue, right cheek pain, mild head and facial pressure, nasal congestion, and purulent nasal discharge for 3 days. Vitals reveal a temperature 100°F (37.8°C). Which of the following is considered the most appropriate next step in the management of this patient?
a. Oral Amoxicillin
b. Oral Amoxicillin-clavulanic acid
c. Non contrast CT of the Maxillofacial bones
d. Ibuprofen, intranasal sterile saline spray, and reassess in 1 week
e. Water's view radiographs

17. A 15-year-old boy presents to the clinic with fatigue, nausea, weight loss, and diffuse myalgias for 3 months. Review of systems is positive for dizziness upon standing. He has no significant past medical history. Vitals are blood pressure 84/52 mmHg, heart rate 94 bpm, respiratory rate 17 breaths/min, and temperature 98.6°F (37°C). On physical examination, proximal muscle weakness of the distal extremities are noted. Initial laboratory evaluation reveals a serum sodium of 128 mEq/L (135-145) and serum potassium 5.6 mEq/L (3.5-5). Which of the following would most likely be seen on physical examination of this patient?
a. Acanthosis nigricans involving the neck and the axillae
b. Hyperpigmentation of the palmar creases, knees, and elbows
c. Nontender goiter with a bruit in the neck
d. Wide, purple-colored abdominal striae
e. Loss of the outer third of the eyebrows

18. A 32-year-old male presents to the outpatient GI department to establish care. He denies any GI symptoms but is concerned because his brother was diagnosed with Colorectal cancer at 45 years of age. Physical examination is unremarkable and routine lab testing is within normal limits. Which of the following is the recommended colorectal cancer screening in this patient?
a. Colonoscopy at 35 years; then every 5 years thereafter
b. Colonoscopy at 40 years; then every 5 years thereafter
c. Colonoscopy at 40 years; then every 10 years thereafter
d. Colonoscopy at age 45; then every 5 years thereafter
e. Colonoscopy at 50 years; then every 10 years thereafter

19. A previously healthy 5-month-old boy presents to the clinic with a nonproductive cough. For 48 hours, he was experiencing sneezing, clear rhinorrhea, and nasal congestion. This morning, his parents states he has been "breathing heavy". Vitals reveal a respiratory rate of 38 breaths per minute, oxygen saturation is 90% on room air, and heart rate 146 beats per minute. There is nasal flaring, grunting, moderate subcostal retractions, scattered rhonchi, crackles, and bilateral expiratory wheezes. Which of the following is the first-line management of choice?
a. Nebulized Epinephrine and supplemental oxygen by nasal cannula
b. Nebulized Albuterol
c. Supplemental oxygen by nasal cannula, hydration, and nasal suctioning
d. Oral Methylprednisolone and supplemental oxygen by nasal cannula
e. Oral Erythromycin

20. An 8-year-old boy is being evaluated for poor academic performance. His teacher states he has difficulty remaining seated in class, squirms in his chair, constantly blurts out answers when it's not his turn, and hands in assignments late. At home, he is easily distracted, unable to concentrate for long periods of time, often interrupts his mother when she is talking, doesn't follow instructions as if he is not even listening to her, and often loses his belongings. Which of the following is the recommended first line management of choice?
a. Atomoxetine
b. Psychotherapy
c. Guanfacine ER
d. Methylphenidate
e. Clonidine ER

21. A 22-year-old female with no significant past medical history presents to the urgent care clinic in January with abrupt onset of fever, nonproductive cough, sore throat, nasal congestion, and back aches for 3 days. Vitals reveal temperature 38.3°C (101°F), P: 96/min, BP: 126/70 mmHg, and SaO2: 99% on room air. She appears hot and flushed, with oropharyngeal hyperemia. Pulmonary examination is unremarkable. Which of the following is the management of choice in this patient?
a. Azithromycin
b. Oseltamivir
c. Ibuprofen
d. Supplemental oxygen
e. Albuterol

22. A 38-year-old woman comes to the clinic because she has a history of severe heartburn that does not resolve with over-the-counter antacids. She is also complaining of intermittent diarrhea, 5 lb. weight loss, and dry cough. Her fingers lose color when she reaches for food in the freezer. Physical examination is remarkable for tightened, shiny skin with induration over her lower arms, legs distal to her knees, and face. Dry rales in the lungs are auscultated. Telangiectasias are noted on her cheeks. Which of the following antibodies would most likely be positive in this patient?
a. Anti-centromere
b. Anti-signal recognition protein
c. Anti double-stranded DNA
d. Anti-SCL 70
e. Anti-cyclic citrullinated peptide

23. During evaluation of patient, the following is seen on ECG (see photo).

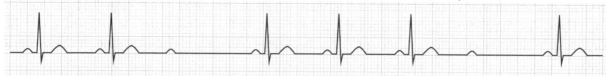

Which of the following is the most likely diagnosis?
a. Sinus bradycardia
b. Mobitz type I second-degree heart block
c. Third-degree heart block
d. Mobitz type II second-degree heart block
e. First-degree heart block

Photo credit:
Shutterstock (used with permission)

24. A 58-year-old male presents to the ED complaining of sudden onset of excruciating, oppressive chest pain between the scapulae radiating to the back for 30 minutes. Associated symptoms include diaphoresis and a doomed feeling. He has a history of uncontrolled hypertension. Vitals reveal a blood pressure of 164/108 mmHg, pulse 118/min, and respirations of 20/min. Physical examination reveals an anxious diaphoretic male. ECG reveals sinus tachycardia and chest radiograph is within normal. Laboratory evaluation reveals a BUN of 18 mg/dL (7-20) and creatinine 0.9 mg/dL (0.6-1.2). Which of the following is the most appropriate next step in management?
a. Administer Aspirin, chewed for faster absorption
b. Obtain a D-dimer
c. Order a Transesophageal echocardiography
d. Order a CT angiogram of the chest
e. Order a Ventilation-perfusion scan

25. A 31-year-old male is being evaluated for Hypertension despite being compliant with Hydrochlorothiazide and Amlodipine. Physical examination is notable for centripetal obesity, abdominal striae, and supraclavicular fat pads. Initial labs reveal an elevated serum glucose. Further workup reveals a serum cortisol of 100 pg/mL (<15), 24-hour urinary cortisol excretion 297 pg/mL (3.5–45), and baseline ACTH 97 pg/mL (9-52). A 48-hour 8 mg Dexamethasone suppression trial results in a serum cortisol level of 32 pg/mL. Which of the following is the most likely etiology of his presentation?
a. Autoimmune adrenal gland dysfunction
b. Exogenous glucocorticoid use
c. Benign Pituitary corticotroph tumor
d. Ectopic ACTH producing tumor
e. Adrenal Tumor

26. An 8-day-old infant is brought to the clinic for right ocular discharge. He was born at home with the aid of a Doula. On examination, copious mucopurulent discharge from both eyes, marked swelling of both eyelids, and thickened conjunctivae (chemosis) are noted. A pseudomembrane adheres to the conjunctivae. Which of the following is the most appropriate treatment of this patient?
a. Topical Silver nitrate
b. Intramuscular Ceftriaxone
c. Oral Azithromycin
d. Ciprofloxacin ophthalmic
e. Erythromycin ophthalmic

27. A 55-year-old male presents to the clinic for malaise, fatigue, decreased appetite, and low-grade fever for the last 5 weeks. He underwent a dental extraction 2 months ago but otherwise has no prior medical conditions. Vitals are temperature 101°F (38.3°C), blood pressure is 120/72 mmHg, pulse 100/min, and respirations 18/min. Nonblanching linear reddish-brown lesions under the nail bed and tender subcutaneous violaceous nodules on the pads of the fingers and toes are noted. Which of the following is the most likely etiology of his presentation?
a. Staphylococcus epidermidis
b. Streptococcus gallolyticus
c. Streptococcus viridans
d. Enterococcus species
e. Eikenella corrodens

28. Which of the following Selective serotonin reuptake inhibitors (SSRIs) has the greatest association with causing a prolonged QT interval?
a. Paroxetine
b. Sertraline
c. Citalopram
d. Fluoxetine
e. Fluvoxamine

29. A 55-year-old male is admitted to the telemetry unit. On day 2, he develops palpitations and confusion. Vital signs reveal a blood pressure is 82/54 mmHg, pulse 120/minute, and respirations 22/minute. The following is seen on the monitor (see photo).

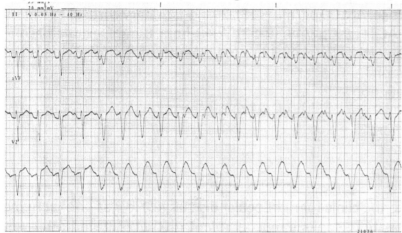

Which of the following is the most appropriate next step in the management of this patient?
a. Synchronized cardioversion
b. Unsynchronized cardioversion
c. Amiodarone
d. Magnesium sulfate
e. Verapamil

Photo credit:
Shutterstock (used with permission)

30. A 31-year-old female presents to the gynecology clinic with intermittent breast tenderness. The tenderness is often associated nodularity that often increases in size prior to the onset of menses. She denies nipple discharge. On examination, there are bilateral mobile masses in the upper outer quadrants of both breasts. There is no skin thickening, edema, discoloration, nipple retraction, discharge, or lymphadenopathy. Based on history and physical examination, which of the following is the most likely diagnosis?
a. Intraductal papilloma
b. Fibroadenoma
c. Paget disease of the breast
d. Infiltrative ductal carcinoma
e. Fibrocystic breast changes

31. A 26-year-old woman is being evaluated for left-sided pleuritic chest pain. Radiographs reveal an acute rib fracture as well as older healed rib fractures. Upon questioning her about these findings, she confides that her boyfriend is physically abusive. Which of the following is the recommended next step in the management of this patient?
a. Call 911 and report the physical abuse
b. Contact her mother to establish an escape plan
c. Speak with the patient's boyfriend regarding his actions towards her
d. Refer her and the boyfriend to couples therapy and him to anger management
e. Provide her information regarding a safety plan should an urgent escape be needed

32. A 5-year-old boy presents to the urgent care clinic with a rash and fever. He has been refusing food due to pain with eating since yesterday. Vitals are blood pressure of 112/72 mmHg, pulse 122/min, T: 102.4°F (39.1°C), respirations 20/min, and SaO2: 98% on room air. There is a diffuse maculopapular rash that blanches with pressure, circumoral pallor, and anterior cervical lymphadenopathy. Which of the following would most likely be seen in this patient?
a. Palpable purpura on the buttocks and lower extremities
b. Erythematous, swollen tongue with a white coating and pronounced papillae
c. Tightly adherent gray pseudomembrane in posterior pharynx
d. Erythematous papules, macules, or ulcers on the soft palate and uvula.
e. Clustered 1-3 mm pale white or blue papules with an erythematous base on the buccal mucosa opposite the second molars

33. A 25-year-old male presents to the clinic for evaluation of flu-like symptoms. While the patient is in the waiting room waiting for his discharge paperwork, the supervising physician realized he forgot to listen to the patient's lung examination. He asks the physician associate to document a normal lung examination in his chart. Which of the following is the most appropriate next step by the physician associate?
a. Document a normal lung examination in the chart
b. Inform the supervising physician to add the normal lung examination in the chart
c. Ask the scribe to add a normal lung examination in the chart
d. Perform the lung examination on the patient and document the findings in the chart
e. Log in using the supervising physician credentials and document a normal lung examination

34. A 37-year-old man presents with a one-month history of persistent dysphagia, odynophagia, coughing, and hoarseness. He has lost 8 kg in the last four months. He denies tobacco or alcohol use. On examination, there is a white patch with an exophytic lesion on the base of the tongue and a neck mass is palpated. Biopsy of the lesion reveals dysplastic cells. Which of the following tests is most likely to detect the most likely etiology of this patient's presentation?
a. Human immunodeficiency virus (HIV) RNA (viral load)
b. Heterophile antibody testing for Epstein-Barr virus (Monospot)
c. Human papillomavirus (HPV) DNA detection assay
d. Real-time Herpes simplex virus (HSV) PCR assays
e. Hepatitis C RNA (viral load)

35. A 45-year-old obese female with type 2 Diabetes mellitus is being evaluated in the clinic. It is decided to place her on injection therapy once weekly with Exenatide extended release to help lower her Hemoglobin A1C to target level and for weight loss. Which of the following questions is essential to ask the patient prior to initiating therapy to reduce complications from therapy?
a. "Do you have a personal or family history of Medullary thyroid cancer or MEN 2 syndrome?"
b. "Do you have Heart failure?"
c. "Do you have recurrent vaginal yeast infections or urinary tract infections?"
d. "Do you have a history of Cirrhosis or hepatic disease?"
e. "Do you have a history of ketosis-prone Type 2 Diabetes mellitus?"

36. A 58-year-old male presents to his primary care provider for progressive dyspnea, loss of balance resulting in recurrent falls, tingling in his hands, impaired depth perception, and changes in his peripheral vision. He has a history of chronic alcohol use disorder. Neurological examination is notable for a wide-based ataxic gait, decreased sensation in the lower extremities, nystagmus, conjugate palsies, and bilateral rectus palsies. A chest radiograph is obtained (see photo).

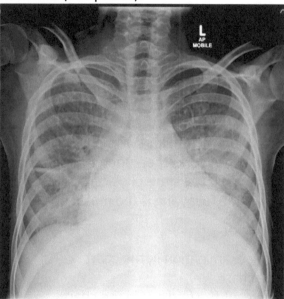

Which of the following nutritional deficiencies is most likely responsible for this patient's presentation?
a. Vitamin B12
b. Vitamin B1
c. Vitamin B6
d. Vitamin B3
e. Vitamin B2

Photo credit:
Case courtesy of Andrew Dixon, Radiopaedia.org, rID: 10666

37. A 16-year-old female presents to the ED with bilateral lower quadrant pain, nausea, and vomiting. She has a history of multiple sexual partners. Vitals reveal a temperature of 102.3°F (39°F), pulse 106/min, and blood pressure 118/74 mmHg. Physical examination is notable for dry mucous membranes and diffuse tenderness in both lower quadrants. External genitalia is normal. Speculum examination shows purulent discharge from the cervical os with cervical motion and adnexal tenderness. There are no palpable adnexal masses. Urine beta hCG is negative. Which of the following is the most appropriate next step?
a. Diagnostic culdocentesis
b. Diagnostic laparoscopy
c. Cervical culture
d. Hospitalization, IV Cefotetan + IV Doxycycline + Metronidazole
e. IM Ceftriaxone, oral Doxycycline, Metronidazole, Naprosyn, follow-up in 2 days

38. A 76-year-old female is brought in by ambulance from a long-term care facility for confusion. 10 days ago, she was experiencing dysuria, urgency, and urinary frequency. On physical examination, she is only alert to person. Vitals are temperature of 103°F (38.3°C), blood pressure 90/40 mmHg, pulse 132/min, respirations 18/min, and SaO2 89% on room air. She appears flushed with warm extremities and bounding pulses. Evaluation of which of the following is most supportive of the most likely diagnosis?
a. White cell count
b. Serum lactic acid
c. Transthoracic echocardiogram
d. Serum glucose
e. Serum creatinine and Blood urea nitrogen

39. A 21-year-old male presents to the clinic for painless swelling of his right testicle over the last 2 months. He has a history of Cryptorchidism during childhood treated with Orchiopexy. Testicular examination reveals a firm mass in the right scrotal area. Initial laboratory evaluation is positive for serum LDH: 498 U/L (140-280), alpha fetoprotein: 3,987 ng/mL (5-10), and Serum ß-hCG: 29,250 IU/L. Which of the following is the most likely etiology of his presentation?
a. Leydig cell testicular tumor
b. Nonseminomatous germ cell tumor
c. Testicular teratoma
d. Seminomatous germ cell tumor
e. Sertoli cell testicular tumor

40. A 50-year-old male presents with dyspnea and palpitations. He has a history of Hypertension. Vital signs reveal a blood pressure of 118/84 mmHg, pulse 150/minute, and respirations 20/minute. The following is seen on the monitor (see photo).

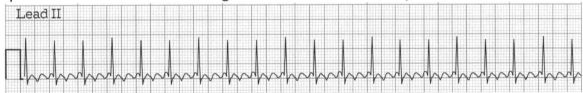

Which of the following is the most appropriate next step in the management of this patient?
a. Synchronized cardioversion
b. Adenosine
c. Amiodarone
d. Digoxin
e. Diltiazem

Photo credit:
Shutterstock (used with permission)

41. A 50-year-old woman presents to the clinic complaining of a frequent need to void at nighttime, which has been disrupting her sleep. She notes embarrassingly that she develops a strong sensation to urinate but is often unable to reach the bathroom quick enough. She experiences urinary leakage throughout the night as well as during the day. She denies dysuria, hematuria, or discharge. Urodynamic testing reveals a residual volume of 20 mL on postvoid analysis (<50). Urinalysis is unremarkable. Which of the following is the recommended management?
a. Vaginal estrogen cream
b. Oxybutynin
c. Bethanechol
d. Urethropexy
e. Advise frequent toileting technique to prevent bladder fullness

42. A 64-year-old male presents with fever, increasing fatigue, and epistaxis. Physical examination is notable for conjunctival pallor, tachycardia, tachypnea, and petechiae on the oral mucosa. Initial laboratory evaluation reveals:
Hemoglobin 8.8 g/dL (13.8-17.2)
WBC 110,000/microliter (5,000-10,000)
Platelets 29,000/microliter (150,000-450,000)
Prolonged PT and PTT, and elevated D-dimer.
Microscopic examination of the peripheral smear reveals schistocytes and the following (see photo).

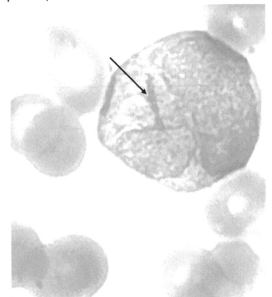

Which of the following is the most likely diagnosis?
a. Acute lymphoblastic leukemia
b. Acute myelogenous leukemia
c. Chronic lymphocytic leukemia
d. Chronic myelogenous leukemia
e. Multiple myeloma

Photo credit:
Shutterstock (used with permission)

43. A 40-year-old male with no past medical history presents to the clinic for constipation, polyuria, bone pain of the right lower leg, and weakness. Physical examination reveals elevated blood pressure, decreased bowel sounds, weakness, and hyporeflexia. Radiographs of the right tibia reveal subperiosteal bone resorption. ECG reveals a short QT interval. Based on the most likely diagnosis, which of the following would most likely be seen on laboratory evaluation?
a. Decreased serum PTH, elevated PTH related protein, elevated serum calcium, decreased serum phosphate
b. Elevated serum PTH, decreased serum calcium, increased serum phosphate
c. Decreased serum PTH, decreased serum calcium, increased serum phosphate
d. Elevated serum PTH, elevated serum calcium, decreased serum phosphate
e. Elevated alkaline phosphatase, normal serum calcium, normal serum phosphate

44. A 22-year-old male with a history of Type I Diabetes mellitus presents to the Emergency department with exquisite right otalgia, otorrhea, right temporal headache, and fever for 8 days. Physical examination is notable for visible granulation tissue in the inferior portion of the external auditory canal at the bone-cartilage junction. Computed tomography (CT) scans of the head and temporal bones revealed small areas of mastoid cell erosion on the temporal bone. IV administration of which of the following is the most appropriate management?
a. Liposomal Amphotericin B
b. Ciprofloxacin
c. Cefazolin
d. Acyclovir
e. Clindamycin

45. A 29-year-old male presents to the clinic with odynophagia and dysphagia. He has a history of Acquired immune deficiency syndrome (AIDS) with last CD4 count of 30/mm^3. Upper endoscopy reveals large shallow esophageal and ulcers and erosions. Histology of the lesions reveal intracytoplasmic and intranuclear inclusions (see photo).

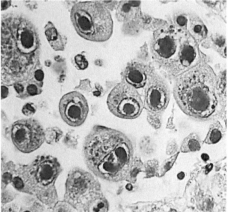

Which of the following is the first line management of this condition?
a. IV Ganciclovir
b. Oral Fluconazole
c. Inhaled Budesonide without spacer use
d. Topical Miconazole buccal
e. IV Acyclovir

46. A 17-year-old male presents to the clinic complaining of pink discoloration of his urine and flank pain since this morning. Associated symptoms include sore throat, "chest cold", and low-grade fever for the last 2 days. Examination of the oropharynx reveals inflamed and enlarged tonsils. Initial laboratory evaluation reveals blood urea nitrogen of 28 mg/dL (7-20) and creatinine of 1.6 mg/dL (0.6-1.2). Urinalysis demonstrated 2+ protein, 20 rbc/hpf, and red cell casts. Which of the following is the most likely diagnosis?
a. Postinfectious glomerulonephritis
b. Membranoproliferative glomerulonephritis
c. IgA Nephropathy
d. Minimal change disease
e. Henoch-Schöenlein purpura

47. A 52-year-old male presents to the clinic complaining of insidious onset of back pain worse with physical activity and generalized malaise for the last 3 months. He denies fever or chills. On examination, there is local tenderness to gentle spinal percussion over T7-T9. Laboratory tests reveal a WBC count of 11,000 cells/10^9/L (5,000-10,000), Erythrocyte sedimentation rate (ESR) 118 mm/h (<20) and C-reactive protein (CRP) 11.4 mg/dL (0.3-1.0). Which of the following is considered a major risk factor for an infective source of his back pain?
a. 20-pack-year smoking history
b. Unilateral radiculopathy
c. Traumatic fall
d. Hemoglobin A1C of 9%
e. Urinary incontinence

48. A 62-year-old female presents to the emergency department complaining of intense left knee pain. Examination of the knee reveals left knee erythema, warmth, and swelling over the knee joint with decreased range of motion. Radiographs are obtained (see photo).

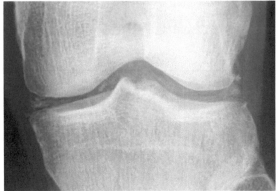

An arthrocentesis is performed. Which of the following would most likely be seen on synovial fluid analysis?
a. WBC count 57,000 and gram-positive cocci in clusters
b. WBC 28,000 and negative gram stain
c. WBC 32,000 negative birefringent needle-shaped crystals
d. WBC count 42,000; gram-negative diplococci
e. WBC 22,000 positive-birefringent rhomboid-shaped crystals

Photo credit:
Case courtesy of Frank Gaillard, Radiopaedia.org, rID: 35840

49. A 62-year-old woman presents to her primary care provider for a 3-month history of aching and stiffness in her neck and shoulders worse in the morning, making it difficult to brush her hair. The stiffness is worse with prolonged activity and is associated with fatigue and malaise. Physical examination is notable for 5/5 strength and decreased active range of motion of her shoulders, especially with abduction. Laboratory investigations revealed an Erythrocyte sedimentation rate (ESR) of 110 mm/h (<20) and C-reactive protein (CRP) 5.2 mg/dL (0.3-1.0). Which of the following is the most likely diagnosis?
a. Adhesive capsulitis
b. Fibromyalgia
c. Polymyositis
d. Spondyloarthropathy
e. Polymyalgia rheumatica

50. A 13-month-old boy is being evaluated for pale skin and fatigue. His mother states he is a finicky eater, as he eats cookies and almost exclusively drinks whole milk. On examination, conjunctival pallor is noted. Initial labs reveal a hemoglobin 8.2 mg/dL (10.9-15), Mean corpuscular volume (MCV): 70 μm^3 (80-100), and serum ferritin 3 ng/mL (7-140). Which of the following would most likely be seen on examination of the child?
a. Splenomegaly
b. Scleral icterus
c. Strawberry tongue
d. Purpura involving the lower extremities
e. Spooning of the nails

51. A 55-year-old female presents to her primary care provider for headache over the right temple area, fatigue, malaise, intermittent fever, jaw pain when she chews, and joint pain. Physical examination is notable for right scalp tenderness and neurological examination is unremarkable. There are no visual changes noted. Laboratory evaluation reveals an Erythrocyte sedimentation rate (ESR) of 118 mm/hr (0-20). Which of the following is the most appropriate next step in management of this patient?
a. Oral Prednisone
b. Anti-Smith antibodies
c. Noncontrast CT scan of the head
d. Temporal artery biopsy
e. Oral Sumatriptan

52. A 19-year-old male presents to the clinic complaining of discomfort with urination and scant discharge at the urethral meatus present on the first morning void. He denies pruritus or skin lesions. He is sexually active with 3 partners. Gram stain of the discharge obtained from the urethra shows 10 WBCs/hpf and no intracellular organisms in the WBCs. Based on the presentation and findings, which of the following is the most effective agent for the management of this patient?
a. Metronidazole oral
b. IM Ceftriaxone
c. Ciprofloxacin oral
d. Doxycycline oral
e. IM Penicillin G

53. A 25-year-old woman at 20 weeks gestation presents to the clinic complaining of a skin rash that has worsened after a recent trip to the beach. On examination, there are symmetric gray-brown hyperpigmented macules and patches on the forehead, nose, chin, and cheeks. Wood lamp examination reveals accentuation of the affected areas. Which of the following is the first line management of choice in this patient?
a. Topical Metronidazole
b. Sun avoidance, sun-protective clothing, and broad-spectrum sunscreen use
c. Hydroquinone 4% cream
d. Topical Fluocinolone, Hydroquinone, and Tretinoin triple combination cream
e. Topical Tretinoin 0.05% cream

54. A 36-year-old male presents to the primary care clinic complaining of increasing fatigue and feeling "cold constantly". Review of systems is positive for 15-lb. weight gain and constipation. Vitals are notable for a heart rate of 48 bpm. Physical examination is notable for dry skin, puffy face with periorbital edema, and slowed relaxation of deep tendon reflexes. Which of the following laboratory abnormalities would most likely be seen in this patient?
a. Decreased TSH and decreased serum free T4 levels
b. Increased TSH and increased serum free T4 levels
c. Diffuse increased radioactive iodine uptake on Thyroid scintigraphy
d. Positive thyroid stimulating immunoglobulins
e. Positive Thyroid peroxidase antibodies

55. A 55-year-old female smoker with 40 pack-year smoking history presents to the clinic with progressive dyspnea, intermittent cough, chest pain, hoarseness, and weight loss. The following is seen on physical examination (see photo).

Labs reveal a serum calcium of 14.4 mg/dL (8.5-10). Chest radiograph is positive for a centrally located cavitary lesion in the left superior sulcus. Which of the following is the most likely diagnosis?
a. Bronchial carcinoid tumor
b. Bronchoalveolar carcinoma
c. Small cell lung cancer
d. Squamous cell carcinoma of the lung
e. Adenocarcinoma of the lung

Photo credit:
Waster, CC BY 2.5 <https://creativecommons.org/licenses/by/2.5>, via Wikimedia Commons

56. A 56-year-old male presents to the ED with severe abdominal pain, vomiting, and diarrhea that was initially nonbloody but became bloody over the last 24 hours. He was recently treated with Levofloxacin for Pneumonia. Vital signs reveal fever, tachycardia hypotension and the patient has altered sensorium. There is abdominal tenderness, marked abdominal distention, and decreased skin turgor. Initial labs reveal leukocytosis of 15,000 cells/µL, hemoglobin level of 7.9 g/dL (14-18), and lactic acid 3.9 (<2). Abdominal radiographs are obtained (see photo).

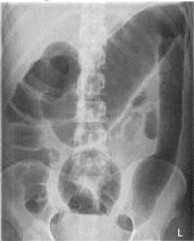

Stool toxins A and B assay and glutamate dehydrogenase (GDH) antigen are positive. Which of the following is the initial management of choice?
a. Bowel rest, IV fluids, Ceftriaxone plus IV Metronidazole 500 mg, Oral Vancomycin 500 mg
b. NPO, IV fluids, Neostigmine 2 mg intravenously
c. Bowel rest, IV fluids, Ceftriaxone plus Metronidazole, IV Ganciclovir 5 mg/kg
d. Subtotal colectomy
e. Bowel rest, IV fluids, Ceftriaxone plus Metronidazole, IV Hydrocortisone 100 mg

Photo credit:
Hellerhoff, CC BY-SA 4.0 <https://creativecommons.org/licenses/by-sa/4.0>, via Wikimedia Commons

57. A 55-year-old obese male presents to the clinic for increased dyspnea, especially on exertion, and persistent productive cough with mucoid expectoration for the last 3 years. He has a 30 pack-year smoking history. Vitals are blood pressure 142/90 mmHg, heart rate 86 bpm, respiratory rate 17 breaths/min, and temperature 98.6°F (37°C), and pulse oximetry with oxygen saturation 84% on room air. Physical examination is positive for scattered rhonchi with a prolonged expiratory phase and increased AP diameter. Labs are significant for a hematocrit of 58% (35-54). Which of the following interventions will have the greatest impact on his survival?
a. Influenza vaccination
b. Pneumococcal vaccination
c. Long-term supplemental oxygen at home
d. Prophylactic antibiotics to decrease frequency of exacerbations
e. Daily use of inhaled corticosteroids and an inhaled antimuscarinic agent

58. A 68-year-old male presents to the clinic with dyspnea on exertion. On examination, there is a late-peaking systolic murmur best heard in the right second intercostal space that increased with the patient sitting up and leaning forward. Which of the following would most likely be seen on physical examination of this patient?
a. Increased murmur intensity with Valsalva maneuver
b. Slow-rising carotid pulse
c. Bounding radial pulses
d. Opening snap and prominent S1
e. Increased intensity of the murmur in the lateral decubitus position

59. A 20-year-old male with Major depressive disorder is still having symptoms of Depression on Fluvoxamine. It is decided to place the patient on Venlafaxine. Which of the following should be monitored prior to and during therapy with Venlafaxine?
a. Thyroid function test
b. Blood pressure
c. Serum glucose
d. Liver function tests
e. Body mass index

60. A 55-year-old male presents to the clinic with intermittent dyspnea on exertion and increasing fatigue. Vitals are blood pressure of 152/92 mmHg, pulse 92/min, T: 98.6°F (37°C), respirations 16/min, and SaO2: 98% on room air. His lungs are clear to auscultation and no peripheral edema is noted. Echocardiography reveals an ejection fraction of 40% (55-70). Which of the following medications is most effective at reducing mortality in this patient?
a. Digoxin
b. Nitroglycerin
c. Enalapril
d. Furosemide
e. Diltiazem

61. A 22-year-old female is being evaluated at 9 weeks gestation. Initial labs reveal:
Serum sodium: 137 mEq/L (135-145)
Serum potassium: 2.6 mEq/L (3.5-5)
Serum chloride: 84 mEq/L (96-106)
An ABG is performed:
pH: 7.55 (7.35-7.45)
pCO2: 51 (35-45)
HCO3-: 45 (22-26)
Which of the following is the most likely etiology of these laboratory findings?
a. Pulmonary embolism
b. Persistent diarrhea
c. Asthma exacerbation
d. Hyperemesis gravidarum
e. Diabetic ketoacidosis

62. A 62-year-old male is brought to the clinic by his wife. She reports her husband has periodic confusion, memory loss, and episodes where he "zones out". Over the last 2 years, he has sometimes mistaken trees for people and will have long conversations with them. He has been walking more slowly. He has recurrent sleep-related vocalization and thrashes during sleep. On examination, he is alert to person and place and can recall 2 of 3 items in 5 minutes. Bradykinesia and cogwheel rigidity are noted. MRI of the brain reveals generalized cortical atrophy. Which of the following is the most likely diagnosis?
a. Parkinson disease
b. Normal pressure hydrocephalus
c. Frontotemporal dementia
d. Dementia with Lewy bodies
e. Alzheimer disease

63. A 7-year-old boy is being evaluated in the neurology clinic for multiple episodes of "staring spells" with associated eye fluttering. The episodes occur throughout the day and last for less than 10-15 seconds, after which he resumes normal activities. He does not experience an aura, lose postural tone, and he does not complain of any symptoms afterwards. He is unaware they happen and is not arousable during the episodes. His parents are concerned because it is affecting his performance in school. During an episode, EEG shows a 3 Hz spike and wave pattern. Which of the following is the first line management of this patient?
a. Gabapentin
b. Phenobarbital
c. Carbamazepine
d. Ethosuximide
e. Phenytoin

64. A 54-year-old male presents to the clinic with yellowing of his eyes for 2 months, associated with dark urine, anorexia, and proximal muscle weakness. Social history is positive for daily consumption of 6 glasses of whiskey for the last 10 months. Physical examination is notable for scleral icterus, proximal muscle wasting, and a palpable liver 7 cm below the right costal margin. Initial labs reveal a total bilirubin of 4.5 mg/dL. Hepatic biopsy reveals microvascular steatosis, hepatocellular ballooning, lobular inflammation, and Mallory-Denk bodies. Which of the following additional laboratory findings is most supportive of the most likely diagnosis?
a. Positive smooth muscle autoantibodies
b. Alanine aminotransferase (ALT)/Aspartate aminotransferase (AST) >2; Serum AST and ALT >500 IU
c. Aspartate aminotransferase (AST)/Alanine aminotransferase (ALT) >2; Serum AST and ALT <300 IU
d. Elevated alkaline phosphatase (ALP) and elevated gamma glutamyl-transferase (GGT)
e. Elevated prothrombin time (PT) and decreased albumin

65. A 25-year-old male presents to the urgent care clinic with gradual onset of localized right-sided scrotal pain and swelling. He denies fever, chills, nausea, or vomiting. Physical examination reveals right scrotal edema and erythema. There is mild relief of pain with scrotal elevation. Testicular Doppler ultrasound reveals increased blood flow on the right side. Which of the following is the most likely diagnosis?
a. Inflammation of the epididymis due to Chlamydia trachomatis
b. Inflammation of the epididymis due to Escherichia coli
c. Fluid accumulation in the scrotal sac
d. Twisting of the testicle on the spermatic cord
e. Torsion of the appendix of the testicle

66. A 57-year-old male presents with a 14-month history of bilateral knee pain, especially right medial knee pain. He denies any knee trauma. The pain is worse with activity and towards the end of the day. Physical examination reveals a mild right knee effusion and crepitus. The knee joint is cool on palpation. His body mass index is 33 kg/m^2. Radiographs are obtained (see photo).

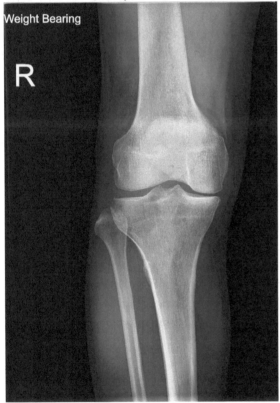

Which of the following is the most appropriate treatment of this patient?
a. Knee arthroscopy
b. Valgus (unloader) knee bracing
c. Total knee replacement
d. Topical knee replacement
e. Weight loss and performing low-impact and aquatic exercise regularly

Photo credit:
Ptrump16, CC BY-SA 4.0 <https://creativecommons.org/licenses/by-sa/4.0>, via Wikimedia Commons

67. An 8-year-old male presents to the ED with easy bruising, fatigue, and abdominal pain. About 7 days ago, he experienced a few episodes of abdominal pain, vomiting, and bloody diarrhea, for which his parents treated with Loperamide. On examination, scleral icterus and petechiae are noted. Initial labs reveal a low platelet count with schistocytes on peripheral smear, increased serum creatinine, and normal prothrombin and partial thromboplastin times. Which of the following organisms is most likely responsible for his presentation?
a. Rotavirus
b. Salmonella spp.
c. Escherichia coli
d. Vibrio cholerae
e. Campylobacter jejuni

68. A 14-year-old male presents to the urgent care clinic with low-grade fever, marked fatigue, and sore throat. Physical examination is notable for palatal petechiae without exudates and posterior cervical lymphadenopathy. He was seen in the urgent care 2 days ago and was given Ampicillin for his symptoms. 2 days later, he developed a blanching maculopapular rash without mucosal lesions. Which of the following would most likely be seen on physical examination of this patient?
a. Enlarged spleen 7 cm below the costal margin
b. Painful mucocutaneous ulcerations
c. Strawberry tongue
d. Grey pseudomembranes on the posterior pharynx
e. Enlarged, warm, and swollen joints (knees, ankles, elbows, wrists)

69. A 22-year-old primigravid female at 35 weeks gestation presents to the labor and delivery department with mild colicky abdominal pain. She felt a sudden gush of fluid followed by regular uterine contractions every 5 minutes for the last 2 hours. Vital signs are stable. Physical examination is notable for cervical dilation of 5 cm, cervical effacement of 85%, and fetal head station at 0 with vertex presentation. Fetal heart tracing reveals variable decelerations with a change of fetal heart rate >20 beats per minute, occur during the onset of contraction and reaches its nadir in <30 seconds. Which of the following is the initial management of choice?
a. Reassurance that it is a normal tracing and no intervention needed
b. Immediate Cesarean delivery
c. Administration of an amnioinfusion via intrauterine pressure catheter placement
d. Maternal repositioning to the right or left lateral decubital position
e. Identify labor progress

70. Which of the following is the most effective contraceptive method?
a. Etonogestrel implant
b. Levonorgestrel IUD
c. Copper IUD (0.8% average failure rate)
d. Depot medroxyprogesterone acetate injection (DMPA) injection
e. Combined oral contraceptive therapy

71. A 14-year-old male presents to the clinic for follow up of an elevated blood pressure reading. Physical examination is notable for weak femoral and posterior tibialis pulses and radio-femoral delay. Which of the following is most associated with the most likely underlying condition?
a. Cyanosis of the lips relieved with squatting
b. Posterior rib notching on chest radiographs
c. Diastolic murmur
d. Upturned apex and concave main pulmonary artery segment with a boot-shaped appearance
e. Cardiomegaly and narrowed mediastinum with the heart appearing globular on chest radiographs with an egg on a string appearance

72. A 20-year-old male presents to his primary care provider for follow up after a recent ED visit for an acute Asthma exacerbation. He has been using his Albuterol pump several times daily with nocturnal awakenings nightly. His home medications include low-dose Fluticasone and Formoterol. PFT shows a Forced expiratory volume (FEV1) of 66% predicted. Which of the following is the most appropriate next step in his management?
a. Switch to medium-dose Fluticasone
b. Discontinue Fluticasone and increase the Salmeterol dose
c. Add Omalizumab
d. Add Montelukast
e. Add Cromolyn sodium

73. A 40-year-old male presents with right arm pain, swelling, and bruising after falling onto the right arm. Radiographs are obtained (see photo).

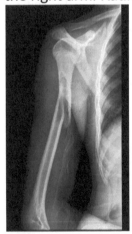

Which of the following would most likely be seen on physical examination of this patient based on his injury?
a. Positive Froment sign
b. Wrist drop
c. Loss of thumb abduction
d. Loss of sensation to the index finger
e. Decreased deltoid pinprick sensation

Photo credit:
Case courtesy of Samir Benoudina, Radiopaedia.org, rID: 22063

74. A 25-year-old primigravid female at 8 weeks gestation is being evaluated for severe nausea and intractable vomiting. Initial labs reveal:
- serum creatinine 2.1 mg/dL (0.6-1.2)
- BUN 62 mg/dL (6-20)
- urine specific gravity of 1.040
- urine osmolality 900 mOsm/kg H_2O (500-850)
- urine sodium 9 mEq/L.
- hyaline casts are seen on microscopic examination of the urine.

Which of the following is the most likely diagnosis?
a. Post obstructive uropathy
b. Acute interstitial nephritis
c. Nephrotic syndrome
d. Acute tubular necrosis
e. Prerenal azotemia

75. A 20-year-old female presents to the emergency department complaining of left midfoot pain for 2 hours. She was playing soccer and when she went to kick the ball, she hyperflexed her foot while it was planted as it got stuck in the turf. She has been unable to bear weight since the injury. On examination, there is swelling and a bruising over the plantar surface of the midfoot. Radiographs are obtained (see photo).

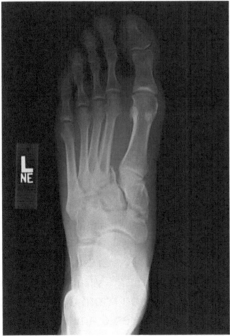

Which of the following is the preferred management of choice in this patient?
a. Rest, ice, elastic bandage, elevation, and non-weight bearing with crutches for 6-8 weeks
b. Resting equinus splint and orthopedic follow-up
c. K-wire pinning followed by open reduction and internal fixation
d. Walking boot for 6-8 weeks
e. Non-weight bearing

Photo credit:
Case courtesy of The Radswiki, Radiopaedia.org, rID: 11581

76. A 17-year-old male with a history of type I Von Willebrand disease is planned to undergo an elective extraction of a wisdom tooth. Which of the following is recommended to reduce his bleeding risk?
a. Factor VIII concentrates
b. Platelet transfusion
c. Plasma exchange therapy (Plasmapheresis)
d. Intravenous immunoglobulin therapy (IVIG)
e. Desmopressin

77. A 40-year-old female presents to the clinic with chronic dry nonproductive cough that is associated with fever, malaise, dyspnea, and fatigue. Over the last 2 days, she has experienced left eye pain. Physical examination of the eye reveals left eye erythema, miosis, and ciliary flush. Chest radiographs are obtained (see photo).

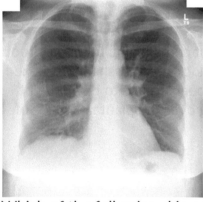

Which of the following skin conditions is most likely to develop in this patient?
a. Erythema multiforme
b. Pyoderma gangrenosum
c. Erythema nodosum
d. Raynaud phenomenon
e. Heliotrope rash

Photo credit:
Case courtesy of Craig Hacking, Radiopaedia.org, rID: 71482

78. A 44-year-old man is admitted to the medical intensive care unit for severe pancreatitis. After 48 hours of admission, he develops increased work of breathing. Vitals reveal a respiratory rate of 30 breaths per minute and oxygen saturation of 81% on room air. A chest radiograph demonstrates bilateral infiltrates with sparing of the costophrenic angles and no evidence of cardiomegaly or pleural effusions. He is placed on mechanical ventilation. Which of the following represents optimal respiratory care for the initial ventilation settings?
a. Low tidal volume ventilation and high PEEP
b. High tidal volume ventilation and high PEEP
c. High tidal volume ventilation and placing the patient supine
d. High tidal volume ventilation, high PEEP, and patient the patient prone
e. Low tidal volume ventilation and high-frequency oscillatory ventilation

79. A 25-year-old male Mycobacteriology lab personnel returns to employee health to follow up on the results of his yearly Tuberculosis screening as part of his routine employment health screening. He denies any symptoms and currently feels healthy. He has a history of HIV (last CD4 count 1,350 cell/mm^3). The site of the PPD (Tuberculosis skin test) placement reveals 6 mm of induration and 7 mm of erythema. Which of the following is the most appropriate next step in this patient?
a. No further management at this time
b. Rifampin daily for 4 months
c. Isoniazid + Vitamin B6 for 6 months duration
d. Chest radiograph
e. Initiate Rifampin, Isoniazid, Pyrazinamide, Ethambutol

80. A 56-year-old male presents to the emergency department with painful swelling to the scrotum and perianal area for 2 days. Vitals are notable for tachycardia and fever. Physical examination reveals tense edema, erythema, and tenderness to the right scrotum with palpable crepitations. There is patchy black area and purulent discharge from the perineum. Which of the following is the most likely predisposing factor for this patient's presentation?
a. Testicular malignancy
b. Diabetes mellitus
c. Sexually transmitted infection
d. Urethral trauma in the setting of urinary infection
e. Human immunodeficiency virus infection

81. A 7-year-old is being evaluated for increase in abdominal girth and rapidly enlarging swelling of his jaw. Abdominal examination reveals marked abdominal distension and shifting dullness. There is a mass in the right mandibular ridge covered by intact overlying mucosa. A biopsy of the mass is performed, and genetic analysis reveals c-myc translocation. Which of the following is the most likely diagnosis?
a. Burkitt lymphoma
b. Acute lymphoblastic leukemia
c. Diffuse large B cell lymphoma
d. Follicular lymphoma
e. Mantle cell lymphoma

82. A 4-week-old infant is being evaluated for multiple episodes of forceful vomiting. The vomitus consists of milk without bile or blood. During examination, peristaltic waves progress across the infant's upper abdomen and then he vomits. A small circular firm mass is palpated at the lateral edge of the rectus abdominis muscle in the right upper quadrant of the abdomen. His mucous membranes are dry, and his fontanelles are sunken. Which of the following is the most likely diagnosis?
a. Physiologic gastroesophageal reflux
b. Hypertrophic pyloric stenosis
c. Duodenal atresia
d. Midgut volvulus
e. Milk-protein allergy

83. A 25-year-old male presents to the clinic with a rash on his palms, soles, and extensor surfaces of the acral extremities. He is sexually active with 1 partner. Physical examination is positive for multiple papular raised lesions. The lesions have a dusky, central area, a dark red inflammatory zone surrounded by a pale ring of edema, and an erythematous halo on the extreme periphery of the lesions. Nikolsky sign is negative. Which of the following is the most common predisposing factor for the development of this rash in this patient?
a. Penicillin
b. Herpes simplex virus
c. Treponema pallidum
d. Human herpesvirus 8
e. Allopurinol

84. A 60-year-old farmer presents to the clinic for a yearly examination. He denies any complaints. He has a skin lesion that has been present for the last 11 months. Physical examination is notable for an erythematous scaly plaque 5 mm in diameter with a rough texture and crust. Which of the following is the patient at highest risk of developing based on the described skin lesion?
a. Malignant melanoma
b. Kaposi sarcoma
c. Squamous cell carcinoma
d. Basal cell carcinoma
e. Seborrheic keratosis

85. A 40-year-old male presents to the clinic complaining of dyspnea on medium exertion for the last 8 months. He has a history of Rheumatic fever during early childhood. Physical examination is notable for a hoarse voice, a low-pitched diastolic rumble, and a loud S1. The murmur is heard best at the apex with the patient lying on the left side in held expiration. An echocardiogram reveals the most likely diagnosis. Which of the following is the most appropriate management in this patient?
a. Beta blockers and Automatic implantable cardioverter defibrillator
b. Mitral valve replacement
c. Aortic valve replacement
d. Aortic valve repair
e. Percutaneous valve balloon commissurotomy

86. A 9-year-old boy presented to the emergency department 2 days ago after he fell off monkey bars. He sustained a supracondylar fracture of his right upper extremity and was placed in a posterior splint. Today, he is complaining of excruciating 10/10 pain. Physical examination reveals swelling to the elbow and the right forearm is tense compared to the left. Which of the following is the most useful sensitive early finding suggestive of Compartment syndrome?
a. Paralysis of the forearm
b. Pallor of the forearm
c. Absence of radial pulses
d. Palpable tenderness of the forearm
e. Pain with passive stretching of the forearm muscles

87. A 62-year-old man with a history of Hypertension and Diabetes mellitus is being evaluated for sudden onset of right arm and facial weakness. On examination, the right arm is weaker than the right leg, he is able to raise both eyebrows, and left gaze preference is noted. When asked to repeat a sentence, he speaks with a long sentence, sometimes using irrelevant words that do not make sense. Which of the following is the most likely diagnosis?
a. Right middle cerebral artery stroke
b. Left vertebrobasilar artery stroke
c. Left middle cerebral artery stroke
d. Right anterior cerebral artery stroke
e. Left anterior cerebral artery stroke

88. A 3-year-old boy presents with a thermal burn. His mother states the child mistakenly got burned by hot water when she tipped over a hot cup of coffee. On examination, there is erythema without blistering with a clean line of demarcation and little tapering of depth at the edges involving the buttocks and area between the anus and the genitals and the upper thighs. Which of the following is the most appropriate management of this patient?
a. Transfer to a burn center
b. Contact social worker for a home visit to assess home safety
c. Consultation with child protective services for suspected abuse
d. Plastic surgery consultation for possible skin grafting
e. Apply Silver sulfadiazine, nonstick gauze, sterile dressing and have the patient follow-up in 24 hours

89. Which of the following is most characteristic of the tremor of Parkinson disease?
a. Postural-action tremor that increases with voluntary muscle contraction and movement
b. Symmetrical and bilateral initially, often involving both hands and arms, head, and voice
c. Most noticeable when affected body part is supported against gravity or not engaged in purposeful activity
d. Worsens when the arms are held outstretched
e. The side that is initially affected tends to be the less affected side throughout the course of the disease

90. A 62-year-old male presents to the office complaining of dull abdominal discomfort. It began initially as right flank a few months ago. Over the last 6 days, he noticed blood in his urine. He denies fever, chills, and dysuria. He has a 30 pack-year smoking history. Physical exam reveals a thin pale male with a firm, homogeneous, nontender right flank mass that moves with respiration and a "bag of worms" feel with palpation of the left scrotum. Urinalysis is positive for red blood cells and negative for leukocytes. Which of the following tests is the preferred diagnostic imaging modality to establish the most likely diagnosis?
a. Computed tomography (CT) of the abdomen and pelvis
b. Abdominal and pelvic ultrasound
c. Urine cytology
d. Cystoscopy
e. Voiding cystourethrogram

91. A 24-year-old woman presents to the gynecology clinic for follow-up of her cytology results from her Pap testing. She denies any symptoms and physical examination is normal. Cytology reveals Atypical squamous cells of undetermined significance (ASC-US). Her last Pap smear at age 21 was normal. Which of the following is the most appropriate next step in the management of this patient?
a. Repeat pap test in 1 year
b. Reflex Human papillomavirus testing
c. Perform Pap smear with HPV cotesting in 3 years
d. Repeat pap test in 3 months
e. Colposcopy

92. A 60-year-old male is being evaluated in the ED after a fall from a standing height. Physical examination is notable for prominent motor weakness in both upper limbs compared to lower limbs. His biceps and triceps reflexes are diminished. There are notable sensory deficits worse in the fingers and distributed along the posterior upper arms and the upper back with pain and temperature sensation deficits in the same distribution. Cervical radiographs are positive for an extension teardrop fracture. Which of the following is the most likely diagnosis?
a. Posterior cord syndrome
b. Anterior cord syndrome
c. Central cord syndrome
d. Brown Sequard syndrome
e. Middle cerebral artery stroke

93. A 32-year-old male brings his girlfriend to the ED after she became semi-responsive. Her breathing became agonal, and she was nodding off, with no reaction even after trying to arouse her. On examination, blood pressure is 112/72 mmHg, pulse 56/minute, respirations 4 breaths per minute and shallow, and oxygen saturation 80% on room air. Her Glasgow Coma Score is 3. Her pupils are constricted. Fingerstick glucose is 108 mg/dL (70 – 110). Which of the following is the most appropriate next step?
a. Naloxone therapy
b. Oropharyngeal airway placement and use of bag–valve–mask ventilation
c. Use of a bag–valve–mask device plus Flumazenil
d. Dextrose 5% in water plus Naltrexone
e. Suboxone therapy

94. A 54-year-old male is complaining of dull chest pressure for 40 minutes that began while shoveling snow. He has a history of Hypertension and Dyslipidemia. Vital signs are stable, and he is diaphoretic. An ECG reveals deep, symmetric T wave inversions in V1 and V2 with T wave flattening. Initial labs reveal a troponin of 0.02 ng/mL (0-0.04). Which of the following is the most likely diagnosis?
a. Non-ST elevation myocardial infarction
b. Anterior wall Myocardial infarction
c. Variant (Prinzmetal angina)
d. Stable angina pectoris
e. Unstable angina

95. A 25-year-old male presents to the clinic for low-grade fever, sore throat, myalgia, diarrhea, and headache. He is sexually active with 4 partners and does not always use condoms. Physical examination is notable for nontender occipital and cervical lymphadenopathy. Pharyngeal edema and hyperemia without tonsillar enlargement or exudate are noted. There are painful sharply demarcated ulcers with white bases surrounded by thin erythema on the oral mucosa. There are well-circumscribed oval deeply red colored maculopapules on his thorax and neck. Which of the following is the most likely diagnosis?
a. Epstein-Barr virus Infectious mononucleosis
b. Cytomegalovirus (CMV) mononucleosis
c. Acute HIV retroviral syndrome
d. Group A Streptococcus pharyngitis
e. Pityriasis rosea

96. A 20-year-old female is complaining of intense shock-like, stabbing pain in her face radiating to her right jaw, lasting a few seconds. The pain is triggered when she washes her face or with strong wind gusts. Associated symptoms include a burning sensation in the legs. On examination, stroking the right face reproduces the pain. There is decreased sensation to light touch in the legs and plantar reflexes are upgoing. Which of the following is the most likely etiology of her presentation?
a. Demyelination of the oligodendrocytes in the central nervous system
b. Demyelination of the Schwann cells in the peripheral nervous system
c. Autoantibodies against the postsynaptic acetylcholine receptor
d. Autoantibodies against the presynaptic voltage-gated calcium channels
e. Motor neuron degeneration and death with gliosis replacing lost neurons

97. A 20-year-old male presents to the clinic. He has been having difficulty with a recent breakup. Since the breakup of his 5-week relationship, he has these overwhelming feelings of intense sadness and emptiness. He has been coping by impulsively going out to clubs, drinking excessively, and engaging in unsafe sex with strangers. He has a history of stormy relationships with his friends, family, and significant others. During the interview, moment to moment fluctuations in his mood, including angry outbursts, laughter, and feelings of worthlessness are noted. Which of the following is the first line management of this patient?
a. Paroxetine
b. Cognitive and behavioral therapy
c. Exposure and response prevention therapy
d. Risperidone
e. Lithium

98. A 35-year-old male returns to the clinic for evaluation of multiple elevated blood pressure readings. His second urinalysis remains positive for microalbuminuria. Basic metabolic panel, including glucose, BUN, and creatinine are within normal limits. Which of the following is the first line antihypertensive of choice in this patient?
a. Lisinopril
b. Hydrochlorothiazide
c. Nifedipine
d. Metoprolol
e. Tamsulosin

99. A 25-year-old woman at 37+2 weeks gestation presents to the labor and delivery department after noticing a gush of clear fluid from her vagina. She denies abdominal cramping, uterine contractions, or bleeding. Examination of the vaginal fluid reveals a vaginal pH of 8 and microscopic examination of fluid is positive for ferning. GBS testing is negative. Nonstress testing is reassuring. Which of the following is the most appropriate next step in the management of this patient?
a. Expectant management
b. Oxytocin induction
c. Nifedipine
d. Digital cervicovaginal examination
e. Cesarean section

100. A 40-year-old male presents to his primary care provider for a 12-day history of anorexia, fatigue, malaise, frothy urine, and swelling around his eyes, worse in the morning. He has a history of Chronic Hepatitis B. Vitals are stable. Laboratory evaluation reveals a serum albumin 2.2 g/dL (3.4-5.4) and serum complement 3.25 mg//dL (75-175). 24-hour protein excretion is 4 g/day. Electron microscopic examination reveals subepithelial electron-dense deposits and a spike and dome appearance of the specimen. Which of the following would most likely be seen on light microscopy?
a. Focal and segmental scarring
b. Kimmelstiel Wilson nodules
c. Mesangial expansion
d. Thickening of the glomerular basement membrane
e. Normal appearing glomeruli

END OF EXAM 1

1. CARDIOLOGY – STRESS CARDIOMYOPATHY [MOST LIKELY]

Stress (Takotsubo) cardiomyopathy [choice C] should be suspected in patients with:

- the presence of new electrocardiographic abnormalities (eg, **ST elevations) and mild troponin elevation**
- **absence of angiographic evidence of obstructive coronary disease or acute plaque rupture**
- **Presence of transient regional wall motion abnormalities (systolic dysfunction),** especially of the left ventricle & usually not in a single coronary distribution,
- exclusion of pheochromocytoma or myocarditis.

Stress cardiomyopathy is a type of nonischemic Dilated cardiomyopathy seen most commonly in postmenopausal women and thought to be triggered by a stress surge of catecholamines.

Choice A [Atherosclerotic heart disease] is excluded by the patent coronary arteries on angiography.

Choice B [Variant (Prinzmetal) angina] can also present with chest pain, ECG changes, and positive enzymes. Vasospasm is usually evident on angiography, and it is not associated with apical hypokinesis.

Choice D (Pheochromocytoma) may present with headache, palpitations, and sweating, but it is associated with positive urine and serum catecholamines.

Choice E (Restrictive cardiomyopathy) is classically associated with normal or slightly increased wall thickness and diastolic dysfunction on echocardiography.

2. PSYCHIATRY AND BEHAVIORAL MEDICINE – PANIC DISORDER/AGORAPHOBIA [CLINICAL INTERVENTION]

Treatment of Agoraphobia independent of Panic disorder is treated the same as Agoraphobia in the setting of Panic disorder with Cognitive behavioral therapy as the preferred initial psychotherapy &/or Selective serotonin reuptake inhibitors (SSRIs) as preferred initial pharmacotherapy [choice D].

Agoraphobia is defined in the American Psychiatric Association's Diagnostic and Statistical Manual of Mental Disorders, Fifth Edition, Text Revision (DSM-5-TR) as fear or anxiety about and/or avoidance of situations where help may not be available or where it may be difficult to leave the situation in the event of developing panic-like symptoms or other debilitating or embarrassing symptoms.

3. RENAL – Autosomal dominant polycystic kidney disease (ADPKD), LABS AND DIAGNOSTIC STUDIES

In patients with an established family history of Autosomal dominant polycystic kidney disease (ADPKD), Ultrasonography [choice D] confirms the diagnosis.

≥2 cysts in patients under age 30 years, >2 cysts in each kidney in patients aged 30–59 years, and >4 cysts in each kidney in patients aged 60 years or older can establish the diagnosis of ADPKD.

These criteria do *not* apply to individuals without a known family history.

Individuals without a family history should be evaluated with CT scan.

In addition to renal manifestations, ADPKD can present with Diverticulosis, Mitral valve prolapse, and Subarachnoid hemorrhage.

Choice A [24-hour urine metanephrines] is helpful in establishing the diagnosis of Pheochromocytoma, which can present with paroxysms of headache, diaphoresis, and palpitations. It is not associated with bilateral palpable flank masses.

Choice B [Radionuclide renal scan] may be used in some people to diagnose Renovascular hypertension but it is not associated with bilateral palpable flank masses.

Choice C [Renal biopsy] is not the next appropriate step as it is invasive.

Choice A (Cystoscopy) is used to establish the diagnosis of Bladder cancer.

4. NEUROLOGY – CRANIAL NERVES [HISTORY AND PHYSICAL]
Functions of the oculomotor nerve (cranial nerve III) [choice B] include:
- **Eye movement: all of the ocular muscles** except for the lateral rectus (CN VI) [LR6] and the superior oblique muscles (CN IV) [SO4].
- **Opens eyelid:** supplies the **levator palpebrae**. Damage can lead to **ptosis**.
- **Pupil constriction** (SLUDD-**C**) and accommodations: **efferent pupillary response** (CN III efferent; CN II afferent).

Pathology of CN III includes:
- unresponsive ipsilateral pupillary constriction on the affected side (the **pupil is fixed and dilated [blown pupil]**) when light is shined in either eye (**efferent pupillary defect**).
- **eye is "down and out"***.
- **Diabetes can cause CN III palsy with pupil sparing.**

Choice A [II] is responsible for visual acuity and visual fields. It is also responsible for the afferent pupillary response.

Choice C [IV] innervates the Superior oblique muscle [SO4]. It depresses the eye when adducted in isolation (down and out).

Choice D [VI] is responsible for Lateral eye motion [LR6]: the lateral rectus muscle functions to abduct the ipsilateral eye (look away from the nose).

Choice E [VII] is responsible for motor innervation of the face, innervates the stapedius muscle, and is sensation of the anterior two-thirds of the tongue.

5. EENT – ANTERIOR EPISTAXIS [CLINICAL INTERVENTION]
Cauterization [choice E] with electrocautery or silver nitrate is recommended in the management of Anterior epistaxis if direct pressure with or without a topical vasoconstrictor fails and the site can be visualized.

Choice A [Foley catheter placement] can be used in the management of Posterior epistaxis.

Choice B [Anterior nasal packing with a nasal tampon] can be used in the management of Anterior epistaxis if direct pressure, vasoconstrictors, & cautery are unsuccessful, if the site cannot be visualized, or if there is severe bleeding.

Choice C [Posterior nasal packing] can be used in the management of Posterior epistaxis.

Choice D {Irrigation with normal saline] is not the management of refractory epistaxis.

6. REPRODUCTIVE – POLYCYSTIC OVARY SYNDROME [HISTORY AND PHYSICAL]
Physical examination findings of Polycystic ovary syndrome include hirsutism [choice D], obesity, acne, acanthosis nigricans, and possible bilateral enlarged ovaries on pelvic examination.

Hirsutism is defined as excessive terminal (course) hairs in male pattern of distribution.

Polycystic ovary syndrome (PCOS) is characterized by:
- hyperandrogenism (eg, hirsutism, moderate-severe acne)
- menstrual irregularity (eg, oligo- or amenorrhea, or irregular bleeding)
- obesity and insulin resistance
- polycystic ovaries on imaging.

Choice A [Cervical motion tenderness] may be seen with Ectopic pregnancy or Pelvic inflammatory disease.
Choice B [Diffusely enlarged (globular), soft, mobile tender uterus] is hallmark for Adenomyosis.
Choice C [Discrete, firm, nontender, asymmetric mobile enlarged masses in the pelvis] is hallmark for Leiomyomas [Uterine fibroids].
Choice E [Adnexal tenderness] is hallmark for Ovarian torsion or Pelvic inflammatory disease.

7. PULMONARY – PULMONARY EMBOLISM [HISTORY AND PHYSICAL]

Tachypnea [choice D] is the most common physical examination finding in Pulmonary embolism, occurring in 54% of patients with Pulmonary embolism.
Other findings include:
- Calf or thigh swelling, erythema, edema, tenderness, palpable cords (47%)
- Tachycardia (24%)
- Rales (18%)
- Decreased breath sounds (17%)
- An accentuated pulmonic component of the second heart sound (15%)
- Jugular venous distension (14%)
- Fever (3%)

8. HEMATOLOGY – TRANSFUSION REACTION/ACUTE HEMOLYTIC TRANSFUSION REACTION [FOUNDATIONAL SCIENTIFIC CONCEPTS]

Acute hemolytic transfusion reaction (AHTR) is a potentially life-threatening reaction caused by acute intravascular hemolysis of transfused red blood cells (RBCs), most commonly due to ABO incompatibility [choice C] or caused by a reaction to alleles in other RBC antigen systems. ABO incompatible transfusion reactions are usually the result of human error, resulting in transfusion of a product not appropriate for the recipient.
AHTR classically presents with fever, chills, flank pain, and oozing from intravenous sites, and discomfort at transfusion sites.

Choice A [IgA deficiency] may result in Anaphylactic transfusion reaction resulting from an allergic reaction due to IgE antibodies in the recipient's blood due to antigens in the donor plasma (eg, IgA).
Choice B [Donor blood products contaminated by bacteria or bacterial byproducts] results in Transfusion-related sepsis, which presents with hypotension, fever, chills, and rigor.
Choice D [Reaction to cytokines stored in the transfused blood] results in Febrile non-hemolytic transfusion reaction. It is characterized by fever, chills, headache, & flushing in the absence of other systemic symptoms 1-6 hours after transfusion initiation.

Choice E [Activation of recipient's neutrophils by antigens & anti-leukocyte antibodies in the transfused donor product] may result in Transfusion-related acute lung injury [TRALI]. TRALI usually presents with acute respiratory distress (eg, dyspnea, tachypnea, hypoxia), hypotension within minutes to 6 hours after transfusion, and a new infiltrate on chest radiography (similar to ARDS).

9. EENT – ORBITAL CELLULITIS [FOUNDATIONAL SCIENTIFIC CONCEPTS]

Although both Preseptal cellulitis and orbital cellulitis classically present with eyelid swelling with or without erythema, findings of ophthalmoplegia, pain with eye movements, and/or proptosis occur only with orbital cellulitis, an infection posterior to the orbital septum [choice B].
Imaging studies, such as CT scan, may be useful in distinguishing between the two if the diagnosis is uncertain based on history and physical examination.

Choice A [Severe bacterial infection of the conjunctiva] is often associated with a purulent ocular discharge.
Choice C [Infection anterior to the orbital septum] is Preseptal cellulitis. Although both Preseptal cellulitis and Orbital cellulitis classically present with eyelid swelling with or without erythema, findings of ophthalmoplegia, pain with eye movements, and/or proptosis occur only with orbital cellulitis
Choice D [Thrombus within the cavernous sinus] and Orbital cellulitis have similar symptoms, including periorbital swelling and ophthalmoplegia, but involvement of the cavernous sinus is associated with headache, visual loss, papilledema, bilateral eye involvement, dilated pupil(s), and cranial nerve V palsy.
Choice E [Mucormycosis fungal infection involving the orbit] is most commonly seen in patients with Diabetes mellitus. Initial symptoms include symptoms of Acute sinusitis, perinasal facial edema; necrosis of the palate, nasal mucosa, or skin (eg, black eschar); and orbital edema, proptosis, blindness, or ophthalmoplegia.

10. DERMATOLOGY – ACNE VULGARIS [PHARMACOLOGY]

Oral Isotretinoin [choice C] is the most appropriate next step in the management of refractory moderate to severe nodulocystic Acne vulgaris.
Oral Isotretinoin is the most effective agent for decreasing the number of lesions of Acne. Common adverse effects of Oral Isotretinoin include dry skin and mucous membranes. It is highly teratogenic.

Choice A [Add topical Clindamycin] may result in small improvement but Oral Isotretinoin is a much more effective agent.
Choice B [Switch to oral Doxycycline] is not the best next step in the management as the patient is on an effective Tetracycline already.
Choice D [Add oral Cephalexin] is not used in the management of Nodulocystic acne as *Propionibacterium acnes* is not responsive to Cephalexin.
Choice E [Add topical Erythromycin] is not the next step in the management of nodulocystic acne.

11. EENT – GONOCOCCAL CONJUNCTIVITIS [PHARMACOLOGY]

Single dose of IM Ceftriaxone, topical Ofloxacin, & oral Doxycycline [choice C] is first-line management of Gonococcal conjunctivitis, along with ophthalmology consult or referral.

Choice A [Bacitracin ophthalmic ointment] is used for gram-positive organisms.
Choice B [Erythromycin ointment] does not cover for *N. gonorrhoeae*.
Choice D [Topical Ofloxacin] is used in patients who are contact lens wearers.
Choice E [Single dose of intramuscular (IM) Penicillin G] is used to treat Syphilis.

12. GI/NUTRITION – SMALL BOWEL OBSTRUCTION [HISTORY AND PHYSICAL]

Prior abdominal surgery [choice B] is the most common risk factor for mechanical Small bowel obstruction (SBO) in the United States.
Other less common causes include abdominal hernias [choice D] and GI malignancy [choice E].

Choice A [Hypokalemia] is a common cause of Adynamic (paralytic) ileus.
Choice C [Chronic constipation] may be associated with Diverticular disease and Sigmoid volvulus.

13. ENDOCRINE – DIABETIC KETOACIDOSIS [CLINICAL INTERVENTION]

The management of patients with DKA and low serum potassium (<3.3 mEq/L) is IV fluids (eg, 0.9% saline and IV potassium) [choice E]; Insulin should be withheld until repeat labs reveal a serum potassium of ≥3.3 mEq/L.
The only indication for delaying the initiation of insulin therapy is if the serum potassium is <3.3 mEq/L since Insulin will worsen hypokalemia by shifting potassium intracellularly.
Insulin therapy lowers serum potassium (K+) concentration by driving K+ into cells both (1) directly and (2) indirectly by reversing hyperglycemia and acidosis (hyperglycemia and acidosis shift K+ extracellularly so reversal of hyperglycemia with insulin therapy also shifts potassium intracellularly).

- If Hypokalemia (<3.3 mEq/L): replace potassium and hold insulin.
- If Hyperkalemia (>5.5 mEq/dL): hold the potassium, give insulin.
- Normal potassium (3.3 and 5.5 mEq/dL): give both potassium and insulin and adjust based on labs monitoring every 1-2 hours

Choice A [Insulin, IV 0.9% sodium chloride, and IV potassium] is therapy for DKA in patients with a normal serum potassium 3.3-5.5.
Choice B [IV Insulin, IV potassium, and IV D5 0.9% sodium chloride] can be used for patients with DKA with a normal serum potassium and serum glucose <250 mg/dL.
Choice C [IV 0.9% sodium chloride] is part of the management but potassium should also be repleted in this patient, making this answer incomplete.
Choice D [IV Insulin and IV 0.9% sodium chloride] is incorrect because Insulin should be withheld in patients with DKA and Hypokalemia.

14. ENDOCRINE – SYNDROME OF INAPPROPRIATE ADH [CLINICAL INTERVENTION]

Fluid restriction [choice A] is the mainstay of the treatment of most patients with SIADH, with a suggested goal intake of <800 mL/day; patients with subarachnoid hemorrhage are an exception since fluid restriction may promote cerebral vasospasm.

Causes of SIADH include any CNS disorder, pulmonary disease (such as Legionella Pneumonia in this patient), or certain medications.

Choice B [IV 3% sodium chloride] is used in the management of Hyponatremia <120 mEq/L, acute (occurring in <48 hours), or severe (obtunded, seizures).

Choice C [IV 0.9% sodium chloride] is used in the management of Hypovolemic hypotonic hyponatremia.

Choice D [Dextrose 5% in water] is used in the management of Hypernatremia. It would be inappropriate in this patient as it could worsen the Hyponatremia.

Choice E [Salt tablets] can be used as an add on to patients with Hyponatremia not responsive to initial management.

15. INFECTIOUS DISEASE – ROCKY MOUNTAIN SPOTTED FEVER [FOUNDATIONAL SCIENTIFIC CONCEPTS]

Rickettsia rickettsii [choice E] is the causative agent of Rocky Mountain spotted fever (RMSF), which presents with nonspecific symptoms, such as fever, headache, malaise, myalgias, arthralgias, and nausea.

A maculopapular rash often begins at the wrists and ankles and can become petechial between the third and fifth days of illness.

Common labs seen in RMSF include thrombocytopenia, hyponatremia, elevations in serum aminotransferases, and prolongation of the partial thromboplastin and prothrombin times.

Although RMSF occurs throughout the US, it is most commonly reported in North Carolina, Tennessee, Missouri, Arkansas, and Oklahoma.

Choice A [Ehrlichia chaffeensis] is associated with a macular, maculopapular (rarely petechial), in a minority of patients. When rash is present, alternative etiologies of rash should be examined.

Choice B [Borrelia burgdorferi] is the causative agent of Lyme disease, which presents with Erythema migrans.

Choice C [Neisseria meningitidis] can present with a petechial rash but is often associated with meningeal signs (nuchal rigidity, positive Brudzinski or Kernig signs).

Choice D [West Nile virus] is associated with Encephalitis.

16. EENT – ACUTE RHINOSINUSITIS [CLINICAL INTERVENTION]

Watchful waiting for a 7-day period and symptomatic management [choice D] is the mainstay of therapy for uncomplicated Acute viral and bacterial rhinosinusitis.

Acute rhinosinusitis usually resolves or begins to improve within 10 days.

Patients who fail to improve after ≥10 days of symptomatic management are more likely to have acute bacterial rhinosinusitis (ABRS) and should be managed as such, which may include antibiotics.

Either Oral Amoxicillin [choice A] or Oral Amoxicillin-clavulanic acid [choice B] may be used in the management of Acute bacterial rhinosinusitis with symptoms >10 days or worsening. The addition of clavulanate to amoxicillin improves coverage for ampicillin resistant *Haemophilus influenzae* as well as *Moraxella catarrhalis*.

Choice C [Non contrast CT of the Maxillofacial bones] is usually not necessary in the workup of Acute uncomplicated Rhinosinusitis. However, when imaging is needed (eg, severe symptoms or suspected intracranial or intraocular infection). CT scan without &/or with contrast is usually performed.

Choice E (Water's view radiographs) is the radiograph view of choice for Acute sinusitis when plain radiographs are indicated.

17. ENDOCRINE – ADRENAL INSUFFICIENCY [HISTORY AND PHYSICAL EXAMINATION]

Hyperpigmentation of the skin [choice B] is a classic finding of longstanding Primary adrenocortical insufficiency (AI), in addition to weight loss.

Hyperpigmentation in Primary adrenal insufficiency is caused by an increased production of α-melanocyte-stimulating-hormone (αMSH). This is because both αMSH and ACTH originate from the pro-hormone peptide pro-opiomelanocortin (POMC).

In primary AI, Hyperkalemia and Hyponatremia reflect decreased aldosterone production (normally aldosterone holds onto sodium and increases renal excretion of potassium and hydrogen ions).

Choice A [Acanthosis nigricans of the neck and the axillae] is most commonly seen in obese patients. Other causes include disorders with insulin resistance, such as Diabetes mellitus, and Cushing syndrome.

Choice C [Nontender goiter with a bruit in the neck] may be seen in patients with Graves' disease.

Choice D [Wide, purple-colored abdominal striae] is hallmark of Cushing syndrome.

Choice E [Loss of the outer third of the eyebrows] is hallmark for Hypothyroidism.

18. GI/NUTRITION – COLORECTAL CANCER [HEALTH MAINTENANCE]

This patient should initiate screening Colonoscopy at 35 years; then every 5 years thereafter [choice A], which is 10 years before his brother was diagnosed.

In patients with a first-degree relative with cancer or advanced polyp <60 years at time of diagnosis: Screening Colonoscopy is performed initially at 40 years OR 10 years before the age the relative was diagnosed (whichever is earlier) then colonoscopy every 5 years.

Choice B [Colonoscopy at 40 years; then every 5 years thereafter] is incorrect because 10 years before his brother was diagnosed would make his screening start at age 35.

Choice C [Colonoscopy at 40 years; then every 10 years thereafter] is used in the screening of patients with a first degree relative ≥60 years age.

Choice E [Colonoscopy at 50 years; then every 10 years thereafter] is used for Colorectal cancer in individuals with average risk.

19. PULMONARY – ACUTE BRONCHIOLITIS [CLINICAL INTERVENTION]

The management of Acute bronchiolitis is supportive care, which includes relief of nasal congestion/obstruction, maintenance of adequate hydration, and monitoring for disease progression [choice C].

Education that Acute bronchiolitis peaks on days 3-5, then gradually resolve over a period of 2-3 weeks is recommended.

Acute bronchiolitis should be suspected in children 2 months-2 years of age that present with upper respiratory tract symptoms for 2-3 days, followed by lower respiratory symptoms and signs (increased work of breathing, wheezing, crackles).

Most children with Acute bronchiolitis do NOT require any specific pharmacological management [eg, bronchodilators (choice B), corticosteroids (choice D), or antibiotics (choice E)] as most recover with supportive management alone.

Choice A [Nebulized epinephrine and supplemental oxygen by nasal cannula] may be required in moderate to severe Croup.

20. PSYCHIATRY AND BEHAVIORAL MEDICINE – ATTENTION-DEFICIT HYPERACTIVITY DISORDER [PHARMACOLOGY]

Stimulants, such as Methylphenidate [choice D] are the first line pharmacotherapy for Attention deficit hyperactivity disorder (ADHD).

Selective norepinephrine reuptake inhibitors, such as Atomoxetine [choice A], are an alternative but are not as effective as the stimulants.

Alpha-2-adrenergic agonists, such as Guanfacine [choice C] and Clonidine [choice E] are options in children unresponsive to a trial of stimulants or selective norepinephrine reuptake inhibitors, have intolerable adverse effects, or have significant coexisting conditions.

Medications with or without behavioral/psychological interventions [choice B] are usually recommended for most school-aged children (≥6 years) and adolescents who meet diagnostic criteria for ADHD.

21. PULMONARY – INFLUENZA [PHARMACOLOGY]

Supportive management without antiviral treatment [choice C] is the first line management of Influenza for outpatients with uncomplicated illness who are not at high risk with symptoms ≥48 hours due to lack of any significant benefit.

For outpatients with uncomplicated illness who are not at high risk who present within 48 hours of symptom onset, antiviral may be used in some to reduce the duration of illness by ~24 hours or supportive management alone may be used.

Choice A [Azithromycin] is not indicated in the management of Influenza.

Choice B [Oseltamivir] is indicated in the management of individuals not at high risk who present within 48 hours or in all high-risk patients regardless of symptom duration.

Choice D [Supplemental oxygen] is not needed as the patient has good oxygenation.

Choice E [Albuterol] is not necessary as the patient has a normal pulmonary examination.

22. MUSCULOSKELETAL – SYSTEMIC SCLEROSIS [LABS AND DIAGNOSTIC STUDIES]

The presence of Anticentromere antibodies [choice A] is classically associated with limited cutaneous Systemic sclerosis, which represents 80% of Systemic sclerosis.

Limited cutaneous Systemic sclerosis is associated with skin thickening restricted to the distal extremities (distal to the knees and elbows) and face (as seen in this patient).

Diffuse cutaneous Systemic sclerosis is associated with skin thickening proximal to the elbow and knees, and the trunk. Diffuse SS is classically associated with Anti-topoisomerase I (anti-Scl-70) antibodies [choice D].

Choice B [Anti-signal recognition protein] antibodies are classically associated with Polymyositis.

Choice C [Anti double-stranded DNA] antibodies are classically associated with Systemic lupus erythematosus.

Choice E [Anti-cyclic citrullinated peptide] antibodies are classically associated with Rheumatoid arthritis.

23. CARDIOLOGY – AV HEART BLOCKS [MOST LIKELY]

Mobitz type II second-degree heart block [choice D] is characterized by a nonconducted P wave that is not preceded by progressive PR interval prolongation (all the PR intervals are the same length/duration). SEE PHOTO

In second-degree heart block, some but not all of the sinus impulses reach the ventricles.

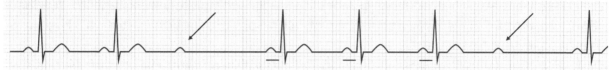

Choice A [Sinus bradycardia] is associated with a slow heart rate <60 bpm but is not associated with nonconducted impulses.

Choice B [Mobitz type I second-degree heart block] is also associated with occasional nonconducted impulses but differs from Mobitz II in that in Mobitz I (Wenckebach), there is progressive lengthening of the PR interval until there is a dropped beat.

Choice C [Third-degree AV block] is associated with AV dissociation, where none of the P waves conduct through the AV node. The P-P intervals and the R-R intervals are regular.

Choice E [First-degree AV block] is associated with a prolonged PR interval > 0.20 seconds but every P is followed by a QRS, reflecting that every atrial beat gets conducted to the ventricles.

24. CARDIOLOGY – AORTIC DISSECTION [LABS AND DIAGNOSTIC STUDIES]

CT angiogram of the chest [choice D] is the first line diagnostic test to establish the diagnosis of Aortic dissection in a patient who is hemodynamically stable.

Aortic dissection should be suspected in patients with a history of Hypertension who present with abrupt onset of chest and back pain, especially if the pain radiates to the back in between the scapulae.

Physical exam findings may include asymmetric upper extremity pulses or blood pressures.

Choice A [Administer Aspirin, chewed for faster absorption] is used in the management of Acute coronary syndrome (eg, MI, UA, NSTEMI). In a patient with Aortic dissection, it can increase the risk of bleeding.

Choice B [D-dimer] is useful in the diagnosis of a Pulmonary embolism, but this patient has classic symptoms of Aortic dissection.

Choice C [Transesophageal echocardiography], performed at the bedside or in the OR, is an alternative to CT angiogram as initial advanced imaging if hemodynamically unstable, impaired renal function (eg, elevated creatinine), or contrast allergy.

Choice E [Ventilation-perfusion scan] is used in the diagnosis of Pulmonary emboli.

25. ENDOCRINE – CUSHING SYNDROME [MOST LIKELY]

Because most pituitary Corticotroph tumors [choice C] are partially sensitive to negative feedback regulation by glucocorticoids, High-dose (8 mg) Dexamethasone suppression tests usually result in serum cortisol level decrease of ≥50%.

In contrast, most nonpituitary tumors associated with the ectopic ACTH production are completely resistant to feedback inhibition, resulting in <50% reduction of cortisol production after a High-dose Dexamethasone suppression test.

Cushing disease (ACTH-producing pituitary tumor) is the most common endogenous cause of Cushing syndrome (signs and/or symptoms of cortisol excess).

Choice A [Autoimmune adrenal gland dysfunction] is the most common cause of Primary adrenal insufficiency.

Choice B [Exogenous glucocorticoid use] is the most common overall cause of Cushing syndrome. Elevated glucose levels would result in a decreased baseline ACTH via negative feedback. This patient's increased baseline ACTH makes this less likely the etiology of CS.

Choice D [Ectopic ACTH producing tumor] is usually completely resistant to feedback inhibition, resulting in <50% reduction of cortisol production after a High-dose Dexamethasone suppression test.

Choice E [Adrenal Tumor] is associated with a decreased baseline ACTH due to negative feedback from the overproduction of cortisol (ACTH-independent).

26. EENT – NEONATAL CONJUNCTIVITIS [PHARMACOLOGY]

Oral Azithromycin [choice C] is the first line management for neonatal *Chlamydia trachomatis* infection of the conjunctiva and pneumonia. Oral Erythromycin base is an alternative.

C. trachomatis conjunctivitis usually presents 5 to 14 days after delivery (up to 23 days). Classic findings of conjunctivitis range from mild swelling with a watery ocular discharge, which becomes mucopurulent, to prominent eyelid swelling and chemosis.

Topical therapy for chlamydial conjunctivitis [choices A, D, and E] is **not** effective, and a high failure rate is correlated with topical use compared with oral therapy in treating Chlamydial conjunctival infection.

Topical therapy also does not eradicate nasopharyngeal infection.

Choice B [Intramuscular Ceftriaxone] or IV Ceftriaxone is used in the management of Neonatal gonococcal conjunctivitis, which usually manifests 2-5 days after birth. It is uncommon for neonatal gonococcal conjunctivitis to occur after day 5.

27. CARDIOLOGY – INFECTIVE ENDOCARDITIS [FOUNDATIONAL SCIENTIFIC CONCEPTS]

Streptococcus viridans [choice C] is the most common cause of Subacute endocarditis (slower disease progression over weeks to months) and is often a complication of dental procedures as it is part of the normal oral flora.

Viridans streptococci has an ability to adhere to diseased endocardium and its frequently implicated in transient bacteremia during dental procedures and routine mouth care.

Choice A [*Staphylococcus epidermidis*] is a common cause of Acute endocarditis in addition to Staphylococcus aureus, especially within the acute period of prosthetic valve placement.

Choice B [*Streptococcus gallolyticus*] is seen with increased incidence in patients with Ulcerative colitis or Colorectal cancer. Patients with Infective endocarditis with *S. gallolyticus* should undergo Colonoscopy.

Choice D [Enterococcus species] is associated with increased incidence in individuals with a history of GI or GU procedure.

Choice E [*Eikenella corrodens*] is one of the fastidious organisms associated with Subacute endocarditis.

28. PSYCHIATRY AND BEHAVIORAL MEDICINE – MAJOR DEPRESSIVE DISORDER [PHARMACOLOGY]

Citalopram [choice C] is associated with the greatest risk of dose-related clinically significant QT prolongation, as well as Escitalopram.

Cardiac effects of Citalopram overdose include QT prolongation (may lead to Torsades de pointes), a type of polymorphic ventricular tachycardia that can result in sudden cardiac death. Citalopram-induced QT-interval prolongation and fatal arrhythmias are presumed to result from one of its metabolites, didemethylcitalopram.

Fluoxetine [choice D], Fluvoxamine [choice E], and Sertraline [choice B] are less likely to cause clinically significant increases in QTc most patients (they have similar low risk for QT prolongation).
Paroxetine [choice A] appears to have the lowest risk.

29. CARDIOLOGY – VENTRICULAR TACHYCARDIA [CLINICAL INTERVENTION]

Urgent synchronized cardioversion [choice A] (following administration of sedation) is recommended for patients with monomorphic Ventricular tachycardia who are hemodynamically unstable (eg, systolic blood pressure in the double digits, altered mental status) with a discernible blood pressure and pulse.

Patients should initially be treated with a synchronized 200 joules shock with subsequent shocks that use increasing energy levels as necessary

Choice B [Unsynchronized cardioversion] is used in the management of Pulseless Ventricular tachycardia and Ventricular fibrillation.
Choice C [Amiodarone] is used in the management of Ventricular tachycardia in patients who are hemodynamically stable.
Choice D [Magnesium sulfate] is used as first-line management of Polymorphic Ventricular tachycardia (Torsades de pointes).
Choice E [Verapamil] is not the management of Ventricular tachycardia.

30. REPRODUCTIVE – FIBROCYSTIC BREAST CHANGES [HISTORY AND PHYSICAL]

Pain, fluctuation in size during the menstrual cycle, and multiplicity of lesions are useful to differentiate Fibrocystic changes [choice E] from Breast carcinoma and Fibroadenoma.
Hallmark findings of Fibrocystic changes include:
- painful, often multiple, often bilateral mobile breast masses
- changes and fluctuation in size of the masses, especially during the premenstrual phase of the cycle.

Choice A [Intraductal papilloma] is classically associated with single or multiple lesions. Nipple discharge, especially bloody nipple discharge, is a frequent clinical presentation.
Choice B [Fibroadenoma] is characterized by a firm, nontender, solitary, smooth, well-circumscribed (discrete), freely mobile, and rubbery lump in the breast.
Choice C [Paget disease of the breast] is usually associated with an eczematous reaction around the nipple.
Choice D [Infiltrative ductal carcinoma] is classically associated with breast changes (eg, nontender fixed mass, change in breast contour, nipple discharge or inversion, skin dimpling, or axillary lymphadenopathy).

31. PSYCHIATRY AND BEHAVIORAL HEALTH – DOMESTIC ABUSE AND VIOLENCE [PROFESSIONAL PRACTICE]

For victims of domestic abuse, establishing a safety plan to keep the patient and children safe from domestic violence is important [choice E].

This may include going to the house of a friend or relative or a domestic violence shelter, an emergency kit that contains essential documents (eg, birth certificate), practicing the escape, knowing having a packed bag ready that is hidden but easy to get to in case escape is necessary.

Choice A [Call 911 and report the physical abuse] is not required and can put the patient at increased risk of danger once the abuser becomes aware that police were notified.

Choice B [Contact her mother to establish an escape plan] violates the patient's confidentiality.

Choice C [Speak with the patient's boyfriend regarding his actions towards her] can result in potential harm to the patient and/or the provider. The abuser should not be directly confronted.

Choice D [Refer her and the boyfriend to couples therapy and him to anger management] is incorrect because when the perpetrator is informed others are notified about the abuse, it can increase the potential violence towards the victim.

32. INFECTIOUS DISEASE – SCARLET FEVER [HISTORY AND PHYSICAL EXAMINATION]

Key features of Scarlet fever include:

- **the "strawberry tongue" begins with a white coating of the tongue with hyperplastic papillae [choice B]**
- circumoral pallor (circumoral area is spared), sore throat, pain with swallowing, and cervical adenopathy.
- blanching, papular rash with a "sandpaper" texture
- Pastia lines are found in the folds of the skin such as the neck, antecubital fossa, and groin.

Choice A [Palpable purpura on the buttocks and lower extremities] can occur with thrombocytopenia or IgA vasculitis, which presents with hematuria, abdominal pain, and arthralgias.

Choice C [Tightly adherent gray pseudomembrane in posterior pharynx] is hallmark of respiratory Diphtheria.

Choice D [Erythematous papules, macules, or ulcers on the soft palate and uvula] are hallmark of Nagayama spots, which can Roseola infantum (Fifth disease).

Choice E [Clustered 1-3 mm pale white or blue papules with an erythematous base on the buccal mucosa opposite the second molars] are hallmark of Koplik spots, which can occur with Rubeola (Measles).

33. PULMONARY – INFLUENZA [PROFESSIONAL PRACTICE]

The most appropriate next step is to complete the lung examination and then document the findings in the patient's chart. [choice D]

Clinicians should not document examinations that are not performed by the person documenting.

Choice A [Document a normal lung examination in the chart] is incorrect because documentation of examination that was not performed should not be done.

Choice B [Inform the supervising physician to add the normal lung examination in the chart] because documentation of examination that was not performed should not be done.

Choice C [Ask the scribe to add a normal lung examination in the chart] because documentation of examination that was not performed should not be done.

Choice E [Log in using the supervising physician credentials and document a normal lung examination] is unethical because documentation should be performed using the provider's own credentials and should not be documented if it wasn't performed.

34. EENT – OROPHARYNGEAL CANCER [LABS AND DIAGNOSTIC TESTS]

Mucocutaneous infection with HPV [choice C] types 6, 11, 16, and 18 is associated with genital warts and precancerous and cancerous lesions of the oropharynx, cervix, vulva, vagina, penis, and anus.

HPV, especially type 16, is associated with increased risk of head and neck cancer, particularly those arising in the base of the tongue and the tonsils

HPV associated oropharyngeal cancers are often seen in younger patients (especially men) who are nonusers of tobacco and alcohol.

Fine needle aspiration (FNA) biopsy is often employed to make an initial tissue diagnosis of a head and neck cancer.

Nasopharyngeal carcinoma is a relatively rare malignancy in most populations but is one of the most common cancers in southern China. It is associated with Epstein-Barr virus [choice B].

Choice D [Real-time Herpes simplex virus (HSV) PCR assay] is incorrect because HSV less corresponds to the development of oral carcinomas compared to HPV and EBV.

Choice E [Hepatitis C RNA (viral load)] is incorrect because Chronic infection with HCV is more commonly associated with the development of hepatocellular carcinoma and some lymphoproliferative disorders (eg, splenic MALT lymphoma).

35. ENDOCRINE – DIABETES MELLITUS [PHARMACOLOGY]

A history of Gastroparesis, Pancreatitis, Medullary thyroid carcinoma, or MEN 2 syndrome [choice A] are contraindications for the use of glucagon-like peptide 1 receptor agonists, such as Exenatide, as well as dual GIP and GLP-1 agonists (eg, Tirzepatide).

Evidence from rodent studies suggested that *GLP-1RAs* may stimulate parafollicular C-cells proliferation, potentially increasing the risk of new-onset Medullary thyroid carcinoma.

Choice B ["Do you have heart failure?"] should be asked prior to the use of Thiazolidinediones as they increase the risk for peripheral edema and Heart failure. In people with type 2 diabetes and established cardiovascular disease (CVD), Metformin, GLP-1 receptor agonists (Liraglutide, Semaglutide, Dulaglutide), and SGLT2 inhibitors reduce the risk of all-cause and cardiovascular mortality & reduce diabetic kidney disease.

Choice C ["Do you have recurrent vaginal yeast infections or urinary tract infections?"] should be asked prior to the start of SGLT2 inhibitors as they increase the risk of these infections due to increased urinary flow of glucose.

Choice D ["Do you have a history of Cirrhosis or hepatic disease?"] should be elicited prior to the start of Biguanides (eg, Metformin) as they can cause hepatic impairment.

Choice E ["Do you have a history of ketosis-prone Type 2 Diabetes mellitus?"] should be elicited prior to the use of SGLT2 inhibitors as they increase the risk of Diabetic ketoacidosis, including Euglycemic DKA.

36. GASTROINTESTINAL/NUTRITION – VITAMIN B1 DEFICIENCY [MOST LIKELY]

Vitamin B1 (Thiamine deficiency) [choice B] can present with any of the 4 following presentations:

- **(1) Dry" beriberi: <u>Nervous system changes</u>: symmetric peripheral neuropathy** of the **distal extremities.**
- **(2) "Wet" beriberi: CHF, dilated cardiomyopathy,** tachycardia.
- **(3) <u>Wernicke encephalopathy</u>: triad of ataxia (walking & balance), global confusion, and ophthalmoplegia.**
- **(4) <u>Korsakoff dementia</u>:** memory loss (especially short-term) anterograde & retrograde & confabulation.

Choice A [Vitamin B12] deficiency can also present with gait abnormalities but is also associated with a macrocytic anemia.

Choice C [Vitamin B6] is associated with peripheral neuropathy.

Choice D [Vitamin B3] is associated with pellagra, which presents with the 3 Ds: diarrhea, dementia, and dermatitis.

Choice E [Vitamin B2] deficiency is associated with the development of oral-ocular-genital syndrome.

37. REPRODUCTIVE – PELVIC INFLAMMATORY DISEASE [PHARMACOLOGY]

Indications for admission for Pelvic inflammatory disease (PID) [choice D] include:

- **severe clinical illness: fever ≥38.5°C [101°F]**
- **nausea and vomiting**
- inability to take oral medications or lack of response to oral medications.
- complicated PID with pelvic abscess (including tubo-ovarian abscess)
- pregnancy.

Choice B [Laparoscopy] may be used to confirm the clinical diagnosis of PID but is not commonly performed in most uncomplicated cases.

Choice A [Diagnostic culdocentesis] is rarely used to confirm pelvic infections or ruptured ectopic pregnancy.

Choice C [cervical culture] may be performed but more useful tests include Nucleic acid amplification tests (NAATs) for *C. trachomatis* and *Neisseria gonorrhoeae*, microscopy of vaginal discharge (where available), and STI screening (eg, HIV & serologic testing for Syphilis).

Choice E [IM Ceftriaxone, oral Doxycycline, Metronidazole, Naprosyn, follow-up in 2 days] can be used in the outpatient management of PID.

38. CARDIOLOGY – SEPTIC SHOCK [LABS & DIAGNOSTIC STUDIES]

An increased serum lactate (eg, >2 mmol/L) [choice B] reflects decreased organ perfusion in Sepsis the presence or absence of hypotension.

A serum lactate level ≥4 mmol/L is consistent with, but not diagnostic of, septic shock.

Serum lactate is an integral part of the initial workup of suspected Sepsis or septic shock.

In this patient, Urosepsis is probably the initiating factor based on her prior UTI symptoms.

Choice A [White cell count] can be elevated, normal, or low in Septic shock.

Choice C [Transthoracic echocardiogram] may be helpful if Endocarditis is the possible source of the infection.

Choice D [Serum glucose] may be increased but is nonspecific.

Choice E [Serum creatinine and Blood urea nitrogen] are often elevated due to renal hypoperfusion but are nonspecific.

39. GENITOURINARY – TESTICULAR CANCER [MOST LIKELY]

Nonseminomatous germ cell tumors [choice B] are classically associated with increased serum alpha-fetoprotein & beta-hCG.

Germ cell tumors (GCTs) account for 95% of testicular cancers.

The 2 main categories of GCTs are [1] pure Seminoma (no nonseminomatous elements present) and all others, known as Nonseminomatous germ cell tumors (NSGCTs).

Choice A [Leydig cell testicular tumor] may produce estrogen or testosterone, leading to feminization (eg, gynecomastia) or precocious puberty, respectively. They do not generate AFP or hCG.

Choice C [Testicular teratomas] are terminally differentiated germ cells that may contain skin or gastrointestinal epithelium, cartilage, and/or neuronal tissue. They are often malignant in adults and may be part of some nonseminomatous germ cell tumors, but they do not usually produce AFP or hCG.

Pure Seminomatous germ cell tumors [choice D] lack the tumor marker alpha fetoprotein.

Choice E [Sertoli cell testicular tumors] are sometimes associated with the excessive production of estrogen but do not usually produce AFP.

40. CARDIOLOGY – ATRIAL FLUTTER [CLINICAL INTERVENTION]

In patients with Atrial flutter with rapid ventricular response, rate control with non-dihydropyridine Calcium channel blockers (eg, Diltiazem, Verapamil) [choice E] or Beta blockers (eg, Esmolol, Metoprolol, Atenolol) are often first line.

The patient is hemodynamically stable with symptoms due to the fast ventricular rate seen on ECG.

Choice A [Synchronized cardioversion] is used in the management of unstable Atrial flutter (eg, systolic blood pressure in the double digits, altered mental status).

Choice B (Adenosine) is first line in the management of stable Supraventricular tachycardia (SVT).

Choice C (Amiodarone) is used in the management of stable wide complex tachycardia.

Choice D (Digoxin) is another option for rate control in Atrial flutter but is usually reserved for patients in whom Beta blockers or CCBs are contraindicated [eg, severe heart failure (New York Heart Association class III or IV), hypotension)] due to its adverse effects and toxicity.

41. GENITOURINARY – URGE INCONTINENCE [PHARMACOLOGY]

Beta-3 adrenergic agonist medications and antimuscarinic agents, such as Oxybutynin [choice B] are the main options for treatment of Overactive bladder (OAB) symptoms (Urge incontinence).

Prior to pharmacological treatment or in conjunction with it, pelvic floor muscle exercises to suppress urgency, lifestyle changes (eg, smoking cessation, weight loss for individuals with obesity), and bladder training (scheduled voiding and bladder reeducation) are essential in the management of OAB.

Choice A [Vaginal estrogen cream] may be used in the management of Genitourinary syndrome of Menopause.

Choice C [Bethanechol] is a medical option for Overflow incontinence.

Choice D [Urethropexy] is a surgical option for Stress incontinence.

Choice E [Advise frequent toileting technique to prevent bladder fullness] is used in the management of Overflow incontinence.

42. HEMATOLOGY – ACUTE MYELOGENOUS LEUKEMIA [MOST LIKELY]
Key features of the Acute promyelocytic leukemia [(APL), t(15;17) or M3], a subtype of Acute myelogenous leukemia [choice B] include:
- **presence of Auer rods (needle like inclusions) that are myeloperoxidase positive**
- **Disseminated intravascular coagulation** (eg, increased PT & aPTT; decreased fibrinogen).
- AML presents with symptoms of pancytopenia.

Choice A [Acute lymphoblastic leukemia] is most commonly seen in children and is associated with TdT positivity.

Choice C [Chronic lymphocytic leukemia] is most commonly associated with large amounts of mature-appearing lymphocytes that don't function well and smudge cells on peripheral smear.

Choice D [Chronic myelogenous leukemia] is associated with Philadelphia chromosome positivity.

Choice E [Multiple myeloma] is associated with anemia, bone pain, and Hypercalcemia.

43. ENDOCRINE – HYPERPARATHYROIDISM [LABS AND DIAGNOSTIC STUDIES]
~80-90% of patients with Primary Hyperparathyroidism will have elevated serum PTH concentrations, Hypercalcemia, and Hypophosphatemia [choice D].

This triad of labs is highly suggestive of Primary hyperparathyroidism, reflecting the functions of Parathyroid hormone.

Primary Hyperparathyroidism is the most common cause of Hypercalcemia. Malignancy is the second most common cause. Both account for ~90% of all cases of Hypercalcemia.

Subperiosteal resorption is classic for Hyperparathyroidism and reflects the effect of PTH pulling calcium from the bone to increase serum calcium levels.

The patient has the classic symptoms of Hypercalcemia: stones, bones (bone pain), abdominal groans (constipation), thrones (polyuria), and increased tones (elevated blood pressure).

Choice A [Decreased serum PTH, elevated PTH related protein, elevated serum calcium, decreased serum phosphate] is hallmark of malignancy, the second most common cause of Hypercalcemia, after Primary hyperparathyroidism.

Choice B [Elevated serum PTH, decreased serum calcium, increased serum phosphate] is hallmark of Secondary Hyperparathyroidism, which is seen in the presence of Chronic kidney disease and liver disease.

Choice C [Decreased serum PTH, decreased serum calcium, increased serum phosphate] is associated with Primary hypoparathyroidism.

Choice E [Elevated alkaline phosphatase, normal serum calcium, normal serum phosphate] is hallmark of Paget disease of the bone, which is associated with lytic and sclerotic lesions on imaging.

44. EENT – MALIGNANT OTITIS EXTERNA [PHARMACOLOGY]
Intravenous (IV) Ciprofloxacin [choice B] is the first line management of Malignant (Necrotizing) otitis externa (MOE) as it has excellent coverage against *Pseudomonas aeruginosa*, the most common organism associated with MOE.

In severe disease, an antipseudomonal beta-lactam may be added to IV Ciprofloxacin.

Malignant Otitis externa is most commonly seen in Diabetics and presents with severe otalgia and otorrhea. Granulation tissue is often seen on otoscopic examination.

Choice A [IV Liposomal Amphotericin B] is the first line therapy for Mucormycosis, which classically presents with erythema, swelling, necrosis, or black eschar on the palate, nasal mucosa, or face.
Choice C [Intravenous Cefazolin] has excellent gram-positive coverage but is ineffective against the gram-negative *Pseudomonas aeruginosa*, the most common cause of MOE.
Choice D [Intravenous Acyclovir] is used in the management of Herpes simplex virus.
Choice E [Intravenous Clindamycin] has excellent gram-positive and anerobic coverage but is ineffective against the gram-negative *Pseudomonas aeruginosa*, the most common cause of MOE.

45. GASTROINTESTINAL/NUTRITION – INFECTIOUS ESOPHAGITIS [PHARMACOLOGY]
Ganciclovir [choice A] is the first line agent for the treatment of AIDS-related CMV gastrointestinal disease (eg, esophagitis and colitis).
Foscarnet is an alternative.
The classic finding of CMV esophagitis are large superficial shallow ulcers and erosions.
The classic histologic finding of CMV is large intranuclear basophilic viral inclusions surrounded by a clear peripheral intranuclear halo with an "owl's eye" appearance.

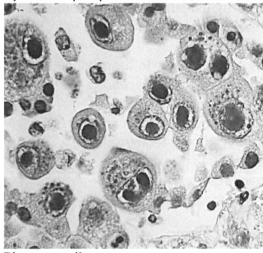

Photo credit:
Yale Rosen from USA, CC BY-SA 2.0 <https://creativecommons.org/licenses/by-sa/2.0>, via Wikimedia Commons

Choice B [Oral Fluconazole] is used in the management of Candida esophagitis, which usually presents with yellow white plaques on endoscopy and budding yeasts and hyphae on histology.
Choice C [Inhaled Budesonide without spacer use] is used in the management of Eosinophilic esophagitis, which usually presents with concentric stacked rings on Upper endoscopy.
Choice D [Topical Miconazole buccal] is used in the management of oropharyngeal Candidiasis.
Choice E [IV Acyclovir] is used in the management of Herpes simplex virus esophagitis which usually presents with deep ulcers and erosions and Type A Cowdry bodies on histology.

46. RENAL – IGA NEPHROPATHY/GLOMERULONEPHRITIS [MOST LIKELY]
IgA Nephropathy [choice C] should be suspected in children or young adults who presents with hematuria within 24-48 hours (<5 days) after the onset of symptoms of Upper respiratory infection or GI infection.

Acute glomerulonephritis is associated with hypertension, flank or abdominal pain, peripheral or periorbital edema, and hematuria.

Labs reveal hematuria, proteinuria, dysmorphic red cells, as well as increased BUN and creatinine.

Choice A [Postinfectious glomerulonephritis] may also present with gross hematuria after an upper respiratory tract infection. However, the time interval between the preceding illness and the development of hematuria is usually longer in PSGN (>10 days versus <5 days in IgAN).

Choice B [Membranoproliferative glomerulonephritis] is usually associated with viral hepatitis, hypertension, HIV, Heroin use, or Bisphosphonates. It can present with a mixed nephrotic-nephritic picture.

Choice D [Minimal change disease] presents with nephrotic range proteinuria (≥3+), hypoalbuminemia, hyperlipidemia, peripheral edema, and fatty casts. It is not associated with nephritic syndrome (eg, hematuria, proteinuria, hypertension, and edema).

Choice E [Henoch-Schöenlein purpura] is associated with hematuria, arthritis, palpable purpura, and abdominal pain.

47. MUSCULOSKELETAL – VERTEBRAL OSTEOMYELITIS – [HISTORY AND PHYSICAL]

Risk factors for Vertebral osteomyelitis include injection drug use, Immunocompromised states (including Diabetes mellitus [choice D], corticosteroid therapy), infective endocarditis, degenerative spine disease, or prior spinal surgery.

Vertebral osteomyelitis classically presents with insidious onset (weeks to months) of localized back pain, worse with activity and percussion over the affected area.

Choice A [20-pack-year smoking history] may delay healing of back diseases due to decreased vascularity but is not correlated with a direct increased risk for Vertebral osteomyelitis.

Choice B [Unilateral radiculopathy] is nonspecific and can be seen with disc disease.

Choice C [Traumatic fall] may be associated with Vertebral fractures.

Choice E [Urinary incontinence] may occur with Cauda equina syndrome.

48. MUSCULOSKELETAL – PSEUDOGOUT/CALCIUM PYROPHOSPHATE DEPOSITION DISEASE [LABS AND DIAGNOSTIC STUDIES]

The presence of positively birefringent rhomboid-shaped calcium pyrophosphate crystals via polarized light microscopy [choice E] is the classic finding on synovial fluid analysis in Calcium pyrophosphate crystal deposition (CPPD) disease.

The classic radiograph finding of CPPD is cartilage calcification (chondrocalcinosis), which appears as punctate or linear radiodensities in articular cartilage.

Choice A [WBC count 57,000 and gram-positive cocci in clusters] is hallmark of Septic arthritis.

Choice B [WBC 28,000 and negative gram stain] is hallmark of inflammatory arthritis.

Choice C [WBC 32,000 negative birefringent needle-shaped crystals] is hallmark of Gout. Classic radiograph findings include punched out lesions with sclerotic overhanging margins.

Choice D [WBC count 42,000; gram-negative diplococci] is hallmark of Septic arthritis.

49. MUSCULOSKELETAL – POLYMYALGIA RHEUMATICA [MOST LIKELY]

Proximal joint and neck pain (aching) and stiffness of the neck, shoulder, and torse, worse with inactivity and in the morning, in addition to restricted range of motion but preserved (normal) muscle strength are hallmark of Polymyalgia rheumatica [choice E].
Polymyalgia rheumatica (PMR) is a disease of the proximal articular and periarticular structures (eg, tendons, bursa) and does not involve the muscles.

Choice A [Adhesive capsulitis] is associated initially with pain worse at night, followed by predominance of stiffness with significant reduction of both active and passive range of motion. ESR and CRP are not usually elevated.
Choice B [Fibromyalgia] presents with widespread muscle pain, aching, stiffness, and fatigue. Physical examination will reveal point tenderness at specific joints and is associated with a normal ESR and CRP.
Choice C [Polymyositis] presents with symmetric proximal muscle weakness with objective muscle weakness on physical examination. Pain and stiffness are not prominent complaints and muscle involvement results in elevated muscle enzymes.
Choice D [Spondyloarthropathy] often presents with pain and stiffness of the axial skeleton, in addition to enthesitis, sacroiliitis, dactylitis, and anterior uveitis.

50. HEMATOLOGY – IRON DEFICIENCY ANEMIA [HISTORY AND PHYSICAL]
Iron deficiency is by far the most common nutritional cause of anemia and koilonychia, (spoon-shaped nails) [choice E].
Koilonychia is characterized by thin, brittle, concave nail (nail appears centrally depressed and everted laterally) as opposed to the normal convex appearance of the nail.
Cow's milk is not a good source of iron and makes it harder for the body to absorb iron. Toddlers can develop iron deficiency anemia if they drink too much cow's milk (more than 24 ounces a day) and do not eat enough foods that are rich in iron, such as green leafy vegetables and red meat.

Choice A [Splenomegaly] may be seen in children with hemolytic anemia or hematologic malignancy.
Choice B [Scleral icterus] can occur with hemolytic diseases.
Choice C [Strawberry tongue] can occur with Kawasaki disease and Scarlet fever.
Choice D [Purpura involving the lower extremities] can be seen with thrombocytopenia or IgA vasculitis.

51. CARDIOLOGY – GIANT CELL ARTERITIS [CLINICAL INTERVENTION]
For all patients with suspected Giant cell arteritis (GCA), the most appropriate next step in management is high dose glucocorticoid therapy [choice A] prior to confirmation of the diagnosis with biopsy, whether the patient presents with or without threatened or established visual loss at diagnosis.
The prompt use of glucocorticoids improves the symptoms and prevents visual loss.

Choice B [Anti-Smith antibodies] are used in the diagnosis of Systemic lupus erythematosus after a positive Antinuclear antibody test.
Choice C [Noncontrast CT scan of the head] is not used in the routine workup of GCA but may be helpful if an intracranial bleed is thought to be the source of the headache.
Choice D [Temporal artery biopsy] is the definitive diagnosis for GCA but biopsy should not prevent or delay treatment of GCA with corticosteroids once GCA is suspected.

Choice E [Oral Sumatriptan] is used in the management of Migraine, which usually presents with unilateral throbbing headache, nausea, vomiting, photophobia, and/or phonophobia.

52. INFECTIOUS DISEASE – NONGONOCOCCAL URETHRITIS/CHLAMYDIA [PHARMACOLOGY]

Doxycycline (100 mg orally twice daily for 7 days) [choice D] is first-line treatment for Chlamydia, the most common cause of Nongonococcal urethritis.
Azithromycin given as a single 1 g oral dose is an alternative if adherence to Doxycycline for 7 days is a concern.
Nongonococcal urethritis (NGU) should be suspected if Gram stain of the discharge shows no gram-negative diplococci in WBC (no evidence of *N. gonorrhoeae*).

Choice A [Metronidazole oral] is used in the management of Bacterial vaginosis and Trichomoniasis.
Choice B [IM Ceftriaxone] is used as a first line agent for Gonococcal urethritis, which would show gram-negative diplococci in WBCs.
Choice C [Ciprofloxacin oral] is not a first line agent for Chlamydia trachomatis urethritis.
Choice E [IM Penicillin G] is the first line management of Syphilis.

53. DERMATOLOGY – MELASMA (CHLOASMA) [CLINICAL INTERVENTION]

Strict photoprotection [choice B], including sun avoidance, sun-protective clothing, and broad-spectrum sunscreens, is a crucial component of the management and prevention for Melasma (Chloasma in pregnancy).
Topical Tretinoin and Hydroxychloroquine, commonly used in the treatment of Melasma, are contraindicated during pregnancy.

Choice A [Topical Metronidazole] is used in the management of Rosacea.
Choice C [Hydroquinone 4% cream] is used in the management of Melasma but is contraindicated in pregnancy.
Choice D [Topical Fluocinolone, Hydroquinone, and Tretinoin triple combination cream] is used in the management of Melasma but Hydroquinone and Tretinoin are contraindicated in pregnancy.
Choice E [Topical Tretinoin 0.05% cream] is used in the management of Melasma but is contraindicated in pregnancy.

54. ENDOCRINE – HYPOTHYROIDISM/HASHIMOTO THYROIDITIS [LABS AND DIAGNOSTIC STUDIES]

In Hashimoto thyroiditis, the most common cause of Hypothyroidism in the US, >90% of patients will have elevated serum concentrations of Thyroid peroxidase (TPO) autoantibodies [choice E] &/or thyroglobulin antibodies.
In primary Hypothyroidism, classic labs are elevated Thyroid stimulating hormone (TSH) and normal or decreased serum free T4 levels.

Choice A [Decreased TSH and decreased serum free T4 levels] are hallmark of central hypothyroidism (presence of pituitary or hypothalamic dysfunction), which is a less common cause of Hypothyroidism in the US.
Choice B [Increased TSH and increased serum free T4 levels] is hallmark of central hyperthyroidism (presence of pituitary or hypothalamic disease).

Choice C [Diffuse increased radioactive iodine uptake on Thyroid scintigraphy] is hallmark of Graves' disease or pituitary TSH-secreting adenoma, both of which are associated with Hyperthyroidism.

Choice E [Positive thyroid stimulating immunoglobulins] are hallmark of Graves' disease, the most common cause of Hyperthyroidism in the US.

55. PULMONARY – LUNG CANCER/SQUAMOUS CELL CARCINOMA OF THE LUNG [MOST LIKELY]

Features suggestive of Squamous cell carcinoma of the lung [choice D] include:
  - **Centrally located cavitary lesion** because it usually begins centrally in the major bronchi or central part of the lung and may undergo partial necrosis.
  - **Hypercalcemia** due to production of parathyroid hormone-related protein. Hypercalcemia is most commonly associated with Squamous cell carcinoma of the lung, occurring in 5-15% (variation depends on the cancer stage).
  - **Horner syndrome (ipsilateral ptosis, miosis, and anhidrosis)** from involvement of the inferior cervical ganglion and the paravertebral sympathetic chain.

SCC is more strongly associated with smoking than any other type of NSCLC.

Although these features are suggestive of SCC of the lung, definitive histological diagnosis is essential.

56. GI/NUTRITION – TOXIC MEGACOLON; C. DIFFICILE COLITIS [CLINICAL INTERVENTION]

Oral Vancomycin [choice A] plus IV Metronidazole is often used in the management of fulminant Clostridioides difficile colitis (eg, hypotension, megacolon).

The patient has positive *C. difficile* stool toxins A and B assay and glutamate dehydrogenase (GDH) antigen positivity.

Common causes of Toxic megacolon include *C. difficile*, CMV, and Ulcerative colitis.

Choice B [NPO, IV fluids, Neostigmine 2 mg intravenously] can be used in the management of Colonic pseudo-obstruction (Ogilvie syndrome).

Choice C [Bowel rest, IV fluids, Ceftriaxone plus Metronidazole, IV Ganciclovir 5 mg/kg] is used in the management of Toxic megacolon due to Cytomegalovirus.

Choice D [Subtotal colectomy] may be indicated in patients with colonic perforation or if peritoneal signs are present.

Choice E [Bowel rest, IV fluids, Ceftriaxone plus Metronidazole, IV Hydrocortisone 100 mg] is used in the management of Toxic megacolon due to Ulcerative colitis.

57. PULMONARY – CHRONIC OBSTRUCTIVE PULMONARY DISEASE [HEALTH MAINTENANCE].

In patients with Chronic obstructive pulmonary disease, home oxygen therapy [choice C] is indicated if:
  - **Oxygen saturation is <88% at rest at baseline** (this patient has a resting SaO2 of 84%)
  - PaO2 <55 mmHg at rest
  - Symptoms, signs, or ECG evidence of cor pulmonale.

Home oxygen therapy is the only "medication" shown to reduce mortality; smoking cessation has the greatest impact on mortality reduction.

Choice A [Influenza vaccination] and choice B [Pneumococcal vaccination] also have mortality benefit but Home oxygen therapy in this patient would have the greatest mortality benefit.

Choice D [Prophylactic antibiotics to decrease frequency of exacerbations] is helpful for symptom reduction.

Choice E [Daily use of inhaled corticosteroids and an inhaled antimuscarinic agent] are for symptom control but they have no mortality benefit.

58. CARDIOLOGY – AORTIC STENOSIS [HISTORY AND PHYSICAL]

A slow-rising, late-peaking, and a low-amplitude carotid impulse, *pulsus parvus et tardus* [choice B], are classic findings in Severe aortic stenosis.

A harsh mid-systolic ejection murmur, heard best over the right second intercostal space, with radiation the carotids is hallmark of Aortic stenosis. The S1 is usually normal in AS.

Maneuvers that decrease LV volume (eg, Valsalva, standing) will diminish the intensity of Aortic stenosis.

Aortic murmurs are accentuated with the patient sitting up and leaning forward.

Choice A [Increased murmur intensity with Valsalva maneuver] is hallmark of Hypertrophic cardiomyopathy, which is best heard along the left sternal border. The murmur of Aortic stenosis decreases in intensity with Valsalva maneuver.

Choice C [Bounding radial pulses] are hallmark of Aortic insufficiency (Aortic regurgitation).

Choice D [Opening snap and prominent S1] are hallmark of Mitral stenosis.

Choice E [Increased intensity of the murmur in the lateral decubitus position] is characteristic of Mitral murmurs (eg, Mitral stenosis and Mitral regurgitation).

59. PSYCHIATRY AND BEHAVIORAL MEDICINE – MAJOR DEPRESSIVE DISORDER [PHARMACOLOGY]

Because Venlafaxine can increase blood pressure [choice B] and cause Hypertension, especially at higher doses, blood pressure should be checked prior to initiation of therapy, and routinely monitored (eg, every 2-6 months).

Because Serotonin and Norepinephrine reuptake inhibitors (SNRIs) affect norepinephrine, they can increase blood pressure.

Other common adverse effects of Serotonin and Norepinephrine reuptake inhibitors (SNRIs) include nausea, diaphoresis, dizziness, headaches, sexual dysfunction, and increased suicidality in individuals <25 years of age.

Choice A [Thyroid function test] is monitored in patients on Lithium therapy, which can cause Hypothyroidism.

Choice C [Serum glucose] may be monitored in patients on second-generation antipsychotics, especially Clozapine and Olanzapine.

Choice D [Liver function tests] is not routinely monitored on SNRIs although they should be used with caution in patients with hepatic impairment. It is not usually routinely monitored

Choice E [Body mass index] does not have to be routinely monitored in patients with SNRI.

60. CARDIOLOGY – HEART FAILURE [HEALTH MAINTENANCE]

Medications associated with mortality reduction in Heart failure with reduced ejection fraction (HFrEF) include:

- **Angiotensin system blockers such as ACE inhibitors [choice C], Angiotensin receptor/neprilysin inhibitors, and Angiotensin II receptor antagonists**
- Beta blockers
- Nitrates + Hydralazine
- Mineralocorticoid antagonist [MRAs (eg, Spironolactone, Eplerenone), and
- SGLT2 inhibitors.

Choice A (Digoxin) is associated with reduced hospitalization in patients maxed out on HF medications but does not have any mortality benefit.

Choice B (Nitroglycerin) has mortality benefit when combined with Hydralazine but not as an individual medication.

Choice D (Furosemide) is useful for control of peripheral and pulmonary edema but has no mortality benefit in the management of chronic HF.

Choice E (Diltiazem) and the other nondihydropyridine Calcium channel blockers have no mortality benefit in HFrEF and may be associated with increased harm due to reduced cardiac contractility.

61. PULMONARY – ACID BASE DISORDERS/METABOLIC ALKALOSIS [MOST LIKELY]

Hyperemesis gravidarum [choice D] and any other cause of excessive vomiting is often associated with a hypokalemic, hypochloremic, metabolic alkalosis.

The loss of hydrochloric acid and potassium from the acid secretions in the stomach leads to the generation of a metabolic alkalosis, hypochloremia, and hypokalemia. Release of aldosterone from hypovolemia further contributes to hypokalemia due to increased renal potassium excretion to compensate for sodium retention.

- Step 1: look at pH: 7.55 (7.35-7.45). Because it is elevated, an alkalosis is present.
- Step 2: look at the pCO2: 51 (35-45). Because it is increased (same direction as pH), it is metabolic in nature. If pCO2 was in the opposite direction of the pH, it would have been respiratory in nature.
- Step 3: look at the HCO3-: 45 (22-26). Because it is increased (same direction as pH), it is metabolic in nature.

Choice A [Pulmonary embolism] causes a respiratory alkalosis due to hyperventilation and tachypnea; in severe cases it may cause a respiratory acidosis.

Choice B [Persistent diarrhea] is associated with development of a normal gap metabolic acidosis.

Choice C [Asthma exacerbation] causes a respiratory alkalosis due to hyperventilation and tachypnea; in severe cases it may cause a respiratory acidosis.

Choice E [Diabetic ketoacidosis] causes a high anion gap metabolic acidosis.

62. NEUROLOGY – DEMENTIA WITH LEWY BODIES [MOST LIKELY]

The 4 "core clinical features" of Dementia with Lewy bodies (DLB) [choice D] include"

- **cognitive fluctuations**
- **visual hallucinations**
- **rapid eye movement (REM) sleep behavior disorder (RBD)**
- **parkinsonism**

Other features may include:

- Sensitivity to neuroleptics
- Autonomic dysfunction

Choice A [Parkinson disease] can also present with tremor, rigidity, and bradykinesia and dementia in the late stages after well-established Parkinsonism and is not usually associated with visual hallucinations and RBD.

Choice B [Normal pressure hydrocephalus] usually presents with the triad of "wobbly, wet, and wacky" (gait abnormalities such as a magnetic wide-based gait, urinary urgency or incontinence, and memory problems).

Choice C [Frontotemporal dementia] is classically associated with early alteration of personality, with marked changes in social behavior and language (aphasia) with preserved visuospatial.

Choice E [Alzheimer disease] is associated with a more gradual progression of memory decline and executive function.

63. NEUROLOGY – ABSENCE SEIZURES [PHARMACOLOGY]

The first-line management of Absence seizures is Ethosuximide [choice D].

Ethosuximide inhibits low-threshold (T-type) Ca^{2+} currents, especially in thalamic neurons, that act as pacemakers to generate rhythmic cortical discharge.

Second-line alternatives for Absence seizures are Valproic acid or Lamotrigine.

Antiseizure medications that should be avoided because they may aggravate Absence seizures include Carbamazepine [choice C], Vigabatrin, Gabapentin [choice A], and Tiagabine.

Phenytoin [choice E] and Phenobarbital [choice E] are ineffective in treating Absence seizures and should also be avoided.

64. GI/NUTRITION – ALCOHOLIC HEPATITIS [LABS AND DIAGNOSTIC STUDIES]

The ratio of the serum aspartate to alanine amino-transferase levels (AST/ALT) is usually greater than 2 in alcoholic hepatitis [choice C]. The elevations of AST and ALT are often mild (usually <500 IU).

Elevation of AST greater relative to ALT in Alcoholic hepatitis is thought to be due to [1] mitochondrial injury from alcohol, which leads to increased release of mAST in the serum and [2] decreased ALT activity often due to B6 depletion in the livers of alcoholics (decreased pyridoxal 5'-phosphate, which is a cofactor for the enzymatic activity of ALT).

Choice A [Positive smooth muscle autoantibodies] is hallmark of Autoimmune hepatitis.

Choice B [Alanine aminotransferase (ALT)/Aspartate aminotransferase (AST) >2; Serum AST and ALT >500 IU] is incorrect because Alcoholic hepatitis is associated with a greater elevation of AST compared to ALT and a mild transaminitis (<500 IU).

Choice D [Elevated alkaline phosphatase (ALP) and elevated gamma glutamyl-transferase (GGT)] is hallmark of cholestasis. In cholestasis the AST/ALT ratio is usually <1.0.

Choice E [Elevated prothrombin time (PT) and decreased albumin] are hallmark of End-stage liver disease and reflect impaired hepatic protein production.

65. GENITOURINARY – EPIDIDYMITIS [MOST LIKELY]

N. gonorrhoeae and C. trachomatis [choice A] are the most common organisms responsible for Acute epididymitis in men under the age of 35 years.

Escherichia coli [choice B], other coliforms, and Pseudomonas species are more common in older men. Men of any age who engage in insertive anal intercourse are also at increased risk for acute bacterial epididymitis from these coliform bacteria in the rectum.

Acute epididymitis should be suspected in males with localized testicular pain with tenderness and swelling on palpation of the affected epididymis.

A positive Prehn sign (relief of the pain with manual elevation of the scrotum) is more often seen with Epididymitis compared Testicular torsion [choice D]. Torsion is also associated with decreased or absent blood flow on Doppler ultrasound.

Choice C [Fluid accumulation in the scrotal sac] is associated with a hydrocele, which would be seen on Scrotal ultrasound.

Choice E [Torsion of the appendix of the testicle] is associated with the "blue dot" sign on examination.

66. MUSCULOSKELETAL – OSTEOARTHRITIS [HEALTH MAINTENANCE]

Nonpharmacologic interventions (eg, weight loss and regular exercise) [choice E] are the mainstay of Osteoarthritis (OA) management and should be tried first, followed by or in concert with medications to relieve pain when necessary.

Nonpharmacologic therapies include weight management if applicable (to reduce the load on the joint), regular exercise, braces, and foot orthoses for patients suitable to these interventions.

For mild OA localized to the knee, topical Nonsteroidal anti-inflammatory drugs (NSAIDs), such as Diclofenac, are often tried prior to oral NSAIDs.

Choice A (Knee arthroscopy), including arthroscopic surgery involving debridement, has been shown to have no significant benefit over standard therapies.

Choice B [Valgus (or unloader) knee bracing] can be employed to shift the load from the medial compartment in patients with medial tibiofemoral (TF) joint OA. It can be used as an adjunct to initial treatment for OA.

Choice C [Total knee replacement] may be considered in severe cases or if refractory to conservative therapy.

Choice D [Topical Capsaicin] may be used for mild OA localized to the knee or a few other joints when other initial treatments are ineffective or contraindicated.

67. GI/NUTRITION – INFECTIOUS DIARRHEA/E. COLI [MOST LIKELY]

Shiga toxin-producing E. coli (STEC) [choice C], especially *E. coli* 0157:H7 is the most cause of Hemolytic uremic syndrome (HUS) in children, and less commonly, Shigella dysenteriae type 1.

Hemolytic uremic syndrome (HUS) is characterized by the simultaneous occurrence of the triad of [1] microangiopathic hemolytic anemia, [2] thrombocytopenia, and [3] acute kidney injury.

Children with STEC-HUS classically have a prodromal illness with abdominal pain, vomiting, and diarrhea (sometimes bloody) that precedes the development of HUS by ~5-10 days.

68. INFECTIOUS DISEASE – INFECTIOUS MONONUCLEOSIS [HISTORY AND PHYSICAL EXAMINATION]

The presence of splenomegaly [choice A], palatal petechiae, and posterior cervical adenopathy are highly suggestive of Epstein-Barr virus (EBV)-associated infectious mononucleosis (IM).

Splenomegaly is seen in 50-60% of patients with IM.

Epstein-Barr virus (EBV)-associated infectious mononucleosis (IM) should be suspected in an adolescent or young adult with sore throat, fever, malaise, lymphadenopathy, and pharyngitis on physical examination.

Choice B [Painful mucocutaneous ulcerations] distinguishes acute HIV infection from EBV Mononucleosis. With the exception of Syphilis, mucocutaneous ulcerations are uncommon in EBV infection.

Choice C [Strawberry tongue] can be seen with Scarlet fever due to Streptococcal infection, which is not usually accompanied by significant fatigue, posterior lymphadenopathy, or splenomegaly on examination.

Choice D [Grey pseudomembranes on the posterior pharynx] is seen in respiratory Diphtheria.

Choice E [Enlarged, warm, and swollen joints (knees, ankles, elbows, wrists)] is a manifestation of Acute rheumatic fever.

69. REPRODUCTIVE – FETAL HEART PATTERN/VARIABLE DECELERATIONS [HISTORY AND PHYSICAL]

The initial management of Variable decelerations is relief of umbilical cord compression with maternal repositioning in the right or left lateral decubitus position [choice D].

Variable decelerations occur due to fetal baroreceptor response to umbilical cord compression, often after acute loss of amniotic fluid from rupture of membranes.

If decelerations do not improve with conservative management, the next step is intrauterine pressure catheter placement and administration of an amnioinfusion [choice C].

Cesarean section [choice B] is performed if late decelerations or significant variable decompressions are unresponsive to the above.

Choice A [Reassurance that it is a normal tracing and no intervention needed} is the management of Accelerations seen on fetal heart tracing.

Choice E [Identify labor progress] can be used in the management of early decelerations seen on Fetal heart tracing.

70. REPRODUCTIVE – CONTRACEPTION [PHARMACOLOGY]

Etonogestrel implant [choice A] is the most effective contraceptive method, with a >99% efficacy (0.05% average failure rate).

In terms of efficacy:
- Etonogestrel implant (most effective contraceptive) >99% efficacy (0.05% average failure rate)
- Vasectomy >99% efficacy (0.3% average failure rate)
- Levonorgestrel IUD [choice B] >99% efficacy (0.1-0.4% average failure rate)
- Tubal ligation >99% efficacy (average failure rate 0.5%)
- Depot medroxyprogesterone acetate injection (DMPA) injection [choice D] perfect use failure rate 0.3%, typical use failure rate of 3-5%
- Copper IUD [choice C]: 0.8% average failure rate.
- Contraceptive pill [choice E] 91% efficacy.

71. CARDIOLOGY – COARCTATION OF THE AORTA [LABS AND DIAGNOSTIC STUDIES]

The 2 classic radiograph findings of Coarctation of the aorta include:

- **Notching of the posterior one-third of the third to eighth ribs [choice B]** due to erosion by the large collateral arteries.
- **The "3" sign**, which describes the indentation of the aortic wall at the site of coarctation with pre- and post-coarctation dilatation.

Coarctation of the aorta should be suspected in

- older infants and children are often asymptomatic but have hypertension &/or systolic murmur often best heard in the infrascapular area
- systolic hypertension in the upper extremities, diminished or delayed femoral pulses (brachial-femoral delay), and decreased arterial blood pressure in the lower extremities.

72. PULMONARY – ASTHMA [PHARMACOLOGY]

In severe persistent Asthma, maintenance with Medium dose inhaled corticosteroids and a long-acting beta blocker is recommended with a reliever agent as needed [choice A].

- **NAEPP guidelines: Medium-dose ICS-Formoterol as maintenance** + reliever (preferred). Alternatives: medium-dose ICS-LABA daily or medium-dose ICS plus LAMA daily or Medium-dose ICS daily plus anti-leukotriene plus SABA as needed.
- **GINA guidelines: Medium-dose ICS-Formoterol as maintenance + reliever (preferred).**

Severe persistent is characterized by <u>any of the following</u>:

- Symptoms all day; nocturnal awakenings nightly
- need for SABA several times/day
- extreme limitation in activity
- FEV1 <60% predicted
- exacerbations ≥2/year.

73. MUSCULOSKELETAL – HUMERAL SHAFT FRACTURE/RADIAL NERVE INJURY [HISTORY AND PHYSICAL]

The most common neurological complication of humeral shaft fractures is a radial nerve injury, which presents as paresthesias of the dorsal hand or weakness of wrist and finger extension, resulting in a wrist drop [choice B].

This is because the radial nerve runs along the humeral shaft and can be damaged with fractures, especially displaced fractures.

Choice A [Positive Froment sign] can be seen with ulnar nerve injuries.
Choice C [Loss of thumb abduction] is associated with median nerve injuries.
Choice D [Loss of sensation to the index finger] is associated with median nerve injuries.
Choice E [Decreased deltoid pinprick sensation] is associated with axillary nerve injury, which is more commonly associated with proximal humerus fractures than with humeral shaft fractures.

74. RENAL – ACUTE KIDNEY INJURY/PRERENAL AZOTEMIA [MOST LIKELY]

In Prerenal azotemia [choice E] due to hypovolemia (vomiting in this case) the kidney responds to the volume loss by volume conservation (retention of both sodium and water).
Volume conservation in Prerenal azotemia is evidenced by:

- **sodium and electrolyte conservation**: **FENA <1%, urine sodium <20** (reflecting an appropriate attempt to retain sodium and volume), and **BUN:creatinine >20:1.**

- <u>water conservation:</u> **high urine specific gravity (>1.020) and increased urine osmolality (>500 mOsm/kg)**

Microscopic examination of the urine in Prerenal azotemia is usually normal or near normal. The presence of a few hyaline casts is normal and is a very nonspecific finding.

Choice A [Post obstructive uropathy] is usually diagnosed by increased post void residual (eg, >200 mL) &/or evidence of Hydronephrosis on Renal ultrasound. Labs are not as helpful in making the diagnosis.

Choice B [Acute interstitial nephritis] is associated with white cell casts with or without eosinophiluria.

Choice C [Nephrotic syndrome] is associated with fatty casts and oval fat bodies on microscopic examination of the urine.

Choice D [Acute tubular necrosis] is associated with granular (muddy brown) and epithelial cell casts on microscopic examination of the urine. Because the cells that normally conserve volume are damaged in ATN, labs usually reflect inability to conserve water (low urine osmolality <500, and low specific gravity <1.015) and inability to conserve electrolytes (eg, FENA: >2%, increased urine sodium >40 mEq/L, and BUN: creatinine ratio <15:1).

75. MUSCULOSKELETAL - LISFRANC INJURY [CLINICAL INTERVENTION]

Surgical intervention [choice C] is indicated in the presence of Lisfranc joint instability, Compartment syndrome, or an open fracture.

The acute management of a Lisfranc injury includes PRICE-M: Protection: Assuming no other injury, the injured foot is immobilized in a short-leg splint or boot, rest, ice, compression, elevation, and medications for analgesia.

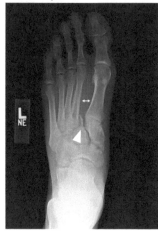

There is **lateral displacement of the lesser metatarsals with respect to the first metatarsal** with **widening of the space between the 1st and 2nd metatarsal base,** with an **intra-articular fracture from the medial margin of the base of the 2nd metatarsal (Fleck sign) [arrow head].**

76. HEMATOLOGY – VON WILLEBRAND DISEASE [HEALTH MAINTENANCE]

The main options for increasing VWF levels for surgical prophylaxis and treatment of mild bleeding are DDAVP (Desmopressin) [choice E] and VWF concentrates.

In most patients with type 1 VWD patients with minor bleeding or undergoing minor procedures, DDAVP is usually effective.

Desmopressin (DDAVP) transiently increases Factor VIII & vWF release from endothelial stores.

Choice A [Factor VIII products] are derived solely to contain purified factor VIII and do not contain any von Willebrand factor.

Choice B [Platelet transfusion] may be used in Von Willebrand disease type 2B, which may be associated with decreased platelets. All of the other types of VWD are associated with normal platelet counts.

Choice C [Plasma exchange therapy (Plasmapheresis)] is used in the management of Thrombotic thrombocytopenic purpura (TTP).

Choice D [Intravenous immunoglobulin therapy (IVIG)] is used in the management of Thrombocytopenic thrombotic purpura.

77. PULMONARY – SARCOIDOSIS [HISTORY AND PHYSICAL EXAMINATION]

The most common early extrapulmonary manifestations include skin lesions (eg, Erythema nodosum [choice C], lupus pernio (pathognomonic of Sarcoidosis), papular Sarcoidosis, nodular Sarcoidosis lesions, and nonspecific rashes (most common skin manifestation).

The classic radiograph finding of stage I Sarcoidosis is bilateral hilar lymphadenopathy (as seen in this patient).

Choice A [Erythema multiforme] is commonly associated with infections (viral, bacterial) and less commonly medications.

Choice B [Pyoderma gangrenosum] is associated with Inflammatory bowel disease.

Choice D [Raynaud phenomenon] is associated with Vasospastic disorders.

Choice E [Heliotrope rash] is pathognomonic of Dermatomyositis.

78. PULMONARY – ACUTE RESPIRATORY DISTRESS SYNDROME [HEALTH MAINTENANCE]

Initial lung protective strategies in Acute respiratory distress syndrome include [choice A]:
- **Low tidal volume ventilation** (4 to 8 mL/kg predicted body weight) to prevent volutrauma (prevents overinflation).
- **High PEEP strategy** (varies but up to 14.6 cm H_2O) is often preferable to a moderate PEEP strategy (5 to 9 cm H_2O), with specific titration of PEEP to target plateau pressures of < 30 cm H_2O. High PEEP is associated with improved lung function, prevents atelectatic collapse (keeps the alveoli open), and reduces duration of mechanical ventilation.

ARDS typically presents with respiratory distress in critically ill patients. Causes may include Pancreatitis (as in this patient), trauma, sepsis, transfusion, etc.

Choice B [High tidal volume ventilation and high PEEP] is incorrect because high tidal volume may result in volutrauma (overdistention of the lungs).

Choice C [High tidal volume ventilation and placing the patient supine] is incorrect because high tidal volume may result in volutrauma (overdistention of the lungs).

Choice D [High tidal volume ventilation, high PEEP, and patient the patient prone] is incorrect because high tidal volume may result in volutrauma (overdistention of the lungs).

Choice E [Low tidal volume ventilation and high-frequency oscillatory ventilation] is incorrect because the use of HFOV has now fallen out of favor since studies have suggest no benefit and possible harm associated with its use.

79. PULMONARY – TUBERCULOSIS [HEALTH MAINTENANCE]

Chest imaging [choice D] is required to rule out active infection in all patients with a positive screening test (eg, PPD/TST or Interferon gamma release assay).

This patient has positive PPD (≥5 mm for HIV positivity; ≥10 mm for Mycobacteriology lab personnel). He has ≥5 mm of induration.

Patients with [1] a positive screening test (PPD or IFGRA) [2] no symptoms, and [3] negative chest imaging for active infection are considered to have Latent TB infection, which is why chest imaging is the best next step for this patient prior to offering treatment for LTBI.

Choice A [No further management at this time] would be indicated if the patient's screening test was negative (<5 mm induration in this patient).

Choice B [Rifampin daily for 4 months] is used in the management of Latent TB infection if this patient's chest imaging showed no evidence of active infection. Therefore, the next step in the evaluation of this patient is to perform chest imaging to rule out active infection.

Choice C [Isoniazid + Vitamin B6 for 6 months duration] is used in the management of Latent TB infection if this patient's chest imaging showed no evidence of active infection. Therefore, the next step in the evaluation of this patient is to perform chest imaging to rule out active infection.

Choice E [Initiate Rifampin, Isoniazid, Pyrazinamide, Ethambutol] is used in the management of Active TB infection if chest imaging is positive for active infection + either a positive NAAT &/or Acid-fast stain.

80. GENITOURINARY – FOURNIER GANGRENE [HISTORY AND PHYSICAL]

Fournier gangrene is most commonly seen in male diabetics over 50 years of age [choice B], often with a history of alcohol abuse.

Fournier's gangrene is a rare necrotizing fasciitis of the perineum which often involves the scrotum. Clinical features may include edema and erythema of the involved skin, blisters/bullae, crepitus, and subcutaneous gas.

Systemic findings (eg, fever, tachycardia, and hypotension) are often present.

Other risk factors include immunocompromised states [choice E], urethral trauma in the presence of urinary infection [choice D], and longstanding indwelling urethral catheters.

81. HEMATOLOGY – BURKITT LYMPHOMA/NONHODGKIN LYMPHOMA [MOST LIKELY]

The nonendemic (sporadic) form of Burkitt lymphoma [choice A] classically presents with a rapidly expanding abdominal mass, often with ascites; 25% have jaw or facial bone involvement.

The typical translocation of c-*myc* into the immunoglobulin heavy chain locus is observed in about 80% of Burkitt's lymphomas.

t(8; 14) translocations may be seen in African Burkitt's lymphoma and pre-B cell ALL [choice B].

The average age of diagnosis in pediatric patients is 3 to 12 years of age.

Choice B [Acute lymphoblastic leukemia] is classically associated with TdT expression.

Choice C [Diffuse large B cell lymphoma] also presents with rapidly enlarging lymph nodes of the neck, abdomen, and groin). It is most common in middle aged adults & the elderly.

Choice D [Follicular lymphoma] is usually associated with t(14:18) mutation

Choice E [Mantle cell lymphoma] is associated with a t(11;14) mutation.

82. GI/NUTRITION – PYLORIC STENOSIS [MOST LIKELY]

Infantile hypertrophic pyloric stenosis [choice B] usually presents with projectile nonbilious vomiting and an olive-shaped mass (hypertrophied pylorus) in the epigastric area in younger infants 3-12 weeks of age.
Despite the vomiting, infants are usually avid feeders.

Choice A [Physiologic gastroesophageal reflux] is associated with mild regurgitation in an otherwise healthy child.
Choice C [Duodenal atresia] usually classically presents with vomiting (usually bilious) within the first 24-38 hours of life after the first feeding, gastric distention, and absent bowel movements.
Choice D [Midgut volvulus] is associated with bilious vomiting, abdominal distension, and high-pitched bowel sounds.
Choice E [Milk-protein allergy] may present with vomiting and diarrhea within 2-4 hours after ingestion of milk, urticaria/angioedema, or anaphylaxis. It is not associated with an olive-shaped abdominal mass.

83. DERMATOLOGY – ERYTHEMA MULTIFORME [FOUNDATIONAL SCIENTIFIC CONCEPTS]

Infections (viral, bacterial, or fungal) account for ~90% of cases of Erythema multiforme, with Herpes simplex virus (HSV) [choice B] as the most commonly identified precipitant.
Mycoplasma pneumoniae infection is an important cause of EM, especially in children.
The target lesion is the hallmark rash of EM, which consists of three concentric zones of color change: [1] a central dusky or blistered area, [2] a dark red inflammatory zone surrounded by a pale ring of edema, and [3] an erythematous peripheral halo.

Medications [choices A and E] account for <10% of cases of Erythema multiforme.
Choice C [Treponema pallidum] is the causative agent of Syphilis.
Choice D [Human herpesvirus 8] is associated with Kaposi sarcoma.

84. DERMATOLOGY – ACTINIC KERATOSIS [HEALTH MAINTENANCE]

Actinic keratoses (AK) are lesions that are on a continuum with Squamous cell carcinoma (SCC) [choice C] as AK can progress to invasive skin cancer.
AKs most commonly present as scaly, erythematous macules or papules on sites of chronic sun exposure (eg, scalp, face, neck, dorsal forearms, and dorsum of the hands).

Choice A [Malignant melanoma] is associated with a hyperpigmented lesion with irregular borders. Actinic keratosis does not progress to MM.
Choice B [Kaposi sarcoma] is associated with Human herpesvirus 8 in patients with advanced HIV disease. It is an AIDS-defining illness.
Choice D [Basal cell carcinoma] classically presents as a translucent lesion with raised borders and central ulceration. Actinic keratosis does not progress to BCC.
Choice E (Seborrheic keratosis) is a different condition from Actinic keratosis and does not arise from it.

85. CARDIOLOGY – MITRAL STENOSIS [CLINICAL INTERVENTION]

In patients with Mitral stenosis with valve obstruction, intervention with percutaneous mitral balloon commissurotomy (PMBC) [choice E] or surgery [surgical repair, commissurotomy, or valve replacement]) improves survival and symptom control.

Although there is a higher rate of reintervention after PMBC (16.3 versus 2.4%), the mortality rate is higher with mitral valve replacement.

Choice A [Beta blockers and Automatic implantable cardioverter defibrillator] may be used in the management of Hypertrophic cardiomyopathy.

Choice B [Mitral valve replacement] is reserved for patients with unfavorable valve morphology. The mortality rate is higher with mitral valve replacement vs. mitral valve repair.

Choice C [Aortic valve replacement] is used in the management of Aortic stenosis.

Choice D [Aortic valve repair] is a possible alternative to AVR in the management of Aortic stenosis.

86. MUSCULOSKELETAL – ACUTE COMPARTMENT SYNDROME [HISTORY AND PHYSICAL]

Pain with passive stretch of muscles within the affected compartment is a sensitive useful and sensitive early finding in Acute compartment syndrome [choice E].

When ACS is suspected, prompt surgical consultation, which may involve measurement of compartment pressures, should be obtained.

If compartment pressures are elevated, emergent fasciotomy is indicated.

Choice A [Paralysis of the forearm] is a late finding of Compartment syndrome.

Choice B [Pallor of the forearm] may occur with Compartment syndrome but is nonspecific and usually occurs later when blood supply is compromised.

Choice C [Absence of radial pulses] may occur with Compartment syndrome but is nonspecific and usually occurs later when blood supply is compromised.

Choice D [Palpable tenderness of the forearm] is not a sensitive or specific finding but often occurs in Compartment syndrome.

87. NEUROLOGY – ISCHEMIC STROKE/MIDDLE CEREBRAL ARTERY STROKE [MOST LIKELY]

Receptive or expressive aphasia is usually seen when Middle cerebral artery strokes involve the dominant hemisphere, which is usually the left hemisphere [choice C].

Key features of Middle cerebral artery stroke include:
- Contralateral facial weakness that spares the forehead
- Contralateral motor weakness (arm > leg), sensory deficit, and hemispatial neglect
- gaze deviation toward the side with the lesion (due to contralateral homonymous hemianopsia)
- Receptive or expressive aphasia is seen when the dominant hemisphere is involved.

Choice A [Right middle cerebral artery stroke] is associated with contralateral (left-sided) motor weakness (arm > leg), sensory deficit, and hemispatial neglect.

Choice B [Left vertebrobasilar artery stroke] is associated with contralateral motor and sensory deficits, vomiting, vertigo, and visual changes.

Choice D [Right anterior cerebral artery stroke] is associated with contralateral (left-sided) motor weakness (leg > arm), sensory deficit, and contralateral homonymous hemianopsia.

Choice E [Left anterior cerebral artery stroke] is associated with contralateral (right-sided) motor weakness (leg > arm), sensory deficit, and contralateral homonymous hemianopsia.

88. PSYCHIATRY AND BEHAVIORAL MEDICINE – CHILD ABUSE [PROFESSIONAL PRACTICE]

When child abuse is suspected, consultation with child protective services for suspected abuse should be done [choice C].

His mother describes the mechanism of the burn as a splash injury, but the burns are consistent with immersion injury (eg, immersion in a tub of hot water).

89. NEUROLOGY – PARKINSON DISEASE [HISTORY AND PHYSICAL]
Key features of the tremor of Parkinson disease include:
- **rest tremor: most noticeable when the affected body part is supported against gravity and not engaged in purposeful activities [choice C].**
- **"pill-rolling" tremor of the upper extremities**
- tremor usually starts unilaterally in the hand and then spreads contralaterally several years after the onset of symptoms
- The side that is initially affected tends to be the more affected side throughout the course of the disease (making choice E incorrect).

Choices A [Postural-action tremor that increases with voluntary muscle contraction and movement, choice B [symmetrical and bilateral initially, often involving both hands and arms, head, and voice] and choice D [worsens when the arms are held outstretched] are hallmark of Essential tremor (ET) and distinguish ET from PD.

90. RENAL – RENAL CELL CARCINOMA [LABS AND DIAGNOSTIC STUDIES]
CT scan of the abdomen and pelvis with and without contrast [choice A] is the recommended diagnostic imaging modality in suspected Renal cell carcinoma, which would reveal a kidney mass.
The diagnosis is confirmed with biopsy, but this is often obtained at the same time as surgical treatment.
The classic triad of flank pain, hematuria, and flank mass is uncommon, presenting in only 10% of patients. When the triad is present, it usually indicates advanced disease.
Some patients may have a left-sided Varicocele (also seen in this patient).

Although ultrasonography [choice B] is less sensitive than CT in detecting a renal mass, it is useful to distinguish a simple benign cyst from a more complex cyst or a solid tumor. If Renal ultrasound shows a solid mass or a complex cyst with septations or nodules, a dedicated CT scan of the kidneys, ureters, and bladder before and after IV contrast with delayed imaging of the entire abdomen and pelvis should be performed.
Choice C [Urine cytology] and choice D [Cystoscopy] are most helpful in establishing the diagnosis of Bladder carcinoma.
Choice E (Voiding cystourethrogram) is helpful in establishing the diagnosis of Vesicoureteral reflux.

91. REPRODUCTIVE – CERVICAL CANCER SCREENING [HEALTH MAINTENANCE]
Because of the lower overall risk of developing Cervical cancer, patients 21-24 years of age with Atypical squamous cells of undetermined significance (ASCUS) can be cared for more conservatively than patients ≥25 years of age, with either:
- **(1) Pap test in 1 year (preferred) [choice A]**

• (2) Reflex HPV testing (acceptable alternative).

Atypical squamous cells of undetermined significance (ASCUS) is the most common abnormal Pap test result.
It is characterized by atypical cells that demonstrate reactive changes but do not meet cytologic criteria for premalignant disease.

Choice B [Reflex Human papillomavirus testing] is the most appropriate next step in the management of ASCUS in women ≥25 years of age.
Choice C [Perform Pap smear with HPV cotesting in 3 years] is used in the evaluation of ASCUS in women ≥25 years of age with ASCUS who are HPV negative after reflex HPV testing.
Choice E [Colposcopy] is performed in women ≥25 years of age with ASCUS who are HPV positive after reflex HPV testing.

92. NEUROLOGY - SPINAL CORD INJURY/CENTRAL CORD SYNDROME [MOST LIKELY]

Central cord syndrome [choice C] is usually occurs after a fall with neck hyperextension (this patient has an extension teardrop fracture).
Classic findings of Central cord syndrome include:
• **significant strength impairments more prominent in the upper extremities (especially the hands) in a shawl like distribution compared to the lower extremities.**
• variable sensory deficits below the level of injury, often in a **"cape-like" distribution across their upper back and down their posterior upper extremities.**
• pain and temperature sensations are often affected; sensation of light touch can also be impaired.
• neck pain at the site of spinal cord injury.

Choice A [Posterior cord syndrome] is associated with sensory ataxia: vibration and fine touch deficits and proprioception deficits – decreased coordination of voluntary movements, leading to poor balance, unsteady gait, and falls. It usually occurs in the setting of B12 deficiency, late Neurosyphilis, or Multiple sclerosis.
Choice B [Anterior cord syndrome] usually occurs in the setting of hyperflexion injury. It classically presents with motor deficits in the lower extremities, +/- bladder dysfunction; sensory deficits: loss of temperature and pain below the lesion (eg, lower extremities), with sparing of proprioception and vibration.
Choice D [Brown Sequard syndrome] usually presents after penetrating injury with ipsilateral motor, vibratory, and proprioception deficits and contralateral pain and temperature deficits.
Choice E [Middle cerebral artery stroke] presents with contralateral motor and sensory deficits of the face and upper extremity greater than the lower extremity.

93. PSYCHIATRY AND BEHAVIORAL MEDICINE – OPIOID INTOXICATION [CLINICAL INTERVENTION]

Once opioid intoxication is suspected, airway protection must be maintained. Assisted ventilation with a bag valve mask [choice E] is utilized until Naloxone reverses the respiratory depression.
Adequate ventilation should be provided before Naloxone [choice A] is given.
Naloxone is a short-acting opioid antagonist that serves as an antidote, ideally administered via the intravenous (IV) route.

The classic signs of Opioid toxicity include:
- **decreased respiratory rate (most specific)**
- **Miotic (constricted) pupils**
- depressed mental status
- decreased bowel sounds

94. CARDIOLOGY – UNSTABLE ANGINA [MOST LIKELY DIAGNOSIS]
Unstable angina (UA) [choice E] is part of Acute coronary syndrome and is defined as:
- symptoms: **chest pain (or equivalent) that is new in onset, not relieved with rest &/or nitroglycerin, or lasts >30 minutes**
- ECG: **ST/T changes - hyperacute T-wave, flattening of the T-waves, inverted T-waves, and/or ST depression**
- enzymes: **negative cardiac enzymes** (reflecting no myocardial cell death).

Choice A [Non-ST elevation myocardial infarction] is associated with similar ECG findings as UA but is associated with positive cardiac enzymes, reflecting some myocardial cell death.
Choice B [Anterior wall Myocardial infarction] is associated with ST elevations in at least 2 contiguous anterior leads (V1 through V4).
Choice C [Variant (Prinzmetal angina)] is associated with chest pain that is classically nonexertional and may be associated with ST elevations.
Choice D [Stable angina pectoris] is associated with chest pain <30 minutes and relieved with rest &/or nitroglycerin.

95. INFECTIOUS DISEASE – ACUTE HIV INFECTION [MOST LIKELY]
The most common symptoms of Acute HIV infection, also known as acute retroviral syndrome [choice C] includes:
- **fever, lymphadenopathy, sore throat, rash, myalgia/arthralgia, and headache.**
- although not always present, **painful mucocutaneous ulcerations is one of the most distinguishing manifestations of acute HIV infection.** With the exception of Syphilis, mucocutaneous ulcerations are uncommon in the other choices listed.
- a **generalized rash** is a common finding in symptomatic acute HIV infection.

Mucocutaneous ulceration and rash are uncommon in EBV mononucleosis (unless antibiotics have been administered) [choice A] and CMV mononucleosis [choice B].
Pharyngeal edema with little associated tonsillar exudate or hypertrophy, and diarrhea, which can be seen in acute HIV, distinguish it from EBV mononucleosis.
The rash of Pityriasis rosea [choice E] can look similar to the rash seen in Acute HIV syndrome but marked constitutional symptoms are uncommon in Pityriasis rosea.
Choice D [Group A Streptococcus pharyngitis] does not usually cause occipital lymphadenopathy and is not usually associated with rash in adults.

96. NEUROLOGY – MULTIPLE SCLEROSIS [FOUNDATIONAL SCIENTIFIC CONCEPTS]
Multiple sclerosis (MS) is an immune-mediated inflammatory demyelinating disease of the central nervous system [choice A].
In MS, there are multifocal areas of demyelination with loss of oligodendrocytes and scarring of the astroglial cells.

MS should be suspected in a young adult with clinically distinct episodes of central nervous system dysfunction, such as optic neuritis, trigeminal neuralgia <40 years of age (as in this patient), upper motor neuron symptoms/signs, or a spinal cord syndrome.

Choice B [Demyelination of the Schwann cells in the peripheral nervous system] is hallmark of Guillain-Barre syndrome, which present with lower motor neuron findings.
Choice C [Autoantibodies against the postsynaptic acetylcholine receptor] is hallmark of Myasthenia gravis, which presents with pure motor weakness without sensory deficits.
Choice D [Autoantibodies against the presynaptic voltage-gated calcium channels] is hallmark of Lambert-Eaton myasthenic syndrome.
Choice E [Motor neuron degeneration and death with gliosis replacing lost neurons] is hallmark of Amyotrophic lateral sclerosis.

97. PSYCHIATRY AND BEHAVIORAL MEDICINE – BORDERLINE PERSONALITY DISORDER [HEALTH MAINTENANCE]
Psychotherapy such a Cognitive behavioral therapy [choice B] is the primary management tool for Borderline personality disorder.
Other therapy options include Dialectical behavior therapy (especially if severe), Transference-focused therapy, Mentalization-based therapy, and Schema-focused therapy.

Unless there is another comorbid condition in which pharmacotherapy would be helpful [choices A, D, and E], medications are not used in the management of most Personality disorders.
Choice C [Exposure and response prevention therapy] is used as the Psychotherapy of choice in patients with Obsessive-compulsive personality disorder.

98. CARDIOLOGY – HYPERTENSION [PHARMACOLOGY]
ACE inhibitors [choice A] and Angiotensin II receptor blockers reduce proteinuria and slow the progression of chronic kidney disease in patients with nondiabetic and diabetic renal disease associated with proteinuria.
They have beneficial effects on intrarenal hemodynamics (eg, reduction of glomerular capillary pressure and efferent arteriole vasodilation), resulting in renoprotective effects in addition to their systemic antihypertensive benefits.

Choice B [Hydrochlorothiazide] is a first line agent for Hypertension with no comorbidities, isolated systolic hypertension, and Hypertension in the elderly.
Choice C [Nifedipine] is a first line agent for Hypertension with no comorbidities.
Choice D [Metoprolol] is useful for Hypertension, especially in the setting of Angina, post MI, and Heart failure with reduced ejection fraction.
Choice E [Tamsulosin] is usually reserved for Hypertension in the setting of Benign prostatic hypertrophy.

99. REPRODUCTIVE – PRELABOR RUPTURE OF MEMBRANES [CLINICAL INTERVENTION].
Prompt induction of labor with Oxytocin [choice B] without preinduction cervical ripening is recommended for the management of term Prelabor rupture of membranes in women ≥37 weeks if there are no contraindications.

Compared with expectant management [choice A], induction of labor is associated with a reduction in maternal and possibly neonatal infection. Expectant management is an option in women who choose this option but there is an increased risk of complications.

Choice C [Nifedipine] is a tocolytic that can be used to delay labor in patients with preterm ROM.

Choice D [Digital cervicovaginal examination] should be avoided in PROM unless delivery is imminent in most cases to avoid introduction of infection.

Choice E [Cesarean section] may be indicated if vaginal delivery would be more harmful than Cesarean section.

100. RENAL – NEPHROTIC SYNDROME/MEMBRANOUS NEPHROPATHY [FOUNDATIONAL SCIENTIFIC CONCEPTS]

Hallmarks of Membranous nephropathy include:

- **light microscopy: diffuse thickening of the glomerular basement membrane (GBM) [choice D].**
- electron microscopy: subepithelial electron-dense deposits on the outer component of the GBM, effacement of the foot processes of the podocyte. Larger deposits causing GBM thickening, along with foot process effacement giving the characteristic "spike and dome" appearance.

Primary Membranous nephropathy can be autoimmune; secondary causes include viral Hepatitis (as in this patient), medications (eg, medications used to treat Rheumatoid arthritis, such as NSAIDs, Penicillamine); malignancy (solid tumors of the breast, lung, colon), and infection (Syphilis, Malaria, Schistosomiasis).

HBV infection and SLE represent the only forms of MN that may be associated with hypocomplementemia.

Choice A [Focal and segmental scarring] on light microscopy is classic for Focal segmental sclerosis, which is more common in people of African descent, HIV, Heroin use, and Hypertension.

Choice B [Kimmelstiel Wilson nodules] on light microscopy is classic for Diabetes mellitus.

Choice C [Mesangial expansion] on light microscopy is classic for Diabetes mellitus.

Choice E [Normal appearing glomeruli] on light microscopy is classic for Minimal change disease, which is the most common cause of Nephrotic syndrome in children.

1. A 70-year-old female presents to the clinic, accompanied by her 20-year-old grandson. Her native language is Haitian creole, but she states she can speak English. She is told she is having symptoms consistent with Stable angina pectoris. While she is being explained the workup needed, it becomes evident to the clinician that she does not fully understand the explanation in English, and she is nodding yes inappropriately. The medical scribe informs the clinician he speaks some Haitian creole. Which of the following is the most appropriate next step?
a. Use the scribe to interpret and then document
b. Explain it to the patient in English using more basic phrases
c. Use the grandson as the interpreter
d. Use the medical interpreter services phone
e. Write down the steps of the workup in English for the patient

2. A 2-year-old boy is brought to the emergency department by his father for cough and difficulty breathing. He was playing outdoor with his toys when he began coughing incessantly for 15 minutes. Vitals are temperature 98.6°F (37°C), pulse 112 bpm, respiratory rate 42 breaths/min, and oxygen saturation 90% on room air. Pulmonary examination is notable for diminished breath sounds, stridor, and monophonic expiratory wheezing. Chest radiograph is positive for hyperinflation of the right lung. Which of the following the most appropriate next step in the management of this patient?
a. CT scan of the chest
b. Thoracotomy
c. Urgent bronchoscopy
d. Nebulized Albuterol
e. Nebulized racemic Epinephrine

3. A 4-year-old boy presents to the clinic with sore throat, cough, reduced appetite, difficulty eating, malaise, and low-grade fever for 48 hours. Vitals are notable for temperature 101°F (38.3°C). Physical examination reveals vesicular lesions on an erythematous base on the tongue and buccal mucosa. There are thin-walled vesicles that contain clear fluid surrounded by a thin halo of erythema on his palms, soles, buttocks, and upper thighs. Which of the following is the most likely etiology of his presentation?
a. Herpes simplex virus
b. Coxsackievirus A16
c. Parvovirus B19
d. Group A streptococcus
e. Varicella virus

4. Which of the following physical examination findings is most specific for left-sided Heart failure?
a. Increased hepatojugular reflux
b. Increased jugular venous pressure
c. Crackles
d. Pitting edema of the legs
e. Abdominal tenderness

5. A 29-year-old female presents to the clinic for a 5-day history of easy bruising and bleeding of her gums when she brushes her teeth. She was recently diagnosed with SARS-CoV-2. Physical examination is notable for a few petechiae scattered over the arms and legs. Initial labs reveal a hemoglobin of 13 g/dL (12.1-15.1), hematocrit 38% (36-48), white blood cell count 8,400/mm3 (5,000-10,000), and platelet count 19,500/mm^3 (150,000-450,000). Which of the following is the most appropriate management?
a. Splenectomy
b. Plasma exchange therapy
c. Platelet transfusion
d. Prednisone
e. Observation

6. A 25-year-old male is referred to the hematology clinic. Review of systems is only positive for occasional fatigue and exertional dyspnea. Physical examination is unremarkable. Initial labs reveal:
- Hemoglobin: 11 g/dL (13-17)
- Mean corpuscular volume (MCV) 65 fL (80-100)
- Red cell distribution width (RDW) within normal limits
- RBC count 7.6 x 10*12/L (4.0-5.9 x 10*12/L)
- Serum ferritin: 480 ng/mL (300-400)
Hemoglobin electrophoresis:
- Hemoglobin A: 87% (96-98%)
- Hemoglobin A2: 8% (2-3.3%)
- Hemoglobin F: 5% (<1%).
Which of the following is the most likely diagnosis?
a. Iron deficiency anemia
b. Beta thalassemia trait (minor)
c. Alpha thalassemia intermedia
d. Alpha thalassemia trait (minor)
e. Beta thalassemia major

7. A 19-year-old female presents to the clinic for a 9-day history of joint pain. The pain was initially in her right ankle, which has since resolved, but is now in the left elbow. On examination, there is warmth and swelling to the wrist joint and there is tenderness along the tendons of the wrist and fingers associated with pain on passive extension. There is a hemorrhagic vesicopustule on the web space of the right hand. There is also a pustule on the sole of the left foot. Which of the following would most likely be in this patient's history?
a. Being outdoors in the woods without the use insect repellant
b. Personal and family history of autoimmunity
c. Injection drug use
d. Recent sore throat not treated with antibiotics
e. Unprotected sexual intercourse

8. A 64-year-old man presents to his primary care physician complaining of hip pain and headaches. His hearing has gotten worse, and his hats he has owned for years are tighter than they were before. Physical examination is notable for leg bowing. Radiographs are positive for osteolytic, osteoblastic, and sclerotic bone changes (see photo).

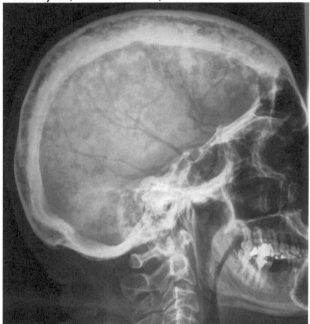

Which of the following laboratory values would most likely be elevated in this patient?
a. Serum vitamin D
b. Serum alkaline phosphatase
c. Serum calcium
d. Intact parathyroid hormone (PTH)
e. Serum phosphate

Photo credit:
Case courtesy of Ashesh Ishwarlal Ranchod, Radiopaedia.org, rID: 178760

9. A 46-year-old woman with no significant medical history presents to the ED with right-sided facial stiffness that began about 40 minutes prior to evaluation. Neurological examination is positive for right-sided facial droop involving the corner of the mouth. No forehead wrinkling is noted on the right side when she is asked to raise her eyebrows. The sclera remains visible when the patient is asked to close the right eye. The rest of the neurological exam is otherwise normal. Which of the following is the most appropriate next step in management in this patient?
a. Emergent CT scan and stat neurology consult
b. Administer Sumatriptan, Prochlorperazine, and Diphenhydramine
c. Obtain a blood glucose level, basic laboratory work, and CT scan of the head
d. Initiate Acyclovir
e. Prednisone, artificial tear drops, eye patch, and follow-up

10. A 22-year-old male presents to the emergency department with headache, vomiting, fever, and lethargy. Vitals are a temperature of 101°F (38.3°C), blood pressure 130/70 mmHg, pulse 120/min, and respirations 20/min. Physical examination is notable for nuchal rigidity, resistance during extension of his knees beyond 135°, and a purpuric rash on the dorsum of his left hand. A lumbar puncture reveals a neutrophilic pleocytosis and decreased CSF glucose. Which of the following is the most likely etiology of his presentation?
a. Streptococcus pneumoniae
b. Listeria monocytogenes
c. Neisseria meningitidis
d. Haemophilus influenzae
e. Group B streptococcus

11. A 60-year-old male presents to the clinic with periumbilical pain, fatigue, and yellowing of his skin. He has a history of chronic alcohol use. Physical examination is remarkable for scleral icterus and a nontender but palpable distended gallbladder at the right costal margin. Based on the most likely diagnosis, which of the following is most useful for indication of disease activity and for prognosis?
a. Alpha-fetoprotein (AFP)
b. Cancer-associated antigen 19-9 (CA 19-9)
c. Carcinoembryonic antigen (CEA)
d. Amylase and lipase
e. Cancer antigen 125 (CA 125)

12. A 10-year-old boy presents to the clinic with a 2-day history of fever, chills, sore throat, and the development of a rash this morning. He developed a maculopapular rash the last time he was given Amoxicillin. Vitals reveal a temperature of 101°F (38.3°C), pulse 116 bpm, and respiratory rate 22 breaths/min. Physical examination reveals diffuse erythematous maculopapular rash with a rough texture that blanches with pressure, circumoral pallor, and an erythematous tongue with hypertrophied papillae. Rapid streptococcal antigen test is positive. Which of the following is the most appropriate management of this patient?
a. Penicillin V potassium
b. Clarithromycin
c. Trimethoprim-sulfamethoxazole
d. Cephalexin
e. Amoxicillin-clavulanate

13. A 22-year-old man presents to the clinic for mild exertional dyspnea. He has no past medical history. On physical examination, there is a high-pitched blowing murmur heard through mid to late systole. The murmur is heard best over the apex and radiates to the axilla. Based on the most likely diagnosis, which of the following physical examination findings would most likely be seen in this patient?
a. Prominent first heart sound (S1)
b. Midsystolic click
c. Hoarseness
d. Weak delayed carotid pulse
e. Increased murmur intensity with inspiration

14. A 4-year-old girl presents to the emergency department with a 6-day history of fever and right knee pain. She denies cough, sore throat, or runny nose. Physical examination is notable for bilateral bulbar conjunctival erythema without purulence, edema of the hands and feet, fissured lips, right anterior cervical lymphadenopathy, a brightly erythematous tongue, and a macular rash on the trunk and extremities. Blood work reveals a white blood cell count of 13,500/mm^3 (5,000-10,000) and platelets 304,000/microliter (150,000-450,000). Which of the following is the initial treatment of choice?
a. Intravenous immunoglobulin (IVIG)
b. Penicillin V potassium
c. Prednisone
d. Doxycycline
e. Ibuprofen

15. A 64-year-old male is brought to the emergency department by ambulance after a brief syncopal episode. Upon arrival, vitals reveal a blood pressure of 80/40 mmHg. He is awake and alert but feels dizzy. The following is seen on the monitor (see photo).

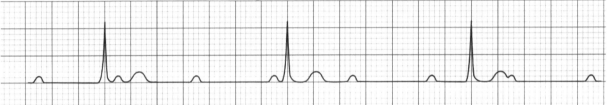

Which of the following treatment modalities is the recommended management of this patient?
a. Synchronized cardioversion
b. Medical cardioversion with Ibutilide
c. Metoprolol
d. Transcutaneous pacing
e. Implantable cardioverter defibrillator

Photo credit:
Shutterstock (used with permission)

16. A 70-year-old male nursing home resident was brought to the ED for altered mental status. He has been experiencing poor oral intake. Physical examination showed stable vital signs, including blood pressure of 124/72 mmHg, and dry mucous membranes. He is alert and able to follow commands but is confused. CT scan is negative. Labs reveal:
- serum potassium: 4.2 mEq/L (3.5-5)
- serum sodium: 166 mEq/L (135-145)
- serum osmolality: 352 mOsm/kg (280-295)
- serum creatinine: 0.9 mg/dL (0.6-1.2)
Which of the following is the first-line management of his Hypernatremia?
a. Dextrose 5% in water
b. 0.9% sodium chloride solution
c. 0.45% sodium chloride solution
d. 3% sodium chloride solution
e. Fluid restriction

17. A 36-year-old woman presents to the clinic with headache and muscle weakness. She has a history of Hypertension treated with 3 different antihypertensives. Vitals reveal a blood pressure of 172/112 mmHg. Initial labs are significant for:
- sodium 144 mEq/L (135-145)
- potassium 2.4 mEq/L (3.5-10)
- bicarbonate 34 mEq/L (22-26)
- Plasma aldosterone concentration (PAC) 29.6 ng/dl (1-16)
- Plasma Renin activity (PRA) 0.4 ng/ml/h (0.5-1.9).
- PAC/PRA ratio: 74
- 24-hour urine Vanillylmandelic acid (VMA) 1.8 mg (<13.6 mg]

Which of the following is the most likely etiology of this patient's presentation?
a. Idiopathic bilateral adrenal hyperplasia
b. Unilateral aldosterone-producing adenoma
c. Adrenal carcinoma with aldosterone hypersecretion
d. Ectopic aldosterone secretion from the kidneys or ovaries
e. Benign tumor in the adrenal medulla

18. A 66-year-old female presents to her primary care provider for mild vague epigastric discomfort. On physical examination, a pulsatile abdominal mass that is tender to palpation is noted. An abdominal ultrasound is performed (see photo).

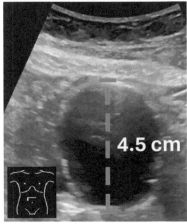

Which of the following is the greatest risk factor for development of her condition?
a. Cigarette smoking
b. Diabetes mellitus
c. Non-White race
d. Female gender
e. Hypertension

Photo credit:
Mikael Häggström, M.D. Author info - Reusing images- Conflicts of interest: NoneMikael Häggström, M.D.Consent note: Written informed consent was obtained from the individual, including online publication., CC0, via Wikimedia Commons

19. A 20-year-old male presents with sudden onset of left-sided pleuritic chest pain while playing football. He denies direct chest trauma. Vitals are blood pressure 92/54 mmHg, pulse 134/min, respirations 32/minute, and SaO2: 89% on oxygen via nasal cannula. Lung examination reveals asymmetrical chest expansion and absent breath sounds on the right hemithorax. Chest radiograph is obtained (see photo).

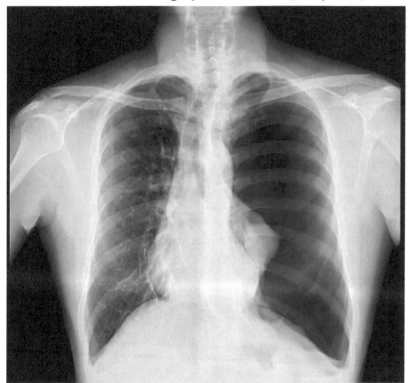

Which of the following is the most appropriate next step in management?
a. Pericardiocentesis
b. Endotracheal intubation
c. Surgical consult for emergent Thoracotomy
d. Needle thoracostomy
e. Video-assisted thoracoscopic surgery (VATS)

Photo credit:
Shutterstock (used with permission)

20. A 29-year-old male presents to the clinic with severe bilateral eye pain, foreign body sensation, photophobia, and inability to open his eyes for 1 hour. On examination, he is rocking back and forth due to severe pain. Physical examination reveals mild reduced visual acuity, which could only be performed after instillation of topical Tetracaine. There is increased tearing, bilateral generalized erythema, conjunctival injection, and chemosis of the bulbar conjunctiva. Instillation of fluorescein reveals diffuse punctate staining of the corneas. Which of the following would most likely be in his history?
a. Welding without the use of protective eyewear a few hours ago
b. Direct eye exposure to lye
c. History of extended wear of daily contact lens
d. Allergies to grass and animal dander
e. History of being in a dark movie theater recently

21. A 32-year-old male presents to the outpatient department complaining of right eye pain and blurred vision. He sees a gap in the center of his right visual field and colors seem "faded", especially red. Ocular examination reveals visual acuity of 20/20 in the left eye and 20/200 in the right eye. There is pain with right eye movement and direct response to light is more sluggish in the right eye. Funduscopic examination is within normal limits. Which of the following is the most likely etiology of his presentation?
a. Retinal detachment
b. Macular degeneration
c. Acute maculopathy
d. Central retinal vein occlusion
e. Optic neuritis

22. A 32-year-old man presents to the emergency department after being burned by hot grease. On examination of the forearm, there is a 4 cm area of skin with blistering. The affected skin is yellow in color and does not blanch. There is decreased pain sensation except with deep pressure and capillary refill is absent. Which of the following is the most likely diagnosis?
a. Fourth degree burn
b. Superficial partial thickness burn
c. Deep partial thickness burn
d. Full thickness burn
e. Superficial burn

23. A 42-year-old male presented to the clinic with an enlarged painful lower anterior neck lump with the pain radiating up to the jaw. He was hospitalized 3 weeks ago for SARS-CoV-2 infection that required sedation, intubation, and invasive ventilation in the intensive care unit (ICU) for 5 days. Physical examination is remarkable for slightly asymmetrically enlarged tender thyroid gland. Initial labs are significant for:
Serum TSH: 0.008 mIU/L (0.4-4)
Serum free T4: 32.1 pmol/L (5-12)
Erythrocyte sedimentation rate 112 mm/hr (1-10)
WBC count 9,000 cells/mcL (5,000-10,000).
Which of the following is the most likely etiology of his presentation?
a. Graves' disease
b. Subacute thyroiditis
c. Suppurative thyroiditis
d. Riedel thyroiditis
e. Euthyroid sick syndrome

24. Which of the following is associated with a decreased risk of Ovarian cancer?
a. Nulliparity
b. Infertility
c. Long-term oral contraceptive use
d. Increasing age
e. Early menarche

25. A 60-year-old woman presents to the ED complaining of palpitations and mild confusion. She has a history of Peptic ulcer disease for 20 years treated with high-dose Pantoprazole. Physical examination is notable for positive Trousseau sign and increased deep tendon reflexes. An ECG is obtained (see photo).

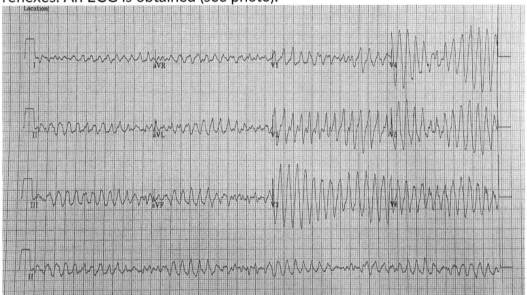

Which of the following is the first line management of this patient?
a. IV Calcium gluconate
b. IV Potassium chloride
c. IV Magnesium sulfate
d. Oral Potassium chloride
e. IV Sodium bicarbonate

26. A 45-year-old male is complaining of darkening of his vision, palpitations, dizziness, and mild confusion. He has a history of Type 2 Diabetes mellitus. On examination, he is diaphoretic, pale, and tachycardic. Fingerstick reveals a glucose of 42 mg/dL (70-110). Which of the following medications is most likely responsible for his current presentation?
a. Metformin
b. Pioglitazone
c. Glyburide
d. Semaglutide
e. Acarbose

27. A 35-year-old male presents to the clinic complaining of intermittent headache. Review of systems is positive for decreased libido. Physical examination reveals a visual field defect in both outer visual fields. A pituitary MRI is performed, revealing a pituitary macroadenoma. Which of the following is the most likely etiology of his presentation?
a. Corticotroph adenoma
b. Somatotroph adenoma
c. TSH adenoma
d. Lactotroph adenoma
e. Glucagonoma

28. A 14-year-old male is being evaluated for learning difficulties. He was diagnosed with Autism spectrum disorder. As a child, he had developmental delay in motor, speech, and language skills. On examination, he has a long narrow face with prominent forehead and chin. He also has protruding ears. Hand flapping and gaze aversion are noted. Which of the following would most likely be seen on physical examination?
a. Gynecomastia, centripetal obesity, and hyperphagia
b. Smooth indistinct philtrum, thin vermillion border, and small palpebral fissures
c. Pale retina with a cherry red macula
d. Dislocation of the lens, tall stature, and arachnodactyly
e. Macroorchidism and hyperextensible finger joints

29. A 32-year-old male is admitted to the hospital for Thyroidectomy for Papillary thyroid carcinoma. On hospital day 2, he is complaining of perioral numbness, muscle cramps, and paresthesias of the hands and feet. ECG reveals a prolonged QT interval. Based on the most likely diagnosis, which of the following would most likely be seen on physical examination?
a. Contraction of the ipsilateral facial muscles elicited by tapping the facial nerve
b. Decreased or absent deep tendon reflexes
c. Elevated blood pressure >140/90 mmHg
d. Absent bowel sounds
e. Decreased vibratory and position sense of the lower extremities

30. A 25-year-old male presents to the emergency department with worsening shortness of breath. He was recently seen in urgent care, where he was found to be COVID-PCR positive. Vitals are blood pressure of 70/42 mmHg, temperature 98.8°F (37.1°C), pulse 122 bpm, respiratory rate 24 breaths/min, and oxygen saturation 91% on room air. Diaphoresis and distended neck veins are noted. The lungs are clear to auscultation. An ECG is obtained (see photo).

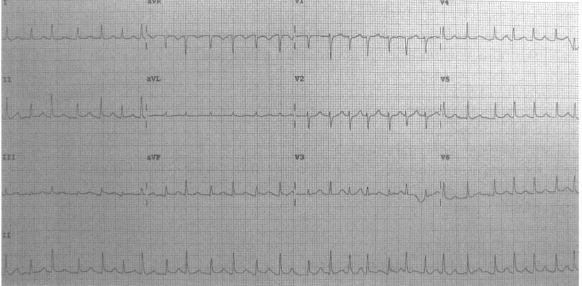

Which of the following is the most appropriate management of this patient at this time?
a. Emergent thoracotomy
b. Needle decompression of the lung
c. Pericardiocentesis
d. High-dose Aspirin and Atenolol
e. Synchronized cardioversion

31. A 30-year-old male presents to the emergency department after sustaining a deep forearm laceration during a construction incident. Immediately after the injury, he irrigated the wound and covered it with gauze. He emigrated to the United States at age 22 and was unvaccinated upon arrival. He only received one Tetanus toxoid vaccine 5 years ago. The wound appears clean without signs of infection at this time. Which of the following is the next best step in the management of this patient?
a. Administer Tetanus immunoglobulin only
b. No further management is needed regarding tetanus immunization/vaccination
c. Administer Tdap vaccine
d. Administer Tdap vaccine and Tetanus immune globulin
e. Administer DTaP vaccine and Tetanus immune globulin

32. A 64-year-old male presents to the clinic complaining of worsening right lower calf cramping and decrease in exercise tolerance, resulting from the right calf discomfort over the last 2 months. The pain begins after he walks about 100 yards and resolves within 2 minutes of rest. He smoked 1 pack of cigarettes daily for 30 years but quit 4 months ago. Physical examination shows no skin changes over the legs or feet. Dorsalis pedis and posterior tibialis pulses are palpable bilaterally and are 1+. Based on history and physical examination, which of the following is the most appropriate next step in the workup of this patient?
a. Exercise treadmill testing
b. Duplex Ultrasound of the lower extremities
c. Venous plethysmography
d. Contrast arteriography of the lower extremities
e. Ankle brachial index

33. A 6-year-old female is brought to the emergency department for decreased urination (she only urinated once today). About 8 days ago, she experienced abdominal cramping and watery diarrhea, which became bloody 2 days later, then spontaneously resolved. Vitals are stable. Physical examination is only notable for conjunctival pallor and petechiae on her legs. Initial labs reveal:
Hemoglobin 9 g/dL (11.9-15)
Platelets 78,000/mm^3 (150,000-450,00)
Creatinine 2.0 mg/dL (0.6-1.2)
Schistocytes are seen on peripheral smear.
Which of the following is the primary pathophysiology of the most likely diagnosis?
a. Decreased ADAMTS13 production
b. Production of Shiga toxin
c. Autoantibody to platelets
d. IgA deposition into the tissues
e. Pathological activation of the clotting cascade

34. A 64-year-old male presents to the clinic with a 5-month history of fatigue, malaise, and weight loss. Physical examination is positive for pallor and splenomegaly.

Labs reveal a hemoglobin of 9.5 g/dL (14-18)

Platelet count 600,000 platelets/mcL (150,000-450,000)

White cell count 115,000 (5,000-10,000)

Leukocyte alkaline phosphatase: low.

Cytogenetic analysis reveals a *BCR::ABL1* fusion gene.

Which of the following is the first-line management?

a. All-trans retinoic acid

b. Dexamethasone, Vincristine, and pegylated Asparaginase

c. Watchful waiting

d. Cytarabine plus Daunorubicin

e. Imatinib

35. A 61-year-old male with longstanding Chronic kidney disease presents with mild right leg pain. Radiographs of the leg reveals the following (see photo).

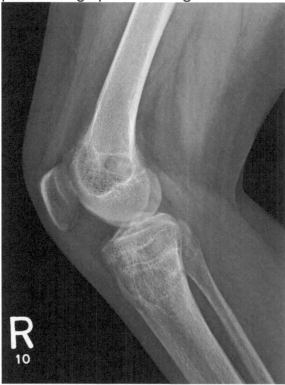

Initial labs reveal a parathyroid hormone level of 184 pg/mL (10-65). Dietary restriction of and decreasing the intestinal absorption of which of the following would most likely benefit this patient?

a. Calcium

b. Iron

c. Magnesium

d. Phosphate

e. Potassium

Photo credit:

Case courtesy of Hani Makky Al Salam, Radiopaedia.org, rID: 12318

36. A 40-year-old female is being evaluated for abnormal vaginal bleeding. She has been having difficulty conceiving. She denies dyschezia or dyspareunia. Physical examination is unremarkable. Transvaginal ultrasound shows a well-defined homogenous lesion of mucosal proliferation with a sharply demarcated vascular pedicle within the narrow stalk that is isoechoic to the endometrium. There is preservation of the endometrial-myometrial interface (see photo).

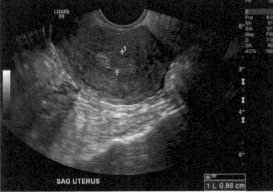

Which of the following is the first-line management in this patient?
a. Expectant management
b. Vaginal estrogen
c. Transcervical polypectomy
d. Leuprolide
e. Uterine artery embolization

Photo credit
Case courtesy of Andrew Ho, Radiopaedia.org, rID: 36694

37. A 20-year-old male is admitted for Cellulitis. The following is seen on monitor (see photo). Which of the following is the most likely diagnosis?

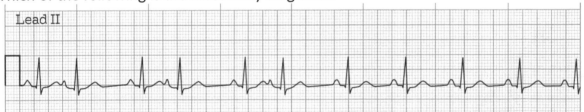

a. Sinus arrhythmia
b. Wolff-Parkinson white
c. Premature atrial complexes
d. First-degree atrioventricular block
e. Mobitz-1 second degree atrioventricular block

Photo credit:
Shutterstock (used with permission)

38. A 24-year-old male recently diagnosed with Hodgkin lymphoma is complaining of swelling of his lower extremities and production of foamy urine for 5 days. Physical examination is notable for 2+ pretibial pitting edema. Initial laboratory workup reveals:
- Serum sodium 136 mEq/L (135-145)
- Serum potassium 4.3 mEq/L (3.5-5)
- Serum albumin 2 g/dL (3.5-5.5)
- Serum creatinine 0.9 mg/dL (0.6-1.2)

Urinalysis reveals:
- Protein: 4+ with oval fat bodies on microscopic examination
- 1 RBC/hpf (<5)

Which of the following is the most likely diagnosis?
a. Membranous nephropathy
b. IgA Nephropathy
c. Focal segmental glomerulosclerosis
d. Amyloidosis
e. Minimal change disease

39. A 41-year-old male presents to the clinic complaining of spiking fever, chills, malaise, dysuria, urgency, perineal pain, cloudy urine, and pain at the tip of the penis. It was preceded by back pain. On examination, the prostate is firm, boggy, and exquisitely tender to palpation. Laboratory evaluation reveals an elevated white blood cell count. Urinalysis reveals pyuria. Which of the following organisms is the most likely etiology of his presentation?
a. Chlamydia trachomatis
b. Escherichia coli
c. Proteus mirabilis
d. Enterobacter species
e. Pseudomonas aeruginosa

40. A 44-year-old male presents with weakness, fatigue, muscle, joint pain, cold intolerance, weight gain, constipation, and decreased libido. Vital reveal a blood pressure of 110/72 mmHg. Sparse pubic and axillary hair are noted. Initial labs reveal:
- serum potassium: 4.0 mEq/L (3.5-5.0)
- serum glucose: 60 mg/dL (80-110)
- serum sodium: 130 mEq/L (135-145)
- serum thyroxine: 3.8 mcg/dL (4.5-11.2)
- serum TSH: 0.1 mIU/L (0.5–5)
- serum luteinizing hormone: 1.4 mIU/L (1.8-8.6).

Which of the following is the most likely etiology of his presentation?
a. Hashimoto thyroiditis
b. Hyperprolactinemia
c. Hypopituitarism
d. Follicular thyroid cancer
e. Medication induced hypothyroidism

41. A 32-year-old male is brought in by his partner. He has become irritable and has developed antisocial behavior. Over the last few weeks, he has developed intermittent involuntary dance-like movements of his face and limbs. His mother had similar symptoms prior to committing suicide. CT scan of the brain shows atrophy of the cerebral cortex and caudate nucleus. Which of the following is most useful to establish the most likely diagnosis?
a. MRI of the brain with gadolinium
b. Brain biopsy
c. Lumbar puncture
d. Single fiber electromyography
e. Number of CAG repeats

42. A 25-year-old male presents with left elbow pain and swelling after falling with his hands outstretched. On examination, there is decreased light touch sensation over the hypothenar eminence and the medial side of the dorsum of the hand, decreased 2-point discrimination involving the fifth finger and the medial side of the fourth finger, and decreased adduction of the thumb. The following is seen on imaging (see photo).

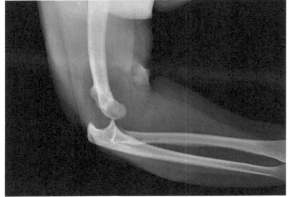

Neuropathy involving which of the following nerves is responsible for these findings?
a. Median
b. Ulnar
c. Radial
d. Axillary
e. Anterior interosseus

Photo credit:
Shutterstock (used with permission)

43. A 22-year-old woman gravida 1 para 0 at 10 weeks gestation presents to the clinic to establish prenatal care. She denies any symptoms and has a history of an allergic reaction to Penicillin. Her initial screening RPR test is positive. Confirmatory fluorescent treponemal antibody absorption test is also positive. Which of the following is the most appropriate next step in the management of this patient?
a. Delay treatment for Syphilis until delivery of the fetus
b. Doxycycline
c. Azithromycin
d. Skin testing, Penicillin desensitization, and then rechallenge
e. Probenecid

44. A 22-year-old male with a history of Type 2B Von Willebrand disease is being transfused with single donor apheresis-derived platelet components obtained 24 hours prior to the transfusion. 20 minutes after the initiation of the transfusion, he develops chills and rigors. He denies respiratory difficulty. Vitals are significant for a pulse of 118/minute, blood pressure 78/42 mmHg (compared to 128/74 mmHg prior to transfusion), and temperature 40°C (104°F). His lungs are clear to auscultation. In addition to discontinuing the platelet transfusion and IV fluids, which of the following is the recommended management?
a. IM Epinephrine
b. Vancomycin plus Piperacillin-tazobactam
c. Mechanical ventilation
d. Furosemide plus supplemental oxygen
e. Acetaminophen

45. A 72-hour-old baby boy born at 38 weeks gestation has been adequately breastfeeding and has had adequate wet diapers. On examination, scleral icterus and yellowing of the skin is noted. Initial labs reveal:
Direct bilirubin: 0.6 mg/dL (0.3-1.0)
Total bilirubin: 9.0 mg/dL (1-12)
8 hours later, repeat total bilirubin is 8.5 mg/dL.
Which of the following is the most appropriate management of this neonate?
a. Exchange transfusion
b. Perform direct antiglobulin (Coombs) testing
c. Observation
d. Phototherapy
e. Discontinue breastfeeding and initiate the use of formula for feedings

46. A 29-year-old male presents to the clinic with fever, night sweats, weight loss, abdominal pain, and nonbloody diarrhea described as 4-5 loose stools daily for the last 12 days. His medical history is significant for HIV infection, but he has been noncompliant with antiretroviral therapy. Vital signs are temperature 102°F (38.8°C), heart rate 102 bpm, and blood pressure 122/72 mm Hg. Laboratory tests show a CD4 count 47/mm^3. Blood cultures reveal Mycobacterium avium complex with a high mycobacterial loads (3 log10 colony-forming units/mL). Which of the following is the first line management in this patient?
a. Clarithromycin plus Ethambutol plus Rifabutin
b. Trimethoprim-sulfamethoxazole
c. Trimethoprim-sulfamethoxazole plus Streptomycin
d. Ciprofloxacin plus Liposomal inhaled Amikacin
e. IV Penicillin G aqueous

47. Which of the following is an indication for the use of irrigation for removal of a foreign body in the external auditory canal?
a. Insects
b. Beans
c. Vegetable matter
d. Button batteries
e. Inorganic object with a perforated tympanic membrane

48. A 54-year-old male is complaining of progressive breathless with exertion over the last 6 months. He denies any recent fevers, chills, cough, sputum production, or night sweats. He has a 20-pack year smoking history, drinks occasionally, and is a plumber. Lung examination reveals bibasilar fine end-expiratory crackles. Pulmonary function testing (PFT) reveals Forced expiratory volume in 1 second (FEV1): 55% of predicted (≥80%) and FEV1-to-forced vital capacity (FVC) ratio: 95% (70-80%). Chest radiographs are obtained (see photo).

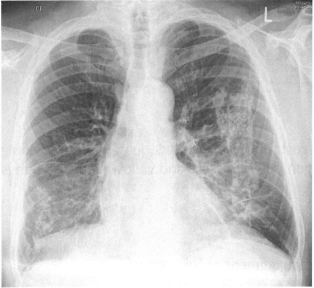

Which of the following is the most likely diagnosis?
a. Asbestosis
b. Emphysema
c. Chronic bronchitis
d. Bronchiectasis
e. Sarcoidosis

Photo credit:
Case courtesy of Roberto Schubert, Radiopaedia.org, rID: 17322

49. A 44-year-old male returns to the clinic for Hypertension despite a trial of diet and exercise. He has a history of Gout, Dyslipidemia, and Diabetes mellitus. Based on his past medical history, which of the following medications is the first line agent for Hypertension in this patient?
a. Prazosin
b. Hydrochlorothiazide
c. Labetalol
d. Furosemide
e. Losartan

50. Which of the following is a contraindication for the use of Bupropion?
a. Management in a patient with Depression who developed sexual dysfunction on Sertraline
b. Management of Seasonal affective disorder
c. Management of Depression in a patient who is obese and fearful of weight gain
d. Patient who desired to quit smoking
e. Management of Depression in a patient with Anorexia nervosa

51. A 22-year-old female presents to the clinic. She is actively trying to get pregnant. She has a history of Epilepsy treated with Valproic acid. Initial labs reveal elevated transaminases 5 times normal values. Her LFTs were normal prior to initiating Valproic acid. The clinician decides to discontinue Valproic acid. This is an example of which of the following principles?
a. Beneficence
b. Nonmalficence
c. Justice
d. Autonomy
e. Caring

52. A 10-year-old male is complaining of sore throat, neck swelling, malaise, and low-grade fever for 2 days. His mother states he never received routine childhood vaccinations. Vitals reveal a temperature of 101°F (38.3°C). Findings include enlarged cervical lymph nodes, neck edema, and a leathery gray leathery exudate on both tonsils and posterior pharynx that bleeds on touch and is difficult to remove. The patient is at greatest risk for the development of which of the following complications due to his present condition?
a. Splenic rupture
b. Glomerulonephritis
c. Myocarditis
d. Hemolytic uremic syndrome
e. Acute rheumatic fever

53. A 20-year-old male presents to the emergency department after a motor vehicle accident. He had brief loss of consciousness at the scene. On examination, his Glasgow coma scale is 15. A Noncontrast CT of the head is performed (see photo).

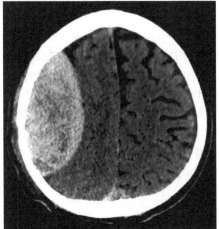

Which of the following is the most likely etiology of his presentation?
a. Rupture of a cortical bridging vein
b. Rupture of a Berry aneurysm
c. Rupture of the penetrating arterioles
d. Arteriovenous malformations
e. Rupture of the middle meningeal artery

Photo credit:
Shutterstock (used with permission)

54. A 64-year-old man presents to the clinic with worsening difficulty swallowing over the past 5 months, associated with a 20-pound weight loss in this time period. He initially had difficulty swallowing large boluses of solid food but now he can only tolerate mashed food and liquids. He has a past medical history of Osteoarthritis for which he takes Naproxen. Vital signs are normal. BMI is 28 kg/m^2. Physical examination is unremarkable. A barium upper GI series reveals a mass in the upper third of the esophagus with marked lumen narrowing. Which of the following risk factors is most likely related to this patient's condition?
a. Cold beverage consumption
b. Long-term Naproxen consumption
c. Gastroesophageal reflux disease and esophagitis
d. Helicobacter pylori infection
e. Alcohol consumption

55. A 43-year-old male presents to the clinic with intermittent abdominal pain after meals. Review of systems is positive for malaise, fever, and weight loss. He denies dyspnea or chest pain. Vitals reveal blood pressure of 148/92 mmHg (his BP is usually 122/70 mmHg). Physical examination is notable for tender cutaneous ulcers and palpable purpuric lesions. Laboratory evaluation is significant for a newly elevated creatinine of 2.1 mg/dL, elevated erythrocyte sedimentation rate, and positive Hepatitis B surface antigen. Antineutrophil cytoplasmic autoantibodies are negative. Urinalysis is positive for 1+ proteinuria and 2 red cells/hpf (0-5) with no red cell casts. Which of the following is the most likely diagnosis?
a. Glomerular basement membrane disease
b. Granulomatosis with polyangiitis
c. Eosinophilic granulomatosis with polyangiitis
d. Polyarteritis nodosa
e. Microscopic polyangiitis

56. A 68-year-old male developed abrupt onset of mild 3/10 cramping left-sided abdominal pain. 24 hours after the onset of the colicky pain, he had a few episodes of bright red blood per rectum and bloody diarrhea. 4 days ago, he underwent elective endovascular repair of an Abdominal aortic aneurysm found on routine screening. He has a history of Myocardial infarction. On examination, there is mild abdominal tenderness without guarding, rigidity, or rebound tenderness. CT scan of the abdomen reveals edema and thickening of the bowl wall in a segmental pattern. Which of the following is the most likely diagnosis?
a. Chronic mesenteric ischemia
b. Ischemic colitis
c. Acute mesenteric ischemia
d. Diverticulitis
e. Infectious colitis

57. A 5-year-old boy returns to the office for follow-up after being treated with high-dose Amoxicillin for 1 week. Although his fever and pain has resolved, he has intermittent fluctuating difficulties with hearing. On examination, there is decreased mobility of the right tympanic membrane and amber-colored middle ear fluid behind a retracted tympanic membrane without erythema. Weber testing reveals lateralization to the right ear and bone conduction greater than air conduction on the right side with a hearing threshold of 10 dB (≤15). He has no speech or language deficits. Which of the following is the first line management of this patient?
a. Urgent ENT referral for myringotomy with tympanostomy tube insertion
b. Oral Cetirizine
c. Watchful waiting
d. Oral Amoxicillin-clavulanate
e. Oral Pseudoephedrine

58. A 20-year-old male presents to the clinic with fever, body aches, fatigue, diarrhea, and myalgias. He is sexually active with 4 partners and does not use condoms. Physical examination is notable for tonsillar hypertrophy and erythema of the posterior pharynx. Bilateral cervical lymphadenopathy is noted. CBC shows a normal white cell count. Monospot testing is negative. A rapid fourth generation antigen/antibody combination HIV-1/2 immunoassay is performed. Which of the following is the most appropriate next step?
a. No further testing is needed if the combination test is negative
b. Diagnose the patient with established HIV infection if combination test is positive
c. Perform a viral load [HIV RNA (RT-PCR)] only if combination test is positive
d. Admission to the hospital if the combination test and confirmatory is positive
e. Perform HIV RNA (RT-PCR); perform HIV-1/HIV-2 antibody differentiation if immunoassay is positive

59. A 20-year-old male presents to the urgent care clinic after sustaining a cat bite to the hand after trying to break up his 2 cats from fighting last night. His last Tetanus booster was 2 years ago. There is a small puncture wound to the dorsum of the hand with localized warmth, erythema, edema, and tenderness. There is no purulent discharge. Which of the following pathogens is most commonly associated with infection resulting from his injury?
a. Pasteurella multocida
b. Bartonella henselae
c. Staphylococcus aureus
d. Streptococcus pyogenes
e. Pseudomonas aeruginosa

60. A 57-year-old woman presents to the clinic with heavy vaginal bleeding. Her last menstrual period occurred when she was 51 years of age. Physical examination is unremarkable. A Transvaginal ultrasound reveals an endometrial stripe of 11 mm. Which of the following is the most appropriate next step?
a. Hysterectomy
b. Progestin add-back therapy
c. Hysteroscopy
d. Endometrial biopsy
e. Repeat Transvaginal ultrasound 4 months

61. A 35-year-old male presents to the clinic with a skin rash. He was recently diagnosed with Atrial fibrillation, for which he was placed on Propranolol. On examination, there are symmetric salmon-colored plaques with overlying silver scales noted on the extensor surfaces of the bilateral elbows and knees. Nail pitting is noted. Which of the following is the initial management of choice in this patient?
a. Oral Prednisone
b. Narrowband ultraviolet B (UVB) phototherapy
c. Betamethasone dipropionate ointment
d. Oral Methotrexate
e. Calcipotriene ointment

62. A 60-year-old man presents to the emergency department due to acute onset of dyspnea, increased productive cough with green sputum, and increased sputum volume for 72 hours. His home medication is a Tiotropium inhaler, and he has a 40-pack-year smoking history. Vitals are blood pressure 142/92 mmHg, pulse is 102/min and regular, and SaO2: 90% on room air. Lung examination reveals diminished breath sounds bilaterally with prolonged expiration. A chest radiograph is obtained (see photo).

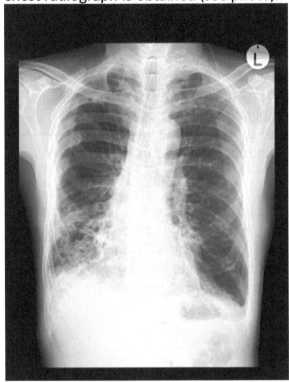

In addition to antibiotics, which of the following would most likely reduce his length of hospital stay and decrease the rate of relapse?
a. Nedocromil
b. Salmeterol
c. Home oxygen therapy
d. Montelukast
e. Prednisone

63. A 40-year-old homeless male with malnutrition presents with increased irritability, insomnia, and apathy. He also reports watery stools, nausea, poor appetite, and painful skin lesions. He has a history of chronic alcohol use. On physical examination, well-demarcated brown discolored skin lesions in a symmetric fashion are seen on the hands, neck, and face. Which of the following is the most appropriate treatment of this patient?
a. Oral Folate
b. Oral Niacin
c. Oral Cobalamin
d. Parenteral Thiamine
e. Parenteral Cobalamin

64. A 23-year-old female presents to the clinic for follow-up. She was placed on antiepileptic therapy for Generalized tonic-clonic seizures. She has not had a seizure in the 6 months since being placed on therapy. On examination, thickened gums that overhang beyond the teeth insertion and increased terminal, coarse, pigmented hairs on her chin and chest are noted. Which antiepileptic medication is most likely responsible for these findings?
a. Phenytoin
b. Carbamazepine
c. Topiramate
d. Lamotrigine
e. Valproic acid

65. A 3-year-old boy presents to the emergency department with fever, severe sore throat, dysphagia, and progressive shortness of breath since last night. Vitals are temperature 104°F (40°C), pulse 124 bpm, respiratory rate 30 breaths/min, and oxygen saturation 94% on room air. He is anxious and agitated. He is seated with slight hyperextension of the neck, an oral breathing pattern, and he refuses to lie supine. Inspiratory stridor is audible. Which of the following is the most appropriate next step in the evaluation of this patient?
a. Tracheostomy
b. Laryngoscopy in the operating room
c. Initiate IV Ceftriaxone after obtaining blood cultures
d. IM Epinephrine and Dexamethasone
e. Direct inspection of the posterior pharynx with a tongue depressor

66. A 55-year-old male is admitted to the hospital after undergoing a knee replacement for Osteoarthritis. On post op day 4, the nurse reports the patient is restless and agitated. He is complaining of seeing insects crawling on his bed sheet and hears the nurses at the nurse's station whispering secrets about him. Vitals are temperature 101°F (38.3°C), blood pressure 178/96 mmHg, pulse 114 bpm, and respiratory rate 24 breaths/min. He is diaphoretic, disoriented, and bilateral fine hand tremors noted. Which of the following is the first-line management for this patient?
a. Disulfiram
b. Haloperidol
c. Naltrexone
d. Flumazenil
e. Chlordiazepoxide

67. A 27-year-old nurse returns to employee health for reading of a Tuberculin skin test (TST) that was placed 48 hours ago. She has no significant medical conditions and denies any symptoms. Vital signs are normal and physical examination is unremarkable. The site where the TST was placed shows 11 mm of induration. A chest radiograph is obtained and is unremarkable. Which of the following is the most appropriate next step in the management of this patient at this time?
a. Place the employee in respiratory isolation and induce sputum for acid-fast bacilli staining and Nucleic acid testing (NAAT)
b. Repeat the Tuberculin skin test (TST) to assess for booster phenomenon
c. Isoniazid and Rifampin daily for 4 months
d. Order CT chest without contrast
e. Initiate Rifampin therapy daily for 4 months

68. A 36-year-old female presents to the clinic with exertional dyspnea and fatigue. Physical examination is notable for wide splitting of the second heart sound. ECG shows right ventricular hypertrophy and increased P wave amplitude in lead II. Echocardiogram revealed pulmonary artery pressure (PAP) of 60 mmHg. Intraoperative administration of IV Adenosine decreases PAP to 30 mmHg. Which of the following is the first line pharmacological therapy in this patient?
a. Bosentan
b. Sildenafil
c. Metoprolol
d. Epoprostenol
e. Nifedipine

69. A 24-year-old female presents with vaginal spotting and right-sided pelvic pain. She denies dizziness, nausea, vomiting, shoulder pain, or syncope. She is sexually active and has an implanted copper intrauterine device. Vitals are stable. There is right lower quadrant tenderness. Serum hCG is 1,140 mIU/mL. Transvaginal ultrasound is performed and does not identify an intrauterine pregnancy or other abnormalities. There is no free fluid noted. Which of the following is the most appropriate next step?
a. Repeat hCG and Ultrasound in 48 hours
b. Salpingostomy
c. CT scan of the abdomen and pelvis
d. Methotrexate administration
e. Uterine aspiration

70. A 17-year-old female presents to the emergency department with severe right knee pain. She was playing soccer when she suddenly decelerated to make a quick cut and run maneuver. Immediately afterwards, she heard a "snapping" sound, followed by abrupt knee pain and swelling. Physical examination is positive for hemarthrosis of the knee. Which of the following tests is most sensitive test to confirm the most likely diagnosis?
a. Straight leg raise test
b. Anterior drawer test
c. Posterior sag test
d. Valgus stress test
e. Lachman test

71. A 42-year-old male presents to the ED. He was playing tennis when he pivoted on his right foot and felt a "pop" in his right ankle followed by severe pain. He was diagnosed with Prostatitis 5 days ago, for which he is taking Ciprofloxacin. On examination, there is exquisite tenderness over the distal aspect of the right lower leg and squeezing of the calf muscle does not produce plantar flexion of the foot. Which of the following is the recommended initial management of this patient?
a. Activity modification, ice application, and Nonsteroidal anti-inflammatory drugs
b. Short-leg splint in dorsiflexion, non-weightbearing with crutches, and orthopedic follow-up
c. Place in a walking boot (air cast) with protected weight bearing and orthopedic follow up
d. Short-leg splint in plantarflexion, non-weightbearing with crutches, & orthopedic follow-up
e. Ice, elastic bandage wraps, keep elevated, weight bearing as tolerated ortho follow up in 7 days

72. A 27-year-old male presents to the clinic with a 48-hour history of back pain. The pain began when he was putting items on a shelf. He denies nocturnal pain, fever, chills, morning stiffness, urinary/bowel changes, or radiation. On examination, there is reproducible paravertebral tenderness over the lower lumbar region. There is no bony tenderness and straight leg raise is negative. Neurological examination is unremarkable. Which of the following is not appropriate part of the management during this visit?
a. Early range of motion exercises
b. Lumbar spine radiographs
c. Ibuprofen
d. Resumption of ordinary activity as tolerated
e. Warm compresses to the affected area

73. A 60-year-old woman presents to the emergency department for nausea, vomiting, and abdominal discomfort than began 45 minutes ago. Initially, the pain improved when she rested but shortly, the abdominal pain returned. She has a history of GERD, Hypertension, Diabetes mellitus, and a 20-pack-year smoking history. Vitals are stable. Physical examination is remarkable for mild abdominal discomfort on palpation. Cardiac and pulmonary examination are within normal limits. Which of the following is the most appropriate next step in the management of this patient?
a. Amylase, lipase, and liver function tests
b. Troponin I and creatine kinase-MB levels
c. Electrocardiogram
d. CT abdomen and pelvis without contrast
e. Ultrasound of the right upper quadrant

74. A 7-year-old boy is being evaluated in the clinic. On examination, there are 8 café au lait macules that are 6-8 mm in diameter, freckling in the axillary or inguinal regions, and tan colored dome-shaped papules projecting from the surface of the iris. Visual acuity is intact. Which of the following is the most likely diagnosis?
a. Neurofibromatosis type 1
b. Noonan syndrome
c. Neurofibromatosis type 2
d. Peutz-Jegher syndrome
e. Tuberous sclerosis

75. A 25-year-old male presents to his primary care provider for a six-week history of intrusive images and nightmares after he and his family were involved in a car wreck 5 weeks ago. The thoughts were triggered when he saw a picture of the car accident. Since then, he has tried to occupy his mind playing sports. However, when he has free time, he is troubled with visual images of being at the wreckage and wakes up in a cold sweat. During the day, he feels disconnected and numb. Which of the following is the first line adjunct to psychotherapy?
a. Buspirone
b. Sertraline
c. Risperidone
d. Trazodone
e. Diazepam

76. A 35-year-old man presents to an urgent care clinic for cough, fever, chills, and myalgias. He is an archeologist and has been exploring ancient caves outside of Pittsburgh, Pennsylvania. Physical examination is positive for fever and rales. PPD is negative. Chest radiographs show patchy pulmonary infiltrates and enlarged hilar lymphadenopathy without cavitations. A sputum sample under microscopy shows macrophages with intracellular narrow-based, ovoid, budding cells, measuring 2-5 micrometers in diameter. Which of the following is the most likely diagnosis?
a. Tuberculosis
b. Histoplasmosis
c. Coccidioidomycosis
d. Cryptococcosis
e. Blastomycosis

77. A 44-year-old male is admitted to the hospital for Pulmonary embolism and was started on Unfractionated Heparin. On hospital day 6, he develops fever, chills, and dyspnea. CT scan shows new Pulmonary emboli. Laboratory evaluation shows a platelet count of 78,000 platelets/mcL (150,00-450,000). His admission platelet count was 410,000. There is no active bleeding currently. Serotonin release assay is 100%. In addition to discontinuing Unfractionated Heparin, which of the following is the recommended management of choice?
a. Enoxaparin
b. Fondaparinux
c. Warfarin
d. Argatroban
e. Platelet transfusion

78. A 9-year-old boy presents to the clinic with episodes of sneezing, rhinorrhea, nasal congestion, and postnasal drip. On examination, scant clear rhinorrhea a pale bluish hue to the nasal mucosa, and turbinate edema are noted. A nasal polyp is noted. In addition to avoidance of known allergens, which of the following is the most effective single maintenance therapy for this patient's condition?
a. Intranasal Oxymetazoline
b. Oral Cetirizine
c. Intranasal Azelastine
d. Cromolyn sodium nasal spray
e. Intranasal Mometasone

79. A 56-year-old male is being evaluated in the clinic after numerous falls due to difficulty with balance and symmetric paresthesias to the legs. He has a longstanding history of alcohol use disorder. Physical examination is notable for an unsteady ataxic gait, symmetric decreased sensation, 2-point discrimination of the lower extremities, decreased vibratory, tactile, and position senses over the dorsum of the feet and ankles, diminished deep tendon reflexes, and a positive Babinski sign. Which of the following is the most likely diagnosis?
a. Cobalamin (vitamin B12) deficiency
b. Guillain-Barre syndrome
c. Amyotrophic lateral sclerosis
d. Type 2 Diabetes mellitus
e. Anterior cerebral artery stroke

80. A 23-year-old primigravid female at 10 weeks gestation presents for her initial prenatal visit. She is complaining of vulvar itching, soreness, and vaginal discharge for 4 days. She was recently seen in an ED for Asthma exacerbation, for which she was placed on Prednisone. Physical examination is significant for vulvar erythema and edema. There is a clumpy white discharge adherent to the vaginal walls without an odor with a normal appearing cervix. Vaginal pH is normal. Based on the most likely diagnosis, which of the following is the first line management for this patient?
a. Oral Fluconazole
b. Topical Metronidazole gel
c. Topical Clotrimazole
d. Nystatin pessary
e. Oral Metronidazole

81. A 14-month-old boy is being evaluated in the urology clinic for recurrent febrile urinary tract infections. On examination, the external genitalia is unremarkable. A Urinalysis reveals pyuria. Urine culture is positive for Proteus mirabilis. Renal ultrasonography reveals dilatation of the drainage system of the renal calyces and pelvis. Which of the following should be performed next in this patient?
a. Intravenous pyelogram
b. Radionuclide cystogram
c. Dimercaptosuccinic acid (DMSA) renal scan
d. Voiding cystourethrography
e. Computed tomography of the abdomen and pelvis

82. A 38-year-old female presents to the clinic to establish care. She denies any complaints, except mild dyspnea on exertion. Physical exam is notable for a soft holosystolic ejection murmur best heard over the left second intercostal space. There is a widely split and fixed second heart sound (S2). Which of the following is the most likely diagnosis?
a. Still murmur
b. Atrial septal defect
c. Ventricular septal defect
d. Coarctation of the aorta
e. Mitral regurgitation

83. A 21-year-old man presents to the clinic with periods of depression and mood swings for the last 3 years. He has episodes of sadness, hypersomnia, loss of interest in his hobbies, and eating a lot, which last a few weeks. Other times, he has euphoric mood, decreased need for sleep, increase in goal-directed activities, and enhanced creativity. On examination, his speech is loud and rapid, but he is easy to interrupt. Laboratory evaluation and urine toxicology are negative. Based on the most likely diagnosis, which of the following is the first line management of choice for his condition?
a. Buspirone
b. Nortriptyline
c. Valproic acid
d. Sertraline
e. Bupropion

84. A 32-year-old male presents to the emergency department with increasing breathlessness, cough, and pleuritic chest pain. Physical examination is positive for dullness to percussion and decreased fremitus. Chest radiograph is positive for a moderate right Pleural effusion. A thoracentesis is performed, revealing pleural fluid protein of 4.5 g/dL, serum protein 5.9 g/dL [ratio 0.76]; pleural lactate dehydrogenase (LDH) 51 U/L and serum LDH 72 U/L [ratio 0.7]. Which of the following is the most likely etiology of this patient's Pleural effusion?
a. Atelectasis
b. Decompensated heart failure
c. Pneumonia
d. Nephrotic syndrome
e. Cirrhosis

85. A 24-year-old female at 11 weeks gestation presents to the ED for abdominal cramping and vaginal spotting over the last 2 hours that has become increasingly heavy. Vitals are stable. Speculum examination reveals a moderate amount of bleeding and clots in the vaginal vault. The cervical os is dilated. Urine beta-hCG is positive. Transvaginal ultrasound is notable for intrauterine products of conception and no fetal cardiac activity. Which of the following is the most likely diagnosis?
a. Inevitable abortion
b. Missed abortion
c. Threatened abortion
d. Incomplete abortion
e. Complete abortion

86. A 34-year-old female presents with acute right-sided low back pain radiating from the right gluteus muscle into the right posterior leg. On examination, decreased plantar flexion and decreased sensation to the plantar surface of the foot are noted. Walking on her toes is more difficult than walking on her heels. There is loss of the ankle jerk reflex. Physical examination is otherwise unremarkable. Which of the following is the most likely diagnosis?
a. Cauda equina syndrome
b. L5 – S1 lumbosacral radiculopathy
c. L3 – L4 lumbosacral radiculopathy
d. L4 – L5 lumbosacral radiculopathy
e. Acute lumbosacral strain

87. A 55-year-old male presents to his primary care provider complaining of urinary frequency. He wakes up 4-5 times nightly to urinate. He experiences post-void dribbling, hesitancy, difficulty initiating a stream of urine, and a weak urinary stream. He denies any difficulty maintaining an erection or perineal pain. On digital rectal exam, his prostate is uniformly enlarged, smooth, firm, and nontender without nodules. Sphincter tone is normal. Which of the following medications is indicated as first-line therapy for this patient?
a. Oxybutynin
b. Mirabegron
c. Sildenafil
d. Tamsulosin
e. Finasteride

88. A 52-year-old man with a longstanding history of alcoholism and Hepatitis C presents to the ED after 2 episodes of vomiting bright red blood. He denies abdominal pain, constipation, or diarrhea. Physical examination is notable for bulging flanks, shifting dullness, hepatosplenomegaly, and spider angiomata. He is stabilized and taken urgently for an Upper endoscopy, which revealed bleeding from dilated esophageal veins. Which of the following is the recommended next step?
a. Endoscopic sclerotherapy and Vasopressin
b. Placement of Transjugular intrahepatic portosystemic shunt (TIPS)
c. Endoscopic banding and Octreotide
d. Insertion of a modified Sengstaken-Blakemore (Minnesota) tube for compression
e. Surgical esophageal devascularization of the varices

89. A 20-year-old male presents to the emergency department with hallucinations and agitation. He was at a party where he was using drugs. Vitals are temperature 101°F (38.3°C), blood pressure 180/92 mmHg, pulse 122 bpm, and respiratory rate 22 breaths/min. He is combative and despite having a bony deformity of the forearm, he denies arm pain. His pupils are 4 mm bilaterally, multidirectional nystagmus, and involuntary conjugate upwards deviation of the eyeballs are noted. Urine toxicology confirms the most likely diagnosis. Which of the following substances did he most likely ingest?
a. Marijuana
b. Diazepam
c. Cocaine
d. Phencyclidine
e. Amphetamines

90. A woman has a 70% greater risk of being killed by her domestic abuser at which of the following periods?
a. When she leaves the abusive partner
b. During the physical altercation
c. When she seeks medical care for trauma perpetrated by the abuser
d. When she returns to the abuser after leaving him
e. When the abuser totally isolates her from her support systems

91. A 41-year-old female presents to the clinic complaining of bilateral hand and wrist stiffness and swelling for 3 months. She has difficulty moving the joints after getting out of bed, but the stiffness improves in the afternoon. Review of systems is positive for malaise and fatigue. On examination, there is erythema, tenderness, and swelling to the metacarpophalangeal, proximal interphalangeal, and wrist joints. Initial labs are positive for Anti-citrullinated peptide antibodies. Which of the following medications has the greatest efficacy in reducing progression of the most likely diagnosis?
a. Methotrexate
b. Naproxen
c. Colchicine
d. Prednisone
e. Triamcinolone intraarticular injection

92. A 22-year-old female presents to the clinic to be evaluated for depression. Upon questioning, she admits that she consumes large amounts of snack foods and pasta in a short amount of time at least twice a week. She feels guilty afterwards, and then vomits and/or exercises for hours to feel better. Her BMI is 26 kg/m^2. Which of the following medications is FDA-approved and the best studied medication for the management of Depression in the setting of her underlying condition?
a. Bupropion
b. Trazodone
c. Sertraline
d. Fluoxetine
e. Desipramine

93. A 48-hour neonate is being evaluated for poor feeding and bilious vomiting. He has not had passage of stool since birth. Physical examination is notable for abdominal distention and firmness. There is a tight anal sphincter with expulsion of gas and stool with digital rectal examination. Plain abdominal radiographs reveal distended loops of bowel and an absence of gas in the rectum. Which of the following is the most likely etiology of his presentation?
a. Invagination (telescoping) of a part of the intestine into itself
b. Persistence of the vitelline (omphaloenteric) duct
c. Congenital absence of ganglion cells in the distal rectum and part of the sigmoid colon
d. Narrowing or blockage of the duodenum
e. Part of the intestine protrudes through the umbilical opening in the abdominal muscle

94. A 32-year-old male with a history of Obesity returns to the clinic for follow-up. He has not met his weight loss goals of at least 5% body weight in 6 months despite being compliant with a low-fat, hypocaloric diet and 180 minutes of exercise weekly. He has a history of Nephrolithiasis. His current BMI is 32 kg/m^2. Which of the following is first-line therapy for weight loss in this patient?
a. Bariatric surgery
b. Orlistat
c. Phentermine-Topiramate
d. Tirzepatide
e. Sertraline

95. A 20-year-old male is complaining of progressive tingling and numbness in both legs. He has since developed mild incoordination, making it difficult to walk. 2 weeks ago, he had sore throat, sneezing, and rhinorrhea that spontaneously resolved. Physical examination is notable for flaccid proximal and distal arm and leg weakness (predominant in the legs) and 1+ knee reflexes. Sensory loss was variable in the feet and hands. A lumbar puncture is performed, which of the following would most likely be seen on Cerebrospinal fluid (CSF) analysis?
a. Elevated protein, normal leukocyte count, normal RBC, normal glucose
b. Increased opening pressure with otherwise normal CSF parameters
c. Normal glucose, increased protein, increased white cells (predominantly lymphocytes)
d. Increased IgG and IgG oligoclonal bands
e. Decreased glucose, increased protein, increased white cells (predominantly neutrophils)

96. A 54-year-old female returns to the clinic for follow-up after undergoing bone densitometry. She eats a balanced diet and exercises 4 days a week. She has no past medical history and underwent menopause 3 years ago. She takes over-the counter Cholecalciferol (D3). She drinks a glass of red wine daily and does not smoke. Her mother had an osteoporotic hip fracture at age 83. Her BMI is 26 kg/m^3. Physical examination is unremarkable. Bone densitometry reveals a T score of -0.9 in the femoral neck, and 0.7 in the lumbar spine. Which of the following is the best next step in the management of this patient's bone density?
a. Advise her to switch to low-impact aerobic activities
b. Recommend cessation of alcohol
c. Prescribe Alendronate
d. Prescribe Raloxifene
e. Reassure and advise no additional therapy

97. A 7-year-old male presents to the clinic for evaluation of a limp. Initially, he has activity intermittent related left hip and groin pain over the last 5 weeks. The pain has subsided, but he has a persistent limp that is not painful. Vital signs are within normal limits. On examination, there is significant limitation of range of motion of the hip, especially with internal rotation and abduction of the left hip and a Trendelenburg gait is noted. There is no erythema or warmth present over the hip joint. Radiographs of the hip are unremarkable. Which of the following is the most likely diagnosis?
a. Juvenile idiopathic arthritis
b. Septic arthritis
c. Slipped capital femoral epiphysis
d. Legg-Calves Perthes disease
e. Developmental dysplasia of the hip

98. A 5-month-old male is being evaluated for an empty and poorly rugated right hemiscrotum. The left testicle appears normal and is in the scrotum. The child otherwise appears to be healthy. He was born preterm. Which of the following is the most appropriate management for this patient?
a. Surgical referral for orchiectomy
b. Observation and reassurance that most undescended testicles will spontaneously resolve within 1 year of age
c. Surgical referral for orchiopexy
d. Gonadotrophin-releasing hormone nasal spray to facilitate descension
e. Luteinizing hormone-releasing hormone (LHRH) agonist and urine-derived human chorionic gonadotropin [hCG] and reassure parents it will descend

99. A 13-year-old girl presents to the clinic. She confides she wishes she were a boy, prefers to dress like a boy, and often plays stereotyped "boy" games with other boys. Since she was 5, she always felt she was trapped in the wrong body. She has been feeling increasingly distressed after developing larger breasts and used chest banding to conceal her breasts from showing. She is scared to tell her parents because "I don't want to disappoint them". Which of the following is most appropriate management of this patient?
a. Inform her parents of her desires so they can determine the next best appropriate steps
b. Reassure her that this is age-appropriate behavior
c. Ask if she feels comfortable and secure in her family dynamics and at home
d. Surgical referral for gender reassignment therapy
e. Endocrinologist referral to initiate testosterone hormonal therapy

100. A 66-year-old female presents with palpitations. She has a history of Hypertension and Type 2 Diabetes mellitus. She has no history of bleeding. The following is seen (see photo).

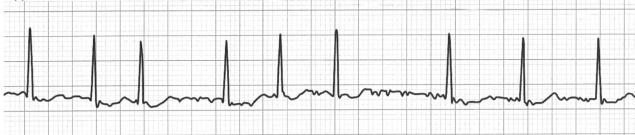

Which of the following is the preferred treatment option?
a. Ticagrelor
b. Aspirin
c. Rivaroxaban
d. Dipyridamole
e. Aspirin and Clopidogrel

END OF EXAM 2

1. CARDIOLOGY – ACUTE CORONARY SYNDROME [PROFESSIONAL PRACTICE]

In nonemergent situations, certified medical interpreters [choice D] are most appropriate for patient-provider interactions to ensure patients have a full understanding in the language they are most comfortable in.

These interpreters are trained in medical terminology, allows for more accurate histories, and improves overall effective communication.

Family members [choice C] should be used only in medical emergencies.

2. PULMONARY – FOREIGN BODY ASPIRATION [CLINICAL INTERVENTION]

In children with known or strongly suspected Foreign body aspiration (FBA), Rigid bronchoscopy [choice C] is the procedure of choice to locate and remove the object.

The object should be removed as soon as possible as it can cause life-threatening obstruction. FBA should be suspected in children with dyspnea, cyanosis, stridor, abrupt onset of cough and wheezing (often focal and monophonic), and/or unilaterally decreased breath sounds.

Choice A [CT scan of the chest] can be used in patients with moderate suspicion of FBA in which chest radiograph is inconclusive. This patient is hypoxic and has a high risk for FBA.

Choice B [Thoracotomy] can be used in the rare instance the foreign body that is visualized cannot be removed via Rigid bronchoscopy.

Choice D [Nebulized albuterol] is used in the management of Asthma.

Choice E [Nebulized racemic Epinephrine] can be used in the management of stridor associated with moderate to severe Croup.

3. EENT – HAND, FOOT, AND MOUTH DISEASE [APPLYING FUNDAMENTAL CONCEPTS]

Coxsackievirus type A16 [choice B] and enterovirus A71 are the serotypes most commonly associated Hand, foot, and mouth disease (HFMD) and Herpangina.

Coxsackievirus type B is most commonly associated with Myocarditis and Pericarditis.

HFMD is characterized by a painful oral enanthem that involves vesicles &/or ulcers in the anterior oral cavity. It is often associated with flu-like symptoms (eg, low-grade fever, cough, malaise).

The exanthem is characterized by vesicles or erythematous papules on the palms, soles, legs (especially upper thighs), arms, and buttocks.

Choice A [Herpes simplex virus] is associated with Primary herpes simplex gingivostomatitis, which can also present with oral vesicles &/or ulceration. If HSV stomatitis is associated with a rash, it is usually unilateral (eg, Herpetic whitlow) unlike the bilateral rash of HFMD.

Choice C [Parvovirus B19] causes Erythema infectiosum, which is associated with facial erythema with sparing of the perioral region (slapped cheek appearance), followed by a lacy reticular rash on the extremities.

Choice D [Group A streptococcus] can be associated with sore throat but less associated with vesicles and GAS is usually not associated with cough (this patient has a cough) or viral symptoms.

Choice E [Varicella virus] can cause an asynchronous rash (macules, papules, vesicles, crusted lesions) simultaneously.

4. CARDIOLOGY – HEART FAILURE [HISTORY AND PHYSICAL]

Left-sided Heart failure presents with pulmonary symptoms (eg, crackles) [choice C] resulting from increased pulmonary venous pressure from fluid backing up into the lungs (Think L for Lungs and L-sided).

Common findings include progressive dyspnea, orthopnea, paroxysmal nocturnal dyspnea, and fatigue.

Chronic, nonproductive cough or productive with pink, frothy sputum, worse in the supine position or at night, may also be seen.

Right-sided Heart failure is associated with systemic symptoms of peripheral and abdominal congestion due to increased systemic venous pressure.

This results in peripheral edema (eg, pitting edema of the legs), increased body weight, jugular venous distention (due to increased jugular venous pressure), GI & hepatic congestion: anorexia, loss of appetite, nausea, vomiting, hepatojugular reflux (increased JVP with liver palpation), hepatosplenomegaly, and ascites.

5. HEMATOLOGY – IMMUNE THROMBOCYTOPENIC PURPURA (ITP) [PHARMACOLOGY]

Administration of a glucocorticoid, such as IM Dexamethasone or oral Prednisone [choice D] is the first line management of Immune thrombocytopenic purpura (ITP) with minor bleeding or severe thrombocytopenia (platelet count <30,000 without bleeding).

Glucocorticoids help to raise the platelet count and reduce the rate of platelet destruction by reducing the number of platelet autoantibodies.

Both IVIG and Glucocorticoids raise platelet levels. Both have similar efficacy, but Glucocorticoids are easier to administer, less expensive, and can be given on an outpatient basis.

IVIG is an infusion but works more rapidly (1-3 days) vs. 2-14 days with glucocorticoids.

In adults, the 4 main therapies for ITP include:
- Mild bleeding + platelet count <50,000: Glucocorticoids
- Severe bleeding (CNS/GI): Platelet transfusion [choice C] + IVIG + glucocorticoids.
- No bleeding + platelet count >30,000: Observation [choice D]
- No bleeding + platelet count <30,000: Glucocorticoids

Choice A [Splenectomy] can be used in refractory cases.
Choice B [Plasma exchange therapy] is not used in the management of ITP.

6. HEMATOLOGY - THALASSEMIA [MOST LIKELY]

Beta thalassemia minor (trait) [choice B] should be suspected in patients with:
- **Hemoglobin electrophoresis: increased Hb F and Hb A2 (to compensate for decreased Hb A production)**
- **No symptoms (most common) or mild to moderate anemia.**

Beta thalassemia minor (trait) is the most common type of Beta thalassemia.
In Beta thalassemia minor (trait), there is only one point mutation (heterozygous).

Choice A [Iron deficiency anemia] is also associated with a microcytic anemia but IDA is associated with a decreased RBC count, decreased serum ferritin, and a normal Hb electrophoresis.

Choice C [Alpha thalassemia intermedia/Hemoglobin H disease] is usually symptomatic at birth and is associated with Hemoglobin H on electrophoresis.

Choice D [Alpha thalassemia trait (minor)] presents similar to Beta thalassemia but is associated with normal Hb ratios on electrophoresis.

Choice E [Beta thalassemia major] is a transfusion-dependent thalassemia. By adulthood, he would have a history of multiple transfusion and may have the stigmata of a major thalassemia (frontal bossing, chipmunk facies, splenomegaly, etc.).

7. MUSCULOSKELETAL – DISSEMINATED GONOCOCCAL INFECTION [HISTORY AND PHYSICAL EXAMINATION]

Unprotected sexual activity [choice E] can result in Disseminated gonococcal infection, (DGI), which may present with either [A] purulent arthritis or [B] Arthritis-dermatitis syndrome, which is characterized by the triad of:

- [1] <u>migratory polyarthralgia</u> involving the small or large joints
- [2] <u>tenosynovitis</u>: involving multiple tendons simultaneously (eg, toes, ankles, wrists, and fingers); may be worse with passive extension
- [3] <u>dermatitis</u>: painless pustular or vesiculopustular lesions, most common on the distal extremities; usually does not involve the face.

Fever, chills, and generalized malaise are also common.

Choice A [Being outdoors in the woods without the use insect repellant] increases the risk for Lyme disease or Rocky mountain spotted fever. Although both are associated with a rash, the vesiculopustular or pustular lesions distinguish DGI from these tick-borne diseases.

Choice B [Personal and family history of autoimmunity] can increase the risk of autoimmune-related arthritis.

Choice C [Injection drug use] can increase the risk for Septic arthritis, which is usually monoarticular or oligoarticular and not associated with vesiculopustular lesions.

Choice D [Recent sore throat not treated with antibiotics] can increase the risk of Acute rheumatic fever, which is not classically associated with pustular or vesiculopustular lesions.

8. MUSCULOSKELETAL – PAGET DISEASE OF THE BONE [LABS AND DIAGNOSTIC STUDIES]

In Paget disease of the bone (PDB), markers of increased bone turnover include serum alkaline phosphatase (sAP) [choice B] and bone-specific alkaline phosphatase (bAP).

Because most patients are asymptomatic, the diagnosis is often made as incidental finding in a patient with elevated isolated serum alkaline phosphatase.

Isolated PDB is usually associated with normal serum phosphate, calcium, parathyroid hormone, and vitamin D levels in most patients.

Although most patients are asymptomatic, symptoms include bone and/or joint pain or bony deformity (eg, bowing of the legs).

Skull involvement can cause hearing loss due to narrowing of the auditory foramen where cranial nerve 8 traverses.

The classic skull radiograph findings of PDB is mixed sclerotic and lucent areas, often described as the "cotton wool" appearance (as seen in the photo).

9. NEUROLOGY – BELL PALSY [CLINICAL INTERVENTION]

Short-term oral glucocorticoid [choice E] is the mainstay of pharmacologic therapy for Bell's palsy, along with supportive management.

Eye care is also important for individuals who have incomplete eye closure.

In severe acute cases, antiviral therapy [choice D] may be given with glucocorticoids to reduce complications.

Choice A [Emergent CT scan and stat neurology consult] is not necessary in Bell's palsy unless there are neurological deficits that warrant neuroimaging.

Choice B [Administer Sumatriptan, Prochlorperazine, and Diphenhydramine] can be used in the management of Migraine headache.

Choice C [Obtain a blood glucose level, basic laboratory work, and CT scan of the head] is used in the management of suspected Transient ischemic attack or Stroke.

10. NEUROLOGY – BACTERIAL MENINGITIS/MENINGOCOCCAL MENINGITIS [APPLYING FOUNDATIONAL CONCEPTS]

A rapidly spreading petechial rash (purpura fulminans) is characteristic of Meningococcal infection [choice C].

Neisseria menigitidis is the most common in older children (10 years–19 years of age) and is the second most common bacterial cause in adults.

Choice A [*Streptococcus pneumoniae*] is the most common cause bacterial in adults of all ages & children ages >3 months–10 years. It is not classically associated with a petechial rash.

Choice B [*Listeria monocytogenes*] is seen with increased incidence in neonates, >50 years, & immunocompromised states (eg, history of glucocorticoid use, alcoholism, pregnant, AIDS or HIV, chemotherapy).

Choice D [*Haemophilus influenzae*] is associated with reduced incidence since widespread *H. influenzae* vaccination.

Choice E [Group B streptococcus] is the most common bacterial cause in neonates <1 month (part of the vaginal flora) & infants <3 months.

11. GASTROINTESTINAL/NUTRITION – PANCREATIC CANCER [LABS AND DIAGNOSTICS]

Although not specific, cancer-associated antigen 19-9 (CA 19-9) [choice B] is the most useful serum marker for Pancreatic cancer.

CA 19-9 is also helpful to monitor disease activity if elevated at initial diagnosis.

The patient has a history of alcohol use and presents with the classic symptoms and findings of Pancreatic cancer: abdominal pain, jaundice, weight loss, and Courvoisier's sign (a palpable nontender gallbladder).

Choice A [Alpha-fetoprotein (AFP)] is a tumor marker for Hepatocellular carcinoma and Nonseminomatous germ cell testicular cancer.

Choice C [Carcinoembryonic antigen (CEA) is a tumor marker most useful for Colorectal cancer.

Choice D [Amylase and lipase] are useful for Acute pancreatitis.

Choice E [Cancer antigen 125 (CA 125)] is most useful for Ovarian cancer.

12. INFECTIOUS DISEASE – SCARLET FEVER [PHARMACOLOGY]

In patients with Streptococcal infections with mild, non-IgE-mediated reactions to Penicillin (eg, maculopapular rash beginning days into therapy), narrow-spectrum 1st-generation Cephalosporin (eg, Cephalexin) [choice D].

If mild, possibly IgE-mediated reactions (eg, urticaria or angioedema but NOT anaphylaxis), 2nd or 3rd generation Cephalosporin with a side chain dissimilar to PCN (Cefdinir, Cefpodoxime, Cefuroxime) can be used.

In cases of severe angioedema and/or anaphylaxis or with serious delayed reactions or for patients who cannot take cephalosporins, Macrolides [choice B] can be used. Clindamycin is an alternative.

Choice A {Penicillin V potassium] is not recommended in a patient with a Penicillin allergy as in this patient. Otherwise, Penicillin or Amoxicillin is the first line treatment for Scarlet fever.
Choice C [Trimethoprim-sulfamethoxazole] is inappropriate because TMP-SMX does not have adequate Streptococcal coverage.
Choice E [Amoxicillin-clavulanate] is broad spectrum and Scarlet fever is caused by one organism. The patient has a Penicillin allergy.

13. CARDIOLOGY – MITRAL REGURGITATION/MITRAL VALVE PROLAPSE [HISTORY AND PHYSICAL]

When the cause of Mitral regurgitation (MR) is Mitral valve prolapse (MVP), a Midsystolic click [choice B] (correlating with the maximal prolapse and tension on the chordae) may be auscultated and the murmur may start in mid to late systole.
Degenerative mitral valve disease (including Mitral valve prolapse) is the most common cause of primary MR in resource-rich countries.

The hallmark features of MR include
  • holosystolic apical murmur best heard at the apex and radiates to axilla
  • systolic thrill; S3 heart sound may be heard
  • S1 is diminished.

Choice A [Prominent first heart sound (S1)] is hallmark of Mitral stenosis. In Mitral regurgitation, S1 is diminished, due to insufficient apposition of the mitral leaflets as LV pressure becomes greater than left atrial pressure.
Choice C [Hoarseness] is associated with Mitral stenosis, known as Ortner syndrome.
Choice D [Weak delayed carotid pulse] is hallmark of Aortic stenosis.
Choice E [Increased murmur intensity with inspiration] is hallmark of right-sided murmurs (eg, Tricuspid and Pulmonic murmurs), known as Carvallo's sign.

14. CARDIOLOGY – KAWASAKI DISEASE [CLINICAL INTERVENTION]

The first line management of Kawasaki disease in children include Intravenous immune globulin (IVIG) [choice A] and Aspirin during the acute phase of illness.
IVIG is most effective when started within 10 days of fever onset to reduce the risk of coronary artery aneurysm from ~25% to <5%.

Clinical manifestations of Kawasaki disease include the mnemonic "warm cream":
- **Warm** – fever ≥5 days, plus 4 of the following 5:
- **C**onjunctivitis – bilateral, nonpurulent, perilimbic sparing
- **R**ash – generalized nonvesicular (commonly maculopapular, morbilliform)
- **E**xtremity changes – erythema and edema of hands and feet, followed by desquamation
- **A**denopathy – anterior cervical with at least one palpable node ≥1.5 cm
- **M**ucous membrane changes – cracked red lips, "strawberry" tongue.

Although not part of the criteria up to 1/4 of patients with KD also experience arthritis.

Choice B [Penicillin V potassium] is used in the management of Scarlet fever. Scarlet fever can present with fever and a strawberry tongue similar to KD, however the rash is usually papular with a "sandpaper" texture and Scarlet fever lacks the ocular and articular symptoms seen with KD.
Choice C [Prednisone] can be used in the management of some patients with KD at high risk for IVIG resistance.
Choice D [Doxycycline] is used in the management of Rocky mountain spotted fever.
Choice E [Ibuprofen] can be used in the management of Juvenile idiopathic arthritis, which does not usually present with the conjunctival and oral findings seen with KD. JIA is more commonly associated with Anterior uveitis.

15. CARDIOLOGY – THIRD-DEGREE (COMPLETE) AV BLOCK [CLINICAL INTERVENTION]

Transcutaneous pacing [choice D] is the treatment of choice for any symptomatic patient with Third-Degree Atrioventricular Block (Complete Heart Block) to increase heart rate and cardiac output (or if immediately available, transvenous pacing).

All patients who have third-degree atrioventricular (AV) block (complete heart block) associated with repeated pauses, an inadequate escape rhythm, or a block below the AV node (AVN) should be stabilized with temporary pacing.

Asymptomatic patients should be continuously monitored with transcutaneous pacing pads in place in the event of clinical deterioration.

Treatment with Atropine should not delay intervention with temporary pacing transcutaneous or transvenous) for stabilization &/or a chronotropic medication [eg, Dopamine (if hypotensive) or Epinephrine].
Permanent pacemaker is indicated for most when there is no reversible etiology present.
The ECG shows a third-degree (complete) AV block (see photo).

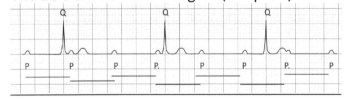

Choice A [Synchronized cardioversion] is used in the management of Unstable tachyarrhythmias and as definitive management for Atrial flutter and Atrial fibrillation.
Choice B [Medical cardioversion with Ibutilide] is an alternative to electrical cardioversion as definitive management of Atrial fibrillation.
Choice C [Metoprolol] is contraindicated in patients with Third-degree (complete) AV block as Metoprolol is an AV node blocker.
Choice E [Implantable cardioverter defibrillator] is used as definitive management of Tachyarrhythmias.

16. RENAL – HYPERNATREMIA [CLINICAL INTERVENTION]

Hypotonic fluids, such as free water or 5% Dextrose in water [choice A] is the first line management of Hyponatremia in most patients.

Hypernatremia results from decreased total body free water so in patients who can tolerate oral intake, ingestion of free water can be used instead of D5W.

In patients with significant hypovolemia (tachycardia, increased BUN/Cr >20:1, hypovolemia), Isotonic fluids [choice B] can be given to expand extracellular volume. The patient should be switched to a hypotonic solution once volume is repleted. This patient has a normal blood pressure and creatinine making hypovolemia less likely.

Choice C [0.45% sodium chloride solution] is another type of Hypotonic solution but free water or D5W is preferred initial management.

Choice D [3% sodium chloride solution] would worsen Hypernatremia. 3% sodium chloride is used in the management of severe Hyponatremia.

Choice E [Fluid restriction] would further increase his serum osmolality and sodium levels as this patient is already at a total free water deficit. Water restriction is used in the management of Isovolemic hypotonic Hyponatremia.

17. ENDOCRINE – PRIMARY HYPERALDOSTERONISM [APPLYING FUNDAMENTAL CONCEPTS]

Idiopathic bilateral adrenal hyperplasia [choice A] or idiopathic hyperplasia are the most common causes of Primary Hyperaldosteronism (PA), accounting for 60-70% of cases.

Unilateral Aldosterone-producing adenomas [choice B] account for 30-40% of cases.

Primary hyperaldosteronism is characterized by the triad of [1] hypertension, [2] hypokalemia, and [3] metabolic alkalosis.

It is also associated with a high plasma aldosterone to renin ratio >20:1.

Less common causes include:
- unilateral hyperplasia or primary adrenal hyperplasia (2%)
- aldosterone-producing adrenal carcinoma (<1%) [choice C]
- ectopic aldosterone secretion from the kidneys or ovaries [choice D], and
- bilateral zona glomerulosa hyperplasia.

Choice E (Benign tumor in the adrenal medulla) characterizes Pheochromocytoma, which is associated with increased plasma metanephrines and Vanillylmandelic acid.

18. CARDIOLOGY – ABDOMINAL AORTIC ANEURYSM [HISTORY AND PHYSICAL]

Cigarette smoking [choice A] is the greatest risk factor for the development of Abdominal aortic aneurysm (AAA).

Smoking cessation is the most effective means of decreasing the rate of Abdominal aortic aneurysm expansion.

Other risk factors include age >50 years, male gender, atherosclerosis (most common risk factor), family history, and Caucasian race.

Non-Caucasian individuals [choice C] and Diabetes mellitus [choice B] are associated with a decreased risk for AAA.

Female gender [choice D] is less commonly associated with AAA (females make up ~20% of all AAA cases). However, females present more commonly with rupture compared to males.

19. PULMONARY – TENSION PNEUMOTHORAX [CLINICAL INTERVENTION]

Patients with a Tension pneumothorax who are hemodynamically unstable should undergo needle decompression with a catheter thoracostomy [choice D], followed by chest tube thoracostomy.

Chest tube thoracostomy may be performed without needle decompression in some.

Choice A [Pericardiocentesis] is performed for a Cardiac tamponade, which would have normal lung sounds and symmetrical chest expansion.

Choice B [Endotracheal intubation] can be used if the airway needs to be maintained. The most important step in this patient is needle decompression.

Choice C [Surgical consult for emergent Thoracotomy] is a more invasive option in the management of a Tension pneumothorax.

Choice E [Video-assisted thoracoscopic surgery (VATS)] is not commonly employed in the management of Tension pneumothorax. VATS may be indicated if there is persistent leak after chest tube placement or no regression with chest tube, persistent or recurrent pneumothoracies.

20. UV KERATITIS – EENT [HISTORY AND PHYSICAL]

Welder's arc burns (welder's flash) [choice A] and snow blindness are the most common conditions associated with Photokeratitis (UV keratitis), but other exposures include tanning bed and industrial UV light.

Ultraviolet keratitis may occur if protective glasses are not applied tightly to the face, resulting in exposure to excess UV light.

Classic findings on slit lamp examination includes diffuse punctate corneal edema, and instillation of Fluorescein reveals diffuse punctate corneal abrasion-like lesions.

UK Keratitis often occurs within 6-12 hours after exposure and healing often occurs in 24 to 36 hours.

Choice B [Direct eye exposure to lye] is associated with liquefactive necrosis and chemical burn injuries.

Choice C [History of extended wear of daily contact lens] may result in Bacterial keratitis, which would reveal corneal ulcers on slit lamp examination. Bacterial keratitis is usually unilateral and usually results in a single large corneal ulcer.

Choice D [Allergies to grass and animal dander] can result in Allergic conjunctivitis. Ocular pruritis is the hallmark feature of Allergic conjunctivitis.

Choice E [History of being in a dark movie theater recently] is a predisposing factor for the development of Acute angle-closure glaucoma.

21. OPTIC NEURITIS – EENT [MOST LIKELY]

Key features of Optic neuritis [choice E] include:
- **Vision loss, especially central visual acuity (central scotoma)**
- **Periocular pain worse with ocular movements**
- **Color desaturation**

Physical examination often reveals:
- decreased visual acuity
- funduscopy: 2/3 normal; 1/3 papillitis (optic disc pallor and/or optic disc swelling)
- relative afferent pupillary defect (Marcus Gunn pupil): when performing the swinging light test in the affected eye, the pupil will appear to dilate or have a sluggish response.

Choice A [Retinal detachment] causes painless vision loss and is not associated with pain with ocular movement.

Choice B [Macular degeneration] causes Metamorphopsia, where straight lines appear bent in the central vision. Fundoscopic examination reveals drusen body in dry MD and new abnormal blood vessels in wet MD.

Choice C [Acute maculopathy] can also cause central blind spot (scotoma), blurred vision, and vision changes similar to Optic neuritis but is not associated with Marcus Gunn pupil or pain with eye movements.

Choice D [Central retinal vein occlusion] is associated with complete vision loss in the affected eye. Funduscopic examination reveals extensive hemorrhage and exudates with a "blood and thunder" appearance.

22. DERMATOLOGY – THERMAL BURNS [HISTORY AND PHYSICAL]

Deep partial thickness burns [choice C] the affected area is characterized by:
- **skin blistering**
- **pale white to yellow in color of the exposed dermis**
- **no blanching of the burned area**
- **absent capillary refill and absent pain sensation.**

A Deep partial thickness burn extends into the deep dermis (reticular layer).
Healing takes 3 weeks to 2 months; scarring is common.
Surgical debridement and skin grafting may be required to attain maximum function.

Choice A [Fourth degree burn] extend through the skin to the subcutaneous fat, muscle, and may extend to the bone.

Choice B [Superficial partial thickness burn] is associated with skin blistering but the exposed dermis is moist and erythematous. It is extremely painful to touch, and capillary refill is intact.

Choice D [Full thickness burn], formerly known as third degree burn, is characterized by the skin appearing charred, pale, painless, and leathery without blistering.

Choice E [Superficial burn] is characterized by skin erythema, similar to sunburn, without blistering.

23. ENDOCRINE – SUBACUTE (DEQUERVAIN) THYROIDITIS [MOST LIKELY]

Subacute thyroiditis (subacute [DeQuervain] granulomatous thyroiditis) [choice B] is characterized by:
- **neck pain and a markedly tender diffuse goiter most commonly caused by a viral infection or a postviral inflammatory process** (the patient recently had Coronavirus)
- **Hyperthyroidism is most common at presentation (decreased TSH and increased free T4 &/or T3),** followed by euthyroidism, hypothyroidism, and return to normal thyroid function after weeks to months.

Causes of thyroid pain and tenderness include infection (eg, Subacute thyroiditis after viral infection; Suppurative thyroiditis after a bacterial infection), radiation, or trauma.

Autoimmune conditions [choice A], medications, and idiopathic fibrotic conditions [choice D] are usually painless.
Choice C [Suppurative thyroiditis] is also associated with thyroid pain and tenderness but is usually associated with localized tenderness and leukocytosis.
Choice E [Euthyroid sick syndrome] is not associated with a painful thyroid. Euthyroid sick syndrome denotes abnormal thyroid lab studies in a patient with normal thyroid gland function during an acute systemic illness.

24. REPRODUCTIVE SYSTEM – OVARIAN CANCER [HISTORY AND PHYSICAL]

Because combined oral contraceptives [choice C] reduce the number of menstrual cycles, they are protective against both Ovarian and Endometrial cancers.
Factors associated with a decreased risk of Ovarian cancer include combined OCPs, previous pregnancy, history of breastfeeding, use of an intrauterine device, tubal ligation, and hysterectomy.

Factors associated with increased risk of Ovarian cancer include:
- Increased number of ovulatory cycles: eg, early menarche [choice E], late menopause, nulliparity [choice A]
- Increasing age [choice D]
- Infertility [choice B]
- Endometriosis, Polycystic ovary syndrome
- cigarette smoking (for mucinous carcinomas.

25. RENAL – HYPOMAGNESEMIA/TORSADES DE POINTES [PHARMACOLOGY]

IV Magnesium sulfate [choice C] is the first-line management of severe Hypomagnesemia, including the development of Torsades de pointes.
Hypomagnesemia is a serious and potentially life-threatening adverse effect of Long-term Proton pump inhibitor use as PPIs may decrease intestinal magnesium absorption.
Symptoms of Hypomagnesemia include:
- **Neuromuscular manifestations similar to Hypocalcemia**, including neuromuscular hyperexcitability (eg, tremor, tetany, convulsions, Chvostek sign, and Trousseau sign), weakness, delirium, and coma.
- **Cardiovascular manifestations** include widening of the QRS and peaking of T waves, and widening of the PR interval, diminution of T waves, and atrial and ventricular arrhythmias with severe depletion, such as Torsades de pointes.

Choice A [IV Calcium gluconate] is used in the management of severe Hypocalcemia. Calcium gluconate is also used to stabilize the cardiac membrane in severe Hypermagnesemia, and Hyperkalemia.

Choice B [IV Potassium chloride] is used in the management of severe Hypokalemia.

Choice D [Oral Potassium chloride] is used in the management of mild to moderate Hypokalemia.

Choice E [IV Sodium bicarbonate] is used in the management of Wide complex tachycardia associated with Tricyclic antidepressant (TCA) toxicity.

26. ENDOCRINE – DIABETES MELLITUS [PHARMACOLOGY]

Sulfonylureas, such as Glyburide [choice C] and Meglitinides are the medications most commonly associated with hypoglycemia.

Sulfonylureas and Meglitinides are insulin secretagogues which increase insulin release from the pancreas, which can result in hypoglycemia and weight gain.

Choice A [Metformin] and Biguanides have a primary mechanism of action of reduction of hepatic production of glucose, so they are not classically associated with causing Hypoglycemia.

Choice B [Pioglitazone] and other Thiazolidinediones reduce insulin resistance, increasing insulin sensitivity at muscle, hepatic, and adipose tissues.

Choice D [Semaglutide] and other GLP-1 agonists have a small risk of Hypoglycemia. When Hypoglycemia occurs, it is usually in the setting of concomitant use of other hypoglycemic agents.

Choice E [Acarbose] and other alpha glucosidase inhibitors do not have any significant effect on insulin secretion, so they are unlikely to cause Hypoglycemia.

27. ENDOCRINE – PITUITARY ADENOMA/LACTOTROPH ADENOMA (PROLACTINOMA) [MOST LIKELY]

Pituitary lactotroph adenoma (Prolactinoma) [choice D] is the most common type of Pituitary tumor, accounting for 40-50% of all clinically diagnosed pituitary adenomas.

Hyperprolactinemia in males usually present with hypogonadotropic hypogonadism (eg, decreased libido, infertility, gynecomastia).

Headache and bitemporal hemianopsia can be seen with any pituitary tumor.

Galactorrhea is a rare presentation in males.

28. REPRODUCTIVE SYSTEM – FRAGILE X SYNDROME [HISTORY AND PHYSICAL]

Fragile X syndrome, the most common genetic cause of inherited intellectual disability is classically associated with characteristic physical features:
- **Macroorchidism [Testicular enlargement (volume >25 mL after puberty)] [choice E] with normal testicular function**
- **Hyperextensible finger joints and thumbs**
- Long and narrow face with prominent forehead and chin (prognathism)
- Large ears

Fragile X syndrome is an X-linked disorder caused by a loss-of-function variant in the fragile X messenger ribonucleoprotein 1 (*FMR1*) gene located at Xq27.3.

This results in decreased or absent levels of fragile X messenger ribonucleoprotein (FMRP).

Choice A [Gynecomastia, centripetal obesity, and hyperphagia] are associated with Prader-Willi syndrome.

Choice B [Smooth indistinct philtrum, thin vermillion border, and small palpebral fissures] are associated with Fetal alcohol syndrome.

Choice C [Pale retina with a cherry red macula] are associated with Tay-Sachs disease.

Choice D [Dislocation of the lens and tall stature with arachnodactyly] are associated with Marfan syndrome.

29. ENDOCRINE – HYPOPARATHYROIDISM [HISTORY AND PHYSICAL EXAMINATION]

The classic physical findings of acute Hypocalcemia is hyperexcitability of the peripheral neurons and tetany, which can manifest as:
- **Chvostek's sign: facial spasm with tapping of the facial nerve near the ear [choice A]**
- Trousseau's sign: induction of carpal spasm with inflation of a blood pressure cuff.

Primary hypoparathyroidism is the most common cause of Hypocalcemia.

Postsurgical hypoparathyroidism can occur after thyroid, parathyroid, or radical neck surgery for head and neck cancer, and it may be transient, prolonged, or permanent.

Choice B [Decreased or absent deep tendon reflexes] can occur with Hypercalcemia or Hypermagnesemia. Hypocalcemia is associated with Hyperreflexia.

Choice C [Elevated blood pressure >140/90 mmHg] is hallmark of Hypercalcemia. Hypotension may complicate acute Hypocalcemia.

Choice D [Absent bowel sounds] is associated with Hypercalcemia. Hypocalcemia may cause increased bowel sounds due to increased muscle contraction in the bowels.

Choice E [Decreased vibratory and position sense of the lower extremities] can be seen with Cobalamin (Vitamin B12 deficiency].

30. CARDIOLOGY – CARDIAC TAMPONADE [CLINICAL INTERVENTION]

Emergent pericardiocentesis [choice C] is the most appropriate management of Cardiac tamponade in patients who are hemodynamically unstable (eg, systolic blood pressure in the double digits), which can be performed at the bedside, often with visualization by bedside echocardiography (FAST exam).

Emergent pericardial fluid drainage prevents hemodynamic collapse and causes a significant improvement of acute symptoms and hemodynamics.

When present, Electrical alternans with sinus tachycardia is a highly specific sign of Pericardial effusion, often with cardiac tamponade (see photo).

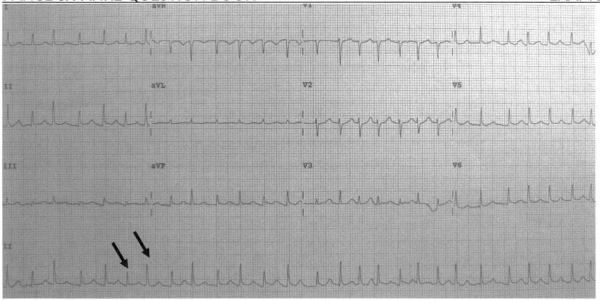

Electrical alternans is characterized by beat-to-beat alternations in the QRS complex amplitude.

Choice A [Emergent thoracotomy] is surgical management of certain conditions in which other approaches are contraindicated or are not feasible.

Choice B [Needle decompression of the lung] can be used in the management of Tension pneumothorax, which would present with absent breath sounds on the affected side. This patient had a clear lung examination, making Tension pneumothorax less likely.

Choice D [High-dose Aspirin and Atenolol] is not indicated in this patient as Beta blockers are contraindicated in patients with hypotension.

Choice E [Synchronized cardioversion] is used in the management of Unstable tachycardia. However, the treatment of stable or unstable sinus tachycardia is to treat the underlying cause.

31. INFECTIOUS DISEASE – TETANUS [HEALTH MAINTENANCE]

In adults with wounds that are not clean or minor, administer Tdap vaccine (with the intent on completing the 3 series for vaccinations in adults) and Tetanus immune globulin [choice D] to protect them until the vaccination series is complete if:
- **(1) <3 prior doses of tetanus toxoid-containing vaccine (as in this patient)**
- **(2) unknown vaccination history, or**
- **(3) the individual has never been vaccinated**

Choice A [Administer Tetanus immunoglobulin only] is incorrect because tetanus immune globulin should be given with a Tetanus toxoid vaccine.

Choice B [No further management is needed regarding tetanus immunization/vaccination] is incorrect because the patient is not fully vaccinated. In adults, full vaccination requires 3 doses of a tetanus toxoid vaccine.

Choice C [Administer Tdap vaccine] is used in someone who is fully vaccinated with a deep wound that is ≥5 years since the last booster.

Choice E [Administer DTaP vaccine and tetanus immune globulin] is used in children <7 years of age who are not fully vaccinated with the 5 doses with a wound that is not clean or minor.

32. CARDIOLOGY – PERIPHERAL ARTERIAL DISEASE [LABS AND DIAGNOSTIC STUDIES]

Ankle-brachial index (with or without exercise) [choice E] is the diagnostic test of choice to confirm the diagnosis of Peripheral arterial disease (PAD) in patients with risk factors, symptoms, &/or signs of PAD.
 An ABI of ≤0.9 establishes the diagnosis of PAD.

Choice A [Exercise treadmill testing] may be used in some patients with suspected PAD with a normal resting ABI (0.91 to 1.30). Abnormal exercise ABIs support a diagnosis of PAD in these patients.

Choice B [Duplex Ultrasound of the lower extremities] is used to establish the diagnosis of Peripheral venous disease, which is associated with leg edema and normal pulses.

Choice C [Venous plethysmography] can be used in the workup of Varicose veins.

Choice D [Contrast arteriography of the lower extremities] can be used as definitive diagnosis of PAD but is rarely indicated in most patients with PAD, unless intervention is planned.

33. RENAL – HEMOLYTIC UREMIC SYNDROME [APPLYING FUNDAMENTAL CONCEPTS]

Shiga toxin-producing E. coli (STEC) [choice B] Hemolytic uremic syndrome (HUS) causes >90% of cases of HUS in children.
HUS presents with the classic triad of
- [1] microangiopathic hemolytic anemia,
- [2] thrombocytopenia, and
- [3] acute kidney injury.
HUS is often preceded by a prodromal illness with abdominal pain and diarrhea by 5-13 days.

Choice A [Decreased ADAMTS13 production] is associated with Thrombotic thrombocytopenic purpura (TTP). TTP is associated with the pentad of [1] microangiopathic hemolytic anemia, [2] thrombocytopenia, [3] acute kidney injury, [4] fever, and [5] neurological symptoms.

Choice C [Autoantibody to platelets] is hallmark of Immune thrombocytopenic purpura (ITP), which is associated with an isolated thrombocytopenia.

Choice D [IgA deposition into the tissues] is hallmark of Henoch Schoenlein purpura (HSP), which is associated with hematuria, joint pain, palpable purpura, and abdominal pain. Coagulation and CBC are within normal limits as the purpura is due to vasculitis and not due to coagulopathy nor thrombocytopenia.

Choice E [Pathological activation of the clotting cascade] is the hallmark of Dissemination intravascular coagulation.

34. HEMATOLOGY – CHRONIC MYELOGENOUS LEUKEMIA [PHARMACOLOGY]

Tyrosine kinase inhibitors (TKIs), such as Imatinib [choice E] are the first-line therapy for most newly diagnosed Chronic myelogenous leukemia (CML).
TKIs inhibit Philadelphia chromosome tyrosine kinase activity & myeloid leukemic cell proliferation implicated in the pathogenesis of CML.
In CML, fusion of 2 genes: BCR (on chromosome 22) & ABL1 (on chromosome 9), result in BCR-ABL1 fusion gene. Translocation between chromosomes 9 & 22 [t(9;22)] = Philadelphia chromosome, which causes hyperactive tyrosine kinase activity.

This causes excessive accumulation of maturing granulocytic cells in blood, marrow, liver, & spleen.

- <u>First generation TKIs:</u> Imatinib
- <u>Second-generation TKI:</u> Dasatinib, Nilotinib, Bosutinib
- <u>Third generation TKI:</u> Ponatinib is used if there is resistance to second line TKIs.

Choice A [All-trans retinoic acid] is used in the management of Acute promyelocytic leukemia.

Choice B [Dexamethasone, Vincristine, and pegylated Asparaginase] are used in the management of Acute lymphoblastic leukemia.

Choice C [Watchful waiting] may be used in the management of Chronic lymphocytic leukemia/Small lymphocytic lymphoma.

Choice D [Cytarabine plus Daunorubicin] is used as induction therapy for Acute myelogenous leukemia.

35. RENAL – CHRONIC KIDNEY DISEASE [HEALTH MAINTENANCE]

Prevention and/or treatment of Osteitis fibrosis cystica & Renal osteodystrophy with predialysis CKD are primarily based on directly suppressing the secretion of PTH (Secondary hyperparathyroidism) via

- **[1] dietary phosphate restriction (800–1,000 mg/day) [choice D],** followed by
- **[2] oral phosphate binders for persistent Hyperphosphatemia** (>5.5 mg/dL) **despite dietary restriction,** &
- **[3]** administration of Calcitriol (or vitamin D analogs) to suppress PTH secretion.

Phosphate retention initially promotes PTH release, which can result in pulling calcium out of the bone, promoting bone disease.

In Chronic kidney disease, secondary hyperparathyroidism from decreased vitamin D production can result in the classic triad:

- [1] Hypocalcemia +
- [2] increased serum phosphate +
- [3] increased serum intact PTH. Calcium levels may be normal early on.

<u>Radiograph:</u> Osteitis Fibrosa Cystica: subperiosteal erosions, bony cysts with thin trabeculum & cortex, "salt & pepper" appearance of the skull (punctate trabecular bone resorption in the skull).

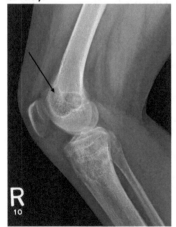

36. REPRODUCTIVE SYSTEM – ENDOMETRIAL POLYP [CLINICAL INTERVENTION]

Surgical removal (eg, transcervical Polypectomy) [choice C] is the recommended management for pre- and postmenopausal patients with an endometrial polyp with bleeding &/or complications (eg, abnormal uterine bleeding, postmenopausal bleeding, infertility).

Because symptomatic polyps have a higher risk for malignancy compared asymptomatic polyps, Polypectomy is often performed to [1] detect potential malignancy & [2] relieve symptoms.

Medical treatment has not been shown to be effective for management of Endometrial polyps.

Choice A [expectant management] is a possible option for pre- and postmenopausal patients with an endometrial polyp but without bleeding, spotting, or other indications for removal.

Choice E [Uterine artery embolization] is an option for the management of Uterine fibroids.

37. CARDIOLOGY – PREMATURE ATRIAL COMPLEX (PAC) [MOST LIKELY DIAGNOSIS]

Premature atrial complexes [choice C] are seen on ECG as a P wave that occurs earlier than expected in the cardiac cycle before the next sinus P wave should occur, often with a different morphology from the sinus P wave (see photo).

Sometimes the abnormal P wave may occur within the T wave, resulting in a "camel hump" or higher T wave than normal.

Premature Atrial Contractions (PACs)

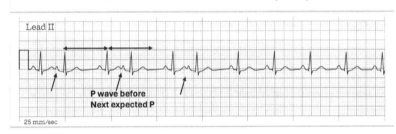

Choice A [Sinus arrhythmia] is associated with a regularly irregular rhythm, in which the rate increases with inspiration and decreases with expiration.

Choice B [Wolff-Parkinson white] is associated with a short PR interval, a delta wave, and often, a wide WRS complex.

Choice D [First-degree atrioventricular block] is associated with a prolonged PR interval ≥5 small boxes (≥0.2 seconds).

Choice E (Mobitz-1 second degree atrioventricular block) is associated with progressive lengthening of the PR interval with occasional nonconducted beats.

38. RENAL – NEPHROTIC SYNDROME/MINIMAL CHANGE DISEASE [MOST LIKELY]

Minimal change disease (MCD) [choice E] is the most common cause of Nephrotic syndrome in individuals with Lymphoma (Hodgkin and NonHodgkin lymphoma).

MCD is also the most common cause of Nephrotic syndrome in children.

Nephrotic syndrome is characterized by high-level proteinuria (>3-3.5 g/day), hypoalbuminemia, edema, hyperlipidemia, and thrombosis.

Choice A [Membranous nephropathy (MN)] is cause of Nephrotic syndrome most commonly seen in middle-age White nondiabetics, viral hepatitis (HBV, HCV), and Systemic lupus erythematosus. MN is more commonly associated with solid tumors than lymphoproliferative malignancies.

Choice B (IgA Nephropathy) is the most common cause of Acute glomerulonephritis, which classically presents with hematuria, dysmorphic red cells, and red cell casts on UA.

Choice C [Focal segmental glomerulosclerosis] is a cause of Nephrotic syndrome most commonly seen in Black nondiabetics, IV heroin use, Hypertension, and HIV infection. It is less commonly associated with HL.

Choice D [Amyloidosis] is an uncommon cause of Nephrotic syndrome most commonly associated with Multiple myeloma.

39. GENITOURINARY – ACUTE PROSTATITIS [APPLYING FOUNDATIONAL CONCEPTS]
Gram-negative coliform bacteria, with *Escherichia coli* being the most common [choice B], followed by *Proteus* species, are the most common causes of Acute prostatitis in men >35 years of age.

The microbiology of Acute prostatitis in men >35 years of age include:
- *E. coli*: 55-88%
- *Proteus* species [choice C]: 3-7%
- *Klebsiella*, *Enterobacter* [choice D], and *Serratia* species: 3-10%
- *Pseudomonas aeruginosa* [choice E]: 3-8%.

In men <35 years of age, *Chlamydia trachomatis* [choice A] & *Neisseria gonorrhoeae* are the most common pathogens. Sexually transmitted urogenital infections (eg, Epididymitis, Urethritis) may extend to involve the prostate.

40. ENDOCRINE – HYPOPITUITARISM, HYPOTHYROIDISM [MOST LIKELY]
Hypopituitarism [choice C] should be suspected in patients with labs that reveal deficient secretion of pituitary hormone (eg, decreased ACTH, TSH, FSH, LH), resulting in decreased secretion of their corresponding target organ hormone levels as well (eg, decreased cortisol, free T4, estrogen, & testosterone).

Each pituitary hormone must be tested separately since there is a variable pattern of hormone deficiency in individuals with hypopituitarism.

This patient has symptoms of Hypothyroidism and hypogonadotropic hypogonadism (decreased libido).

Choice A [Hashimoto thyroiditis] is a primary (target organ) cause of Hypothyroidism, which would result in a low free T4 and/or T3, with a resultant high serum TSH in response.

Choice B [Hyperprolactinemia] can cause decreased libido but would not explain the other findings as well.

Choice D [Follicular thyroid cancer] and other thyroid malignancies are classically associated with a euthyroid profile.

Choice E [Medication induced hypothyroidism] is a primary (target organ) cause of Hypothyroidism, which would result in a low free T4 and/or T3, with a resultant high serum TSH in response.

41. NEUROLOGY – HUNTINGTON DISEASE [APPLYING FOUNDATIONAL CONCEPTS]

Molecular genetic testing for number of CAG repeats [choice E] in each of the HD alleles is diagnostic of Huntington disease (HD).

The increased number of CAG repeats also has prognostic significance as more CAG repeats are associated with earlier onset and more aggressive disease.

HD is an autosomal dominant genetic disease caused by a cytosine-adenine-guanine (CAG) trinucleotide repeat expansion in the huntingtin gene on chromosome 4p.

Huntington disease is a progressive neurodegenerative disorder characterized by "mood, movement, and memory" abnormalities: psychiatric problems, choreiform movements, psychiatric problems, and dementia.

MRI shows atrophy of caudate and putamen, as well as general cerebral atrophy.

In the era of molecular testing, neuroimaging [choice A] is no longer used in confirming the diagnosis of HD. However, neuroimaging studies are generally used to rule out other structural disorders.

42. NEUROLOGY – ULNAR NEUROPATHY/ELBOW DISLOCATION [HISTORY AND PHYSICAL]

Ulnar neuropathy [choice B] occurs in 10% of all posterior elbow dislocations and may be associated with medial epicondyle entrapment.

Ulnar neuropathy may result in:

- Sensory deficits: cutaneous innervation to the medial forearm, medial wrist, the fifth finger, and the medial side of the fourth finger.
- Motor deficits: adductor pollicis of the thumb is innervated by the ulnar nerve (may have thumb adduction deficits if damaged): Froment's sign (when pinching a piece of paper between the thumb & index finger against resistance, the thumb IP joint will flex if the adductor pollicis is weak), Jeanne's sign, problem with index finger abduction (scissors motion). Weakness in the wrist and finger flexion.
- Claw hand if severe: atrophy of the hand intrinsic muscles and clawing of the fourth and the fifth digits.

In addition to ulnar nerve injury, one must rule out brachial artery; median, or radial nerve injuries with Posterior elbow dislocations.

Choice A [Median] neuropathy presents with decreased thumb abduction and decreased sensation to the first 3 and the radial side of the fourth finger.

Choice C [Radial] neuropathy presents with wrist drop and decreased sensation to the first webspace of the dorsum of the hand.

Choice D [Axillary] neuropathy presents with decreased deltoid pinprick sensation and decreased shoulder abduction.

Choice E [Anterior interosseus] neuropathy, as a branch of the median nerve, presents with weakness of the flexor digitorum profundus muscle to the index (and sometimes the middle) finger, the flexor pollicis longus muscle to the thumb and the pronator quadratus of the distal forearm. AIN also has large sensory nerve to the volar wrist bones and compression of the AIN branch of the median nerve at the elbow can cause referred pain in the volar wrist/distal volar forearm.

43. INFECTIOUS DISEASE – SYPHILIS [CLINICAL INTERVENTION]

In pregnant patients with Syphilis who are allergic to Penicillin, they should be managed with an allergist consultation so they can be desensitized or rechallenged and managed with Penicillin [choice D].

This is because Penicillin G benzathine is the only effective therapy for managing Syphilis during pregnancy and reducing transmission to the fetus.

Choice A [Delay treatment until delivery of the fetus] can result in fetal development of Congenital Syphilis.

Choice B [Doxycycline] is an alternative first line treatment for early Syphilis in nonpregnant patients with Penicillin allergy.

Choice C [Azithromycin] and Cefixime have some activity against *T. pallidum* but are not usually used in the management of early Syphilis, and not used in pregnancy for this purpose.

Choice E [Probenecid] is not used in the management of Syphilis during pregnancy.

44. INFECTIOUS DISEASE – TRANSFUSION-ASSOCIATED SEPSIS/SEPTIC SHOCK [CLINICAL INTERVENTION]

The management of Transfusion-associated sepsis includes broad-spectrum antibiotics and hemodynamic support [choice B].

Broad-spectrum antibiotics should cover gram-positive and gram-negative organisms.

Although rare, Transfusion-transmitted bacterial infection (TTBI) is greatest with platelet transfusion.

TTBI occurs when a bacterial pathogen from a transfused blood component causes symptomatic disease in the recipient of the transfusion and may include endotoxin transfer from the blood product.

Initial presentation of TTBI may include fever, chills, rigors, and hypotension.

Choice A [IM Epinephrine] can be used in Transfusion-associated anaphylaxis, which can also present with a significant drop in blood pressure (>30 mmHg) but is also associated with respiratory symptoms (eg, respiratory difficulty, wheezing, stridor, angioedema, and pruritus), all of which are absent in this patient.

Choice C [Mechanical ventilation] can be used in the management of Transfusion-associated lung injury [TRALI]. Like TTBI, TRALI can be associated with fever, chills, and a significant drop in blood pressure, but TRALI is associated with respiratory difficulty (dyspnea, tachypnea, and hypoxia) and abnormal lung findings on auscultation.

Choice D [Furosemide plus supplemental oxygen] is used in the management of Transfusion-associated circulatory overload (TACO). TACO is associated with respiratory difficulty, crackles on lung examination, and Hypertension (not Hypotension as seen in this patient).

Choice E [Acetaminophen] can be used in the management of Febrile nonhemolytic transfusion reaction, which is characterized by fever, chills, headache, & flushing in the absence of other systemic symptoms 1-6 hours after transfusion initiation.

45. GASTROINTESTINAL/NUTRITION – NEONATAL JAUNDICE/PHYSIOLOGIC JAUNDICE [HEALTH MAINTENANCE]

Observation [choice C] is the management of choice for physiologic jaundice of the newborn with total bilirubin <12 mg/dL, as it is a benign self-limited condition.

This patient has mild elevation of unconjugated bilirubin that occurred within 2-5 days, consistent with physiologic jaundice of the newborn.

It is associated with a mild unconjugated (indirect) hyperbilirubinemia: Total bilirubin (TB) rises <5 mg/dL per day, peak on average at 9 mg/dL at 3-5 days of age before decreasing, & total bilirubin is usually ≤15 mg/dL.

Physiologic jaundice of the newborn occurs due to high hemoglobin turnover in the first few days of life, slow development of UDP-glucuronyltransferase activity, and increased enterohepatic circulation of bilirubin.

Bilirubin usually peaks on average at 9 mg/dL at 3-5 days of life and then decreases.

Pathologic jaundice, on the other hand, may present with jaundice in the first 24 hours, total bilirubin >12 mg/dL in a term infant, conjugated bilirubin >2 mg/dL, total serum bilirubin that rises >5 mg/dL/day, or persistent jaundice beyond 10-14 days.

Choice A [Exchange transfusion] is usually reserved for severe cases (eg, hemolysis, ABO incompatibility, Rh isoimmunization), symptomatic infants, severe hyperbilirubinemia (increasing TB), >20 mg/dL, or rapidly rising bilirubin.

Choice B [Perform direct antiglobulin (Coombs) testing] is indicated if immune-mediated hemolytic conditions are suspected, which usually presents with jaundice in the first 24 hours of life.

Choice D [Phototherapy] is used for term infants (≥38 weeks GA) without risk factors, phototherapy is initiated based on total bilirubin: 24 hours of age >12 mg/dL, 48 hours of age >15 mg/dL or 72 hours of age >18 mg/dL.

Choice E [Discontinue breastfeeding and initiate the use of formula for feedings] may be indicated in breastfeeding jaundice. Breastfeeding jaundice is usually associated with inadequate number of wet diapers, weight loss, dark green stools, and usually occurs later in the newborn period (after 6 days of life).

46. INFECTIOUS DISEASE – MYCOBACTERIUM AVIUM COMPLEX [PHARMACOLOGY]

Combination antimicrobial therapy, such as Clarithromycin plus Ethambutol, with a third agent (eg, Rifabutin) added if high mycobacterial load [choice A], is used for patients with AIDS and disseminated or localized MAC infection.

Agents with activity against MAC include Macrolides (eg, Clarithromycin, Azithromycin), Ethambutol, Rifabutin, Aminoglycosides (eg, Streptomycin, Amikacin), and Fluoroquinolones.

Liposomal inhaled Amikacin [choice D] may be added as adjunctive therapy in patients without HIV unresponsive to 6 months of standard MAC therapy.

Choice A [Trimethoprim-sulfamethoxazole] is used in the treatment and prevention of Pneumocystis (PCP) pneumonia.

Choice E [IV Penicillin G aqueous] can be used in the management of Neurosyphilis.

47. EENT – FOREIGN BODY IN THE EAR CANAL [HISTORY AND PHYSICAL]

Irrigation may be used for the removal of small inorganic objects and insects [choice A].

Irrigation is often better tolerated than instrumentation and does not require direct visualization.

Live insects should be killed by instilling mineral oil, 1% Lidocaine, or 2% viscous Lidocaine prior to irrigation.

Contraindications to foreign body removal via irrigation includes organic objects (eg, beans, vegetable matter) [choices B and C] because they may swell as they absorb water, button batteries (increases risk for caustic injury) [choice D], perforated tympanic membranes [choice E], or the presence of tympanostomy tubes.

48. PULMONARY – ASBESTOSIS [MOST LIKELY]

Occupations associated with Asbestos exposure [choice A] include plumbing (as in this patient), pipe fitting, insulation, demolition and repair of old asbestos-containing buildings, and shipbuilding.

The classic radiograph findings include bilateral mid-lung zone parietal pleural thickening or calcification, especially along the lower lung fields and diaphragmatic pleura are hallmark.

The classic PFT findings are consistent with a restrictive lung pattern: [1] decreased lung volumes (RV, TLC, RV/TLC), [2] decreased FEV1, and [3] a normal to increased FEV1/FVC ratio (as seen in this patient).

Choice B [Emphysema] is classically associated with an obstructive pattern: increased lung volumes (RV, TLC, RV/TLC), decreased FEV1, and a decreased FEV1 ratio (≤0.70).

Choice C [Chronic bronchitis] is classically associated with an obstructive pattern: increased lung volumes (RV, TLC, RV/TLC), decreased FEV1, and a decreased FEV1 ratio (≤0.70).

Choice D [Bronchiectasis] is classically associated with an obstructive pattern: increased lung volumes (RV, TLC, RV/TLC), decreased FEV1, and a decreased FEV1 ratio (≤0.70).

Choice E [Sarcoidosis] may also present with a restrictive lung pattern but is usually associated with bilateral hilar lymphadenopathy &/or interstitial lung involvement,

49. CARDIOLOGY – HYPERTENSION [PHARMACOLOGY]

In patients with a history of Gout or hyperuricemia, the ideal antihypertensive with a favorable effect on Gout include Losartan [choice E] or Calcium channel blockers.

Losartan reduces serum uric acid levels by 20-25% by producing a uricosuric effect. This effect is not seen with the other Angiotensin II receptor blockers.

Calcium channel blockers and Losartan are associated with a lower risk of incident Gout among people with hypertension.

Choice A [Prazosin] and other alpha blockers are usually reserved for men with Hypertension and Benign prostatic hypertrophy.

Choice B [Hydrochlorothiazide] and other thiazide diuretics can increase uric acid levels, serum lipids, and serum glucose levels, making Losartan a better choice based on this patient's history of Gout, Diabetes, and Dyslipidemia.

Choice C [Labetalol] and other beta blockers are preferred for Hypertension with a comorbid condition in which Beta blockers would also be helpful (eg, PVCs, Angina, Heart failure, Atrial flutter, Atrial fibrillation). Beta blockers can also increase glucose levels and mask the symptoms of hypoglycemia.

Choice D [Furosemide] and other Loop diuretics can increase uric acid levels, serum lipids, and serum glucose levels, making Losartan a better choice based on this patient's history of Gout, Diabetes, and Dyslipidemia.

50. PSYCHIATRY AND BEHAVIORAL – BUPROPION [PHARMACOLOGY]
Because Bupropion is a CNS stimulant, which lowers the seizure threshold, Bupropion is contraindicated in patients with reduced seizure threshold, which includes:
- **eating disorders, such as Bulimia nervosa and Anorexia nervosa [choice E]**
- Epilepsy or conditions with increased seizure risk
- patients undergoing abrupt discontinuation of alcohol, benzodiazepine, barbiturate, or antiepileptic medications.

Indications for use of Bupropion include:
- smoking cessation
- Seasonal affective disorder
- patients with sexual dysfunction on other antidepressants (Bupropion or Mirtazapine have the least incidence of sexual adverse effects among the antidepressants)
- patients with Depression fearful of weight gain (Bupropion is more commonly associated with causing weight loss than weight gain).

51. NEUROLOGY – VALPROATE [PROFESSIONAL PRACTICE]
An example of a nonmaleficent action would be stopping a medication known to be harmful [choice B] or refusing to give a medication to a patient if it has not been proven to be effective.
Adverse effects of Valproate include teratogenicity and hepatitis.
Of all the antiepileptics, Valproate has the highest incidence of teratogenicity, and she has LFTs consistent with medication-induced Hepatitis.
It is the duty of clinicians who prescribe potentially teratogenic medications to inform the mother about the risks it poses to the child.

Choice A [Beneficence] refers to the principle to act for the patient's benefit and provide benefits for the patient's well-being.
Choice C [Justice] refers to treating others equitably, distribute benefits/burdens fairly.
Choice D [Autonomy] is the ethical principle that all persons have intrinsic and unconditional worth, and therefore, should have the power to make rational decisions and moral choices, and each should be allowed to exercise his or her capacity for self-determination.
Choice E [Caring] emphasizes the importance of emotions, such as sympathy, empathy, and compassion.

52 - INFECTIOUS DISEASE – DIPHTHERIA [HISTORY AND PHYSICAL]
Myocarditis [choice C] and Neuropathy are the most common & most serious complications of Diphtheria.
This is because absorption and dissemination of Diphtheria toxin can result in toxin-mediated damage of the heart and nervous system.

Other complications from direct toxin activity include Acute kidney injury; Non-toxigenic *C. diphtheriae* strains may result in endocarditis, mycotic aneurysms, osteomyelitis, and septic arthritis.

Diphtheria should be suspected in patients with:
- **sore throat, malaise, cervical lymphadenopathy (often prominent), and low-grade fever.**
- **coalescing pseudomembrane** (composed of necrotic fibrin, leukocytes, erythrocytes, epithelial cells, and organisms). in any portion of the respiratory tract, especially tonsillopharyngeal involvement; it is **grey in color, adheres tightly to the underlying tissue, and bleeds when scraped.**

Choice A [Splenic rupture] can result from splenomegaly associated with Infectious mononucleosis.
Choice B [Glomerulonephritis] is a classic complication of Postinfectious glomerulonephritis.
Choice D [Hemolytic uremic syndrome] occurs as complication of Shigella or Enterohemorrhagic *E. coli*.
Choice E [Acute rheumatic fever] is a classic complication of group A Streptococcal infection.

53. NEUROLOGY – EPIDURAL HEMATOMA/HEMORRHAGIC STROKE [APPLYING FOUNDATIONAL CONCEPTS]

Epidural hematomas (EDH) most commonly result from trauma to the skull base, especially temporal bone fracture, associated tearing of the middle meningeal artery [choice E] as it courses through the foramen spinosum.
The classic CT findings of an EDH is a biconvex (lens-shaped) pattern on head CT that does not cross the suture lines.
Most cases of EDH are due to head trauma resulting from traffic accidents, falls, and assaults.

Choice A [Rupture of a cortical bridging vein] most commonly results in a Subdural hematoma.
Choice B [Rupture of a Berry aneurysm] most commonly results in Subarachnoid hemorrhage.
Choice C [Rupture of the penetrating arterioles] most commonly results in Intracerebral hemorrhage.
Choice D [Arteriovenous malformations] are uncommon causes of nontraumatic EDH.

54. GASTROINTESTINAL/NUTRITION – ESOPHAGEAL CARCINOMA/SQUAMOUS CELL CARCINOMA OF THE ESOPHAGUS [HISTORY AND PHYSICAL]

The major risk factors for Squamous cell carcinoma (SCC) of the Esophagus in the United States are smoking and alcohol consumption [choice E].
Worldwide, other risk factors include human papillomavirus (HPV), low intake of fruits and vegetables, and consumption beverages at high temperatures.

The major risk factors for Adenocarcinoma of the esophagus are Barrett's, gastroesophageal reflux disease (GERD) [choice C], smoking, and a high body mass index.

Fiber intake and NSAID [choice B] use have a possible protective effect on Esophageal cancer, Gastric adenocarcinoma, and Colon cancer.

Choice A [Cold beverage consumption] is not associated; hot beverage consumption increases the risk.
Choice D [H. pylori infection] increases the risk of Gastric adenocarcinoma.

55. MUSCULOSKELETAL – POLYARTERITIS NODOSA/VASCULITIS [MOST LIKELY]
Polyarteritis nodosa (PAN) [choice D] is a systemic necrotizing vasculitis that typically affects medium-sized muscular arteries, characterized by:
- **absence of antineutrophil cytoplasmic antibodies (ANCA) and glomerulonephritis**
- **Association with Hepatitis B virus infection**, hepatitis C virus infection, and hairy cell leukemia (secondary PAN).
- systemic symptoms (eg, fatigue, weight loss, weakness, fever, arthralgias)
- skin lesions, hypertension, renal insufficiency, neurologic dysfunction, abdominal pain.
- **absence of lung involvement. Think <u>P</u>ulmonary and <u>ANCA N</u>egative (PAN).**

Choice A [Glomerular basement membrane disease] presents with lung and kidney involvement (hemoptysis and glomerulonephritis).
Choice B [Granulomatosis with polyangiitis] is associated with C-ANCA positivity.
Choice C [Eosinophilic granulomatosis with polyangiitis] is associated with P-ANCA positivity.
Choice E [Microscopic polyangiitis] is associated with P-ANCA positivity.

56. GASTROINTESTINAL/NUTRITION – ISCHEMIC COLITIS [MOST LIKELY]
Patients with Acute colonic ischemia/Ischemic colitis [choice B] typically present with abrupt onset of mild abdominal pain and tenderness over the affected bowel, most often the left colon. Hematochezia &/or bloody diarrhea usually develop within 24 hours of the onset of abdominal pain.
Classic findings of Ischemic colitis on CT imaging include edema and thickening of the bowel wall in a segmental pattern (thumbprinting).
Aortic surgery (as in this patient) can result in Ischemic colitis.

Choice A [Chronic mesenteric ischemia] classically presents with postprandial abdominal pain and weight loss due to less eating in anticipation of postprandial pain.
Choice C [Acute mesenteric ischemia] usually presents with severe abdominal pain, often out of proportion to examination, is not classically associated with bloody diarrhea or hematochezia, and is more often periumbilical than lateral.
Choice D [Diverticulitis] presents with left lower quadrant pain, but hematochezia and bloody diarrhea are not classic features.
Choice E [Infectious colitis] can present with bloody diarrhea and severe abdominal pain, but the patient's medical history, mild pain, and recent aortic surgery makes Ischemic colitis more probable.

57. EENT – OTITIS MEDIA WITH EFFUSION [HEALTH MAINTENANCE]
"Watchful waiting" for 3 months [choice C] is recommended management of Serous otitis media with effusion (OME) for in children not at risk for speech, language, or learning problems with otherwise normal hearing (eg, hearing threshold ≤15 dB).
There is a high rate of spontaneous resolution of OME within the first 3-6 months.
OME can be a precursor to or follow the resolution of Acute otitis media (AOM).
OME is characterized by:
- **Middle ear effusion (often amber or clear fluid)**

- **Neutral or retracted TM without erythema**
- **Absence of ear pain and fever.**

Children at risk for speech, language, or learning problems or those with chronic otitis media with effusion should be referred to otolaryngology for myringotomy with tympanostomy tube insertion evaluation [choice A].

Unproven or ineffective interventions for OME include:
- Antihistamines [choice B] as they are not associated with any benefits
- Decongestants [choice E] as they are not associated with any benefits
- Antibiotics [choice D] as OME is usually unresponsive to antibiotics. In Acute otitis media (eg, bulging or fullness of the tympanic membrane, TM erythema, pain, fever), antibiotics may be helpful.
- Intranasal or oral corticosteroids.

58. INFECTIOUS DISEASE – HIV [LABS AND DIAGNOSTIC STUDIES]
In patients with suspected Early HIV infection, perform combination antigen/antibody immunoassay (screening) + HIV RNA viral load testing (RT-PCR) [choice E]. A confirmation test can be performed in patients with a positive screening immunoassay.
The rational for HIV RNA viral load testing (RT-PCR) in suspected Acute HIV infection is because it may be the only positive marker in the window period.
- A negative screening immunoassay + positive HIV RNA suggests early HIV. A second positive virological test suggests HIV infection.
- A positive HIV screening immunoassay + positive HIV RNA suggests early or established infection.
- If both are negative with high suspicion, repeat both tests within 1-2 weeks.

Acute HIV syndrome (seroconversion syndrome) may present with flu-like symptoms, diarrhea, maculopapular rash, pharyngitis, mucocutaneous ulceration, and other nonspecific symptoms 2-4 weeks after primary exposure.

59. DERMATOLOGY – CAT BITES [BASICS]
***Pasteurella multocida* [choice A] is the most common recovered organism in infected cat and dog bites (although infection is often polymicrobial).**
Infections with *P. multocida* have a characteristic rapid development of infection, often within 24 hours and as early as 3 hours afterwards (earlier than Cellulitis due to the usual pathogens).

Other common organisms include Streptococcus species [choice D], *Staphylococcus aureus* [choice C], and anaerobic bacteria.
For this reason, most infected Cat bites are treated as outpatients with Amoxicillin-clavulanate.

Choice B [Bartonella henselae] is the cause of Cat scratch disease, which presents as a painless papule at the site of inoculation, followed by painful lymphadenopathy weeks later.

60. REPRODUCTIVE SYSTEM – ENDOMETRIAL HYPERPLASIA/CANCER LABS AND DIAGNOSTIC STUDIES
Endometrial biopsy [choice D] is recommended in patients with Postmenopausal bleeding and a thickened endometrial stripe >4 mm to rule out Endometrial cancer.

Individuals with postmenopausal bleeding may be initially evaluated with either [1] an endometrial biopsy or [2] a transvaginal ultrasound, depending on the risk.

The classic finding of Endometrial hyperplasia on histology is widespread endometrial gland crowding. When atypia is present, abnormal nuclei may also be present.

Endometrial cancer is the most common reproductive cancer in women and often presents as postmenopausal bleeding.

Choice A [Hysterectomy] is definitive management if Postmenopausal bleeding is due to Endometrial cancer or Endometrial hyperplasia with atypia, depending on the biopsy findings.

Choice B [Progestin add-back therapy] can be used in select premenopausal patients with Endometrial hyperplasia without atypia on endometrial biopsy with histology.

Choice C [Hysteroscopy] can be used if there is evidence of focal thickening of the endometrium.

Choice E [Repeat Transvaginal ultrasound 4 months] can be used in women with Postmenopausal bleeding with an endometrial strip <4 mm on Transvaginal ultrasound.

61. DERMATOLOGY – PSORIASIS [PHARMACOLOGY]

High-potency topical corticosteroids [choice C] and emollients is the first line management of limited mild-moderate Plaque psoriasis.

Plaque psoriasis, the most common type of Psoriasis, is characterized by erythematous plaques with silver scales. Nail pitting is another common finding.

Beta-blockers (such as Propranolol) can exacerbate Psoriasis (as seen in this patient).

Alternative treatments include Coal tar, topical retinoids (eg, Tazarotene), topical vitamin D (Calcipotriene) [choice E], and Anthralin.

Topical Tacrolimus or Pimecrolimus are alternative steroid-sparing agents.

Narrowband ultraviolet B (UVB) phototherapy,

Choice A [Oral Prednisone] should not be used in the management of Psoriasis as discontinuation can result in the development of Pustular psoriasis.

Choice B [Narrowband ultraviolet B (UVB) phototherapy] can be used in more extensive disease involving more body surface area or in combination with coal tar.

Choice D [Oral Methotrexate] can be used in severe Psoriasis. This patient has mild Psoriasis.

62. PULMONARY – ACUTE EXACERBATION OF COPD [HEALTH MAINTENANCE]

In patients with Acute exacerbation of COPD, systemic glucocorticoids [choice E] are added to bronchodilators to improve lung function, reduce airway inflammation, reverse airflow, limitation, promote shorter hospital stay, & reduce relapse.

Management of COPD exacerbations include

- [1] short course of systemic corticosteroids & aggressive short-acting bronchodilator therapy [SAMA &/or SABA] to reverse airflow limitation
- [2] antibacterial or antiviral agents if indicated,
- [3] oxygen supplementation, &
- [4] ventilatory support.

Choice A [Nedocromil] is used in the management of chronic Asthma.

Choice B [Salmeterol] is used in the long-term management of Chronic Asthma.

Choice C [Home oxygen therapy] can be used if at baseline, the patient has [1] cor pulmonale, [2] resting SaO2 <88%, or [3] PaO2 <55 mmHg.

Choice D [Montelukast] is used in the long-term management of Persistent Asthma.

63. GASTROINTESTINAL/NUTRITION – VITAMIN B3 DEFICIENCY/PELLAGRA [HEALTH MAINTENANCE]

Pellagra is a manifestation of Niacin (vitamin B3) deficiency [choice B], characterized by the "three Ds":

- **diarrhea**
- **dementia**: anxiety, poor concentration, fatigue, and depression can manifest, but dementia and delirium
- **dermatitis:** rash similar to a sunburn on areas exposed to the sun (eg, hands, elbows, knees, and feet).

Choice A [oral folate] presents with fatigue from a macrocytic anemia.

Choice C [oral cobalamin] and choice E [parenteral cobalamin] is used in Vitamin B12 deficiency, which is characterized by macrocytic anemia and subacute degeneration of the spinal cord.

Choice E [parenteral thiamine] is associated with neuropathy, dilated cardiomyopathy, Wernicke's encephalopathy, or Korsakoff dementia.

64. NEUROLOGY – ANTIEPILEPTICS/PHENYTOIN [PHARMACOLOGY]

Gingival hyperplasia and hirsutism are classic adverse effects of Phenytoin [choice A].

Other adverse effects of Phenytoin include nystagmus, ataxia, diplopia, sedation/CNS depression, SLE-like syndrome, osteopenia, megaloblastic anemia (decreased folate absorption), and teratogenicity.

Choice B [Carbamazepine] adverse effects include diplopia, ataxia, Stevens-Johnson syndrome, agranulocytosis, aplastic anemia, hepatotoxicity, SIADH, and teratogenicity.

Choice C [Topiramate] adverse effects include weight loss, sedation, and Nephrolithiasis.

Choice D [Lamotrigine] adverse effects include Stevens-Johnson syndrome.

Choice E [Valproic acid] adverse effects include pancreatitis, hepatotoxicity, and teratogenicity.

65. PULMONARY – ACUTE EPIGLOTTITIS [CLINICAL INTERVENTION]

The most important and critical step in managing a child with Acute epiglottitis is immediate transfer to the operating room for visualization via laryngoscopy and endotracheal intubation [choice B].

Rapid deterioration can occur in patients with Epiglottitis; so prompt and early consultation of specialists proficient in airway management (eg, anesthesiologist, intensivist, and otolaryngologist) is recommended.

Epiglottitis should be suspected in patients with rapid onset high fever and the 3 D's: [1] drooling, [2] dysphagia, and [3] distress (respiratory). In addition, stridor, muffled voice, and sitting in a tripod position often occur.

Choice A [Tracheostomy] may be used to maintain an airway in patients whom Laryngoscopy is unsuccessful or cannot be performed.

Choice C [Initiate IV Ceftriaxone after obtaining blood cultures] is part of the management of Epiglottitis but maintaining the airway is the most important initial step.

Choice D [IM Epinephrine and Dexamethasone] is used in the management of Croup.

Choice E [Direct inspection of the posterior pharynx with a tongue depressor] should not be performed in children with suspected Epiglottitis because it can result in laryngospasm, which can result in closing of the airway, so securing the airway is paramount.

66. PSYCHIATRY AND BEHAVIORAL – ALCOHOL WITHDRAWAL/DELIRIUM TREMENS [CLINICAL INTERVENTION]

Benzodiazepines, such as Diazepam, Lorazepam, or Chlordiazepoxide [choice E] are first line agents for alcohol withdrawal.

Delirium tremens (DT) is a complication of alcohol withdrawal characterized by:

- **delirium (altered sensorium), hallucinations,** agitation; rapid-onset, fluctuating disturbance of attention and cognition (disorientation)
- **Abnormal vital signs** (eg, tachycardia, hypertension, fever, drenching sweats). Patients are often diaphoretic.
- onset: 2–5 days after last drink (most common between 48-96 hours after the last drink).

Choice A [Disulfiram] is used in the management of chronic alcohol use as a deterrent.

Choice B [Haloperidol] is used in the management of Acute psychosis.

Choice C [Naltrexone] is used in the management of Opioid intoxication; it may also be used for maintenance in patients with opioid or alcohol dependence.

Choice D [Flumazenil] is used in the management of Benzodiazepine overdose.

67. PULMONARY – TUBERCULOSIS [HEALTH MAINTENANCE]

Options in the management of Latent Tuberculosis infection (LTBI) include:

(1) Rifamycin-based regimens: (preferred)
- **Rifampin (RIF) daily for 4 months** (4R) **[choice E]**
- **Isoniazid (INH) and Rifampin daily for 3 months** (3HR)
- Isoniazid (INH) and Rifapentine weekly for 3 months (3HP)

(2) Older regimen:
- **Isoniazid monotherapy for 6-9 months.**

Latent TB infection (LTBI) describes someone who is infected with TB but is not infectious to other people, which requires 3 things:

Evidence of TB infection:
- [1] Positive screening test (PPD or IGRA)

No evidence of active infection
- [2] No symptoms of active infection
- [3] Negative chest imaging (no evidence of active infection).

Choice A [Place the employee in respiratory isolation and induce sputum for acid-fast bacilli staining and Nucleic acid testing (NAAT)] is appropriate if the patient has symptoms &/or imaging findings suggestive of active TB infection.

Choice B [Repeat the Tuberculin skin test (TST) to assess for booster phenomenon] is not necessary as the patient already has a positive screening test.

Choice C [Isoniazid and Rifampin daily for 4 months] is incorrect because this regimen is used for 3 months.

Choice D [Order CT chest without contrast] is used in a suspected active TB with a negative chest radiograph.

68. PULMONARY – PULMONARY HYPERTENSION [PHARMACOLOGY]

Patients with suspected Idiopathic pulmonary hypertension and positive vasoreactivity testing (using Adenosine, inhaled Nitric oxide, or Epoprostenol) are candidates for a trial of Calcium channel blocker (CCB) therapy, such as Nifedipine [choice E] or Diltiazem. Amlodipine is an alternative to Nifedipine.

A reactivity test is considered positive if mean pulmonary artery pressure decreases at least 10 mmHg and to a value ≤40 mmHg, with an increased or unchanged cardiac output.

In patients with a nonreactive test, options include Phosphodiesterase 5 inhibitors, such as Sildenafil [choice B], endothelial receptor antagonist, such as Bosentan [choice A], Riociguat, or combination therapy.

Choice D [Epoprostenol] is used as a vasodilator for the vasoreactive test but is not used as long-term initial therapy. It is used as an option for functional class IV (high-risk Pulmonary hypertension).

69. REPRODUCTIVE SYSTEM – ECTOPIC PREGNANCY [LABS AND DIAGNOSTIC STUDIES]

In a hemodynamically stable patient in whom a diagnosis of ectopic pregnancy or IUP cannot be made based on the initial TVUS (eg, beta-hCG <1,500 mIU/mL)), the most appropriate next step is follow-up with serial serum hCG and repeat ultrasound in 2 days [choice A].

An undiagnostic TVUS may be because the gestation is too early to be visualized on ultrasound. It is important to note that institutions and laboratories vary on the beta-hCG levels for the discriminatory zone.

In this case, the patient has a pregnancy of unknown location. Subsequent TVUS can determine if it is an intrauterine or ectopic pregnancy.

Ectopic pregnancy and Threatened abortion have the same presentation.

Although IUDs are used for contraception, if a pregnancy occurs, they increase the risk of Ectopic pregnancies.

Choice B [Salpingostomy] is indicated in the management of a ruptured Ectopic pregnancy. This patient has stable vital signs and denies signs and symptoms of rupture (eg, dizziness, syncope, referred shoulder pain).

Choice C [CT scan of the abdomen and pelvis] can be used if an intrabdominal process is thought to be the cause of the pelvic pain. With the vaginal spotting, a reproductive cause is more likely.

Choice D [Methotrexate administration] can be used in the medical management of an Ectopic pregnancy once the diagnosis is confirmed via TVUS.

Choice E [Uterine aspiration] can disrupt a viable pregnancy.

70. MUSCULOSKELETAL – ANTERIOR CRUCIATE LIGAMENT INJURY [HISTORY AND PHYSICAL]

Of the three tests performed for suspected Anterior cruciate ligament (ACL injuries), the Lachman test [choice E] is the most sensitive for the diagnosis of ACL rupture; the pivot shift test is the most specific and also the most difficult to perform.

In addition to the Lachman test, the Anterior drawer test is performed by most clinicians; sports medicine specialists or those with orthopedic experience may elect to perform the pivot shift test.

The classic presentation of ACL injury is sudden deceleration, change in direction, pivoting, or lateral blow to the knee, followed by a "pop" in the knee, hemarthrosis, and knee instability.

Choice A [Straight leg raise test] is most helpful in assessing a Quadriceps rupture or Patellar tendon rupture.

Choice B [Anterior drawer test] is one of the 3 tests commonly used for ACL, but Lachman is more sensitive.

Choice C [Posterior sag test] is used to assess for Posterior cruciate ligament injury.

Choice D [Valgus stress test] is used to assess for Medial collateral ligament injury.

71. MUSCULOSKELETAL – ACHILLES TENDON RUPTURE [CLINICAL INTERVENTION]

Initial management of Achilles tendon rupture consists of ice application to the area, analgesics, rest (eg, non-weightbearing with crutches), immobilization with the ankle in some plantarflexion (often with a short-leg splint) [choice D], and orthopedic surgeon referral.

Orthopedic surgical referral or consultation should be obtained to determine if surgical or nonoperative management should be implemented.

Fluoroquinolones (this patient is on Ciprofloxacin) has a black box warning of increased risk for Achilles tendinopathy and tendon rupture.

The patient has a positive Thompson test (absence of plantar flexion with calf squeeze).

72. MUSCULOSKELETAL – LUMBAR STRAIN (SPRAIN) [HISTORY AND PHYSICAL]

Radiographs [choice B] are not needed in patients with Lumbar strain (sprain) unless symptoms are persistent, or alarm symptoms are present.

Red flags that may indicate radiographs or other imaging include night pain, fever, chills, bony tenderness, morning stiffness, coagulopathy, extremes of age, saddle anesthesia, urinary or bowel incontinence, or recent spinal instrumentation.

Analgesics (eg, NSAIDs) & resumption of ordinary activity or activity modification is the preferred management of Lumbar sprain or strain.

If not tolerable, BRIEF bed rest (no more than 1-2 days) may be indicated if moderate pain.

Muscle relaxers may help with spasm in some cases.

73. CARDIOLOGY – ACUTE CORONARY SYNDROME [LABS AND DIAGNOSTIC STUDIES]

Because the elderly, women, obese patients, and Diabetics may present with atypical pain (abdominal or shoulder pain instead of typical chest pain), an ECG [choice C] should be obtained initially, followed by cardiac enzymes.

She has cardiac risk factors (elderly, Diabetes, Hypertension, and cigarette smoking history).

An ECG should be obtained within 10 minutes of presentation with symptoms consistent with Acute coronary syndrome.

Choice A [Amylase, lipase, and liver function tests] may be part of the workup to rule out pancreatic and hepatic causes. However, an ECG is still needed prior to CT scan to rule out cardiac causes in patients with increased risk of cardiovascular disease.

Choice B [Troponin I and creatine kinase-MB levels] should be performed but an ECG should be obtained within 10 minutes of presentation with symptoms consistent with Acute coronary syndrome.

Choice D [CT abdomen and pelvis without contrast] may be part of the workup if a cardiac source is not elicited or if her symptomology changes. However, an ECG is still needed prior to CT scan to rule out cardiac causes in patients with increased risk of cardiovascular disease.

Choice E [Ultrasound of the right upper quadrant] can be done to rule out biliary causes of abdominal pain. An ECG should still be performed first to rule out cardiac causes due to her risk factors.

74. DERMATOLOGY – NEUROFIBROMATOSIS [MOST LIKELY]

Neurofibromatosis type 1 [choice A] is characterized by:
- **café au lait macules >5 mm**
- **Lisch nodules on the iris**
- **Axillary and inguinal freckling**
- Neurofibromas
- **Optic glioma**
- **Pheochromocytoma.**

Choice B [Noonan syndrome] is also associated with Café au lait spots, but is also characterized by webbed neck, short stature, and distinct facial features (eg, low-set ears and downward eye slant).

Choice C [Neurofibromatosis type 2] is associated with bilateral acoustic schwannomas, juvenile cataracts, meningiomas, and ependymomas.

Choice D [Peutz-Jegher syndrome] is associated with hyperpigmentation of mucosal surfaces.

Choice E [Tuberous sclerosis] is characterized by collagenomas, ash leaf macules, and angiofibromas.

75. PSYCHIATRY AND BEHAVIORAL – POSTTRAUMATIC STRESS DISORDER [CLINICAL INTERVENTION]

Serotonin reuptake inhibitors, such as SSRIs (eg, Sertraline [choice B] or Citalopram) are first-line alternatives or adjunctive treatment to psychotherapy for Posttraumatic stress disorder (PTSD).

Sertraline and Paroxetine are Food and Drug Administration (FDA)-approved medications for adults with PTSD.

An SNRI (eg, Venlafaxine) is an alternative option.

Clonidine and Prazosin are useful in decreasing prominent trauma-related nightmares or sleep disturbances as an augmenting agent to serotonin reuptake inhibitors (SSRI or SNRI); It can sometimes be used as monotherapy or combined with trauma-focused therapy.

Trazodone [choice D] can also be used for treating insomnia in patients with PTSD as augmentation therapy.

Choice A [Buspirone] can be used as augmentation therapy or monotherapy of Panic disorder.

Choice C [Risperidone] and other second-generation antipsychotics can be used in the management of PTSD with prominent psychosis.

76. PULMONARY – HISTOPLASMOSIS [MOST LIKELY DIAGNOSIS]

The classic finding of *Histoplasma capsulatum* [choice B] on histology are ovoid shaped narrow-based budding yeasts.

Pulmonary histoplasmosis should be considered in patients who traveled to endemic areas with Pneumonia associated with mediastinal or hilar lymphadenopathy.

Histoplasma capsulatum is commonly found in soil contaminated with bird or bat droppings, especially in central & midwestern US, along the Ohio and Mississippi River valleys.

Choice A [Tuberculosis] is in the differential but would show Acid fast bacilli on histology, often with a positive purified protein derivative (PPD).

Choice C [Coccidioidomycosis] is endemic to the Southwestern US and histology findings include spherules with endospores.

Choice D [Cryptococcosis] is associated with encapsulated yeast with budding seen on India ink staining.

Choice E [Blastomycosis] is also endemic to the Mississippi and Ohio river valleys similar to Histoplasmosis, but histology would reveal round, broad-based budding yeast with thick refractile double walls.

77. HEMATOLOGY – HEPARIN INDUCED THROMBOCYTOPENIA [PHARMACOLOGY]

In addition to discontinuing all Heparin products (Unfractionated or low-molecular-weight Heparin), Non-Heparin options in the management of type 2 Heparin induced thrombocytopenia (HIT) include:

- **Parenteral direct thrombin inhibitors Argatroban [choice D] or Bivalirudin as they have a short half-life and would be the most preferred agents to be used first in a patient with acute thrombosis in order to achieve full-dose therapeutic anticoagulation rapidly.**
- Subcutaneous Fondaparinux [choice B] is an alternative but an IV agent would be preferred in a patient with acute thrombosis.
- Direct oral anticoagulants: eg, oral Factor Xa inhibitors (eg, Apixaban, Edoxaban, Rivaroxaban) or oral direct thrombin inhibitor (eg, Dabigatran).

Choice A [Enoxaparin] is incorrect because all Heparin products should be discontinued in HIT. Choice C [Warfarin] is associated with a hypercoagulable state for the first few days after initiation. Therefore, long-term anticoagulation with Warfarin can only be started [1] after other non-Heparin anticoagulation has been started & [2] the thrombosis has decreased because of the initial prothrombotic state normally associated with the first 5 days of the initiation of Warfarin therapy.

Choice E [Platelet transfusion] is usually contraindicated in most patients as platelet transfusion can worsen the hypercoagulable state.

78. EENT – ALLERGIC RHINITIS [PHARMACOLOGY]

Glucocorticoid nasal sprays [choice E] are the most effective single maintenance therapy for Allergic rhinitis and nasal polyps, and cause few adverse effects at the recommended doses.

They reduce the incidence and size of nasal polyps, reduce hypertrophic nasal mucosa, and facilitate nasal drainage.

Adverse effects of Glucocorticoid nasal sprays include scant blood in the nasal mucus, epistaxis, local irritation, and systemic effects with long-term use.

Prolonged use of decongestants, such as intranasal Oxymetazoline [choice A] can result in Rhinitis medicamentosa.
Oral antihistamines [choice B] are useful for pruritus, sneezing, and rhinorrhea but are less effective for nasal congestion compared with glucocorticoid sprays.
Glucocorticoid nasal sprays are usually preferred over antihistamine sprays [choice C].
Choice D [Cromolyn sodium nasal spray] is not used as common as other therapies.

79. HEMATOLOGY – COBALAMIN (VITAMIN B12) DEFICIENCY [MOST LIKELY]
Cobalamin (vitamin B12) deficiency [choice A] can result in subacute combined degeneration of the lateral columns (white matter) of the spinal cord due to demyelination, which results in:
- progressive weakness, gait ataxia, and paresthesias that may progress to spasticity and paraplegia.
- impaired perception of deep touch, pressure and vibration, loss of sense of touch
- decrease or loss of deep muscle-tendon reflexes
- pathological reflexes (eg, Babinski, Rossolimo).

Alcohol use disorder, as seen in this patient, is a risk factor for development of B12 deficiency.

Choice A [Guillain-Barre syndrome] can present with weakness and paresthesias, but as a lower motor neuropathy, it would not present with a positive Babinski.
Choice C [Amyotrophic lateral sclerosis] presents with combined upper and lower motor neuron findings in the absence of an alternative explanation, asymmetric limb weakness, and autonomic symptoms.
Choice D [Type 2 Diabetes mellitus] can present with a symmetric polyneuropathy, usually characterized as a "stocking and glove" distribution.
Choice E [Anterior cerebral artery stroke] can present with lower extremity deficits worse in the leg > arm but would be unilateral (contralateral to the side of the stroke).

80. REPRODUCTIVE SYSTEM – CANDIDA VULVOVAGINITIS [PHARMACOLOGY]
The first line management of Candida vulvovaginitis during pregnancy is topical Imidazoles, such as Clotrimazole [choice C] or Miconazole vaginally for 7 days.
Topical imidazoles are preferred over Nystatin pessary [choice D] or oral Fluconazole [choice A]. Oral Fluconazole can increase the risk for congenital anomalies.

Choice A [Oral Fluconazole] is a first line option in nonpregnant patients. Because she is pregnant, topical therapy is preferred.
Choice B [Topical Metronidazole gel] is not used in the management of Vulvovaginal candidiasis or Trichomoniasis in pregnant women. Oral Metronidazole [choice E] is the first line for Trichomoniasis.

81. GENITOURINARY – VESICOURETERAL REFLUX [LABS AND DIAGNOSTIC STUDIES]
The diagnosis of Vesicoureteral reflux (VUR) is established with contrast voiding cystourethrogram (VCUG) [choice D], showing reflux of urine from the bladder to the upper urinary tract.

VCUG is also used to grade the severity of VUR based upon the degree of retrograde filling and dilation of the renal collecting system.

Contrast voiding cystourethrogram (VCUG) should be obtained in children after a first febrile or symptomatic UTI who have an anomaly on kidney Ultrasound, have Hypertension or poor growth, or have combination of temperature ≥39°C (102.2°F) & a pathogen other than *Escherichia coli* (as in this patient).

Choice A [Intravenous pyelogram] is not routinely used in the diagnosis of VUR.
Choice B [Radionuclide cystogram] is an alternative to VCUG in establishing the diagnosis of VUR but VCUG gives better anatomic detail and Radionuclide cystogram does not accurately outline urethral anatomy in boys.
Choice C [Dimercaptosuccinic acid (DMSA) renal scan] can be used but is not as accurate for detecting Vesicoureteral reflux of all grades in children.
Choice E [Computed tomography of the abdomen and pelvis] is not routinely used in the diagnosis of VUR.

82. CARDIOLOGY – ATRIAL SEPTAL DEFECT [MOST LIKELY]
Atrial septal defect [choice B] is characterized by a soft, systolic ejection murmur over the pulmonic area (second intercostal space) combined with a wide, fixed splitting of S2.
Because Atrial septal defects are frequently asymptomatic, they may go undiagnosed until adulthood, in which they may develop symptoms of dyspnea and Pulmonary hypertension.

Choice A [Still murmur] is characterized by a musical twangy murmur head best at the left lower sternal border and apex.
Choice C [Ventricular septal defect] is characterized by a high-pitched harsh holosystolic murmur best heard at the third or fourth intercostal spaces along the left lower sternal border.
Choice D [Coarctation of the aorta] is not classically associated with a wide fixed split S2.
Choice E [Mitral regurgitation] is associated with a blowing holosystolic murmur that is best heard at the apex.

83. PSYCHIATRY AND BEHAVIORAL – BIPOLAR DISORDER [PHARMACOLOGY]
Mood stabilizers, such as Valproic acid [choice C], Lamotrigine, and Lithium or second-generation antipsychotics (eg, Quetiapine, Lurasidone, Aripiprazole, Olanzapine, Risperidone) are the first line agents for Bipolar II disorder.
The patient has episodes of Major depressive episodes and hypomania, consistent with Bipolar II disorder without manic episodes.

Choice A [Buspirone] is used in the management of Panic disorder alone or as an adjunct to SSRIs.
Choice B [Nortriptyline], choice D [Sertraline] and choice E [Bupropion] and other antidepressants should not be used as monotherapy in Bipolar disorder as they can precipitate mania.

84. PULMONARY – PLEURAL EFFUSION [APPLYING FUNDAMENTAL CONCEPTS]
Causes of an exudative Pleural effusion include [1] infection, such as Pneumonia [choice C], Tuberculosis. or inflammation: malignancies (eg, lung cancer, breast cancer, lymphoma), or other inflammatory disorders.

In an exudative effusion, infection &/or inflammation lead to increased capillary permeability, often via local factors.

Pulmonary embolism can be exudative or rarely transudative.

An exudate effusion meets at least any 1 of the 3 criteria: [1] pleural Total Protein/serum Total Protein ratio >0.5; [2] pleural Lactate dehydrogenase (LDH)/serum LDH ratio >0.6, &/or [3] serum LDH >upper 2/3 of normal limits.

All of the other choices listed are causes of an exudative effusion.

85. REPRODUCTIVE SYSTEM – SPONTANEOUS ABORTION [MOST LIKELY]

An Inevitable abortion [choice A] is defined as vaginal bleeding with progressive dilatation of the cervix but without expulsion of the products of conception prior to 20 weeks of gestation. Patients present with heavy vaginal bleeding, passage of clots, abdominal pain, and cramping. The external cervical os is often dilated.

Choice B [Missed abortion] is defined as fetal demise without expulsion of products of conception.

Choice C [Threatened abortion] is vaginal bleeding with a closed cervix. A threatened abortion is the only type of Spontaneous abortion that is potentially viable.

Choice D [Incomplete abortion] is defined as vaginal bleeding during the first 20 weeks of pregnancy with partial expulsion of products of conception. The cervix is usually dilated.

Choice E [Complete abortion] is defined as vaginal bleeding with complete expulsion of all products of conception before 20 weeks of gestation.

86. MUSCULOSKELETAL – DISC HERNIATION [MOST LIKELY]

Hallmark examination findings of S1 radiculopathy [choice B] include:

- **sacral or buttock pain into the posterior aspect of the patient's leg,** into the foot, or the perineum
- **weakness in plantar flexion**
- loss of sensation along the posterior leg and lateral aspect of the foot.
- **Diminished or absent ankle reflex (S1).**

Choice A [Cauda equina syndrome] may be associated with unilateral or bilateral sciatica, saddle anesthesia, and urinary or bowel incontinence.

Choice C [L3 – L4 lumbosacral radiculopathy] presents with L4 findings of back pain radiating to the anterior aspect of the thigh, sensory loss to the anterior leg and medial ankle, reduced ankle knee jerk reflex, and weakness with ankle dorsiflexion, knee extension, hip adduction, &/or hip flexion.

Choice D [L4 – L5 lumbosacral radiculopathy] is characterized by pain that radiates to the lateral aspect of the leg into the foot, weakness with big toe extension, sensory deficits to the lateral leg and dorsum of the foot and walking on the heels is more difficult than walking on the toes.

Choice E [Acute lumbosacral strain] is not associated with radiation to the leg and is not associated with sensory &/or motor deficits.

87. GENITOURINARY – BENIGN PROSTATIC HYPERPLASIA [PHARMACOLOGY]

Selective alpha-adrenergic receptor blockers, such as Tamsulosin [choice D] are the initial pharmacologic agents of choice for most men with lower urinary tract symptoms (LUTS) due to Benign prostatic hyperplasia (BPH).

Alpha blockers relax the prostatic smooth muscle & the smooth muscle of the bladder neck as well as decrease prostatic urethral resistance.

Many patients see improvement of symptoms within days of initiation of Alpha-adrenergic blockers.

They should be used with caution in men with planned cataract surgery (they can cause floppy iris syndrome) and in some men with specific cardiovascular risk factors.

Beta-3 adrenergic agonists [choice B] or antimuscarinics (anticholinergics) [choice A] are useful for patients with BPH and in whom overactive bladder symptoms (frequency, urgency, and incontinence) are the primary complaints.

Choice C [Sildenafil] and other phosphodiesterase 5 inhibitors are useful for patients with symptomatic BPH and concomitant Erectile dysfunction (this patient denies issues maintaining an erection).

Choice E (Finasteride) and other steroid 5-alpha reductase inhibitors decrease the size of the prostate in 6-12 months, so they are more useful to prevent BPH progression rather than for acute symptom relief.

88. GASTROINTESTINAL/NUTRITION – ESOPHAGEAL VARICES [CLINICAL INTERVENTION]

Combination of medical therapy (Octreotide) & endoscopic therapy (ligation or sclerotherapy) [choice C] is superior to either therapy alone in controlling acute bleeding and decreasing rebleeding in Esophageal varices.

Octreotide is a somatostatin analog that causes vasoconstriction of the portal venous flow, decreasing portal pressure and reducing bleeding.

Endoscopic sclerotherapy is an alternative to banding.

Choice A [Endoscopic sclerotherapy and Vasopressin] is incorrect because although sclerotherapy is a suitable alternative to banding, Vasopressin is a second-line agent. Although Vasopressin decreases portal venous pressure, Vasopressin can cause vasoconstriction in other areas (eg, coronary artery vasospasm, myocardial infarction), & bowel ischemia.

Choice B [Placement of Transjugular intrahepatic portosystemic shunt (TIPS)] can be used for Esophageal varices refractory to endoscopic therapy and tube compression.

Choice D [Insertion of a modified Sengstaken-Blakemore (Minnesota) tube for compression] can be used for Esophageal varices refractory to endoscopic therapy.

Choice E [Surgical esophageal devascularization of the varices] is not the first line management of acute Esophageal varices.

89. PSYCHIATRY AND BEHAVIORAL – PHENCYCLIDINE (PCP) INTOXICATION [HISTORY AND PHYSICAL]

Hallmark features of acute Phencyclidine (PCP) intoxication [choice D] includes:

- **horizontal, vertical, or rotary nystagmus**
- **delusions of super-human strength and diminished pain, even in the setting of trauma** (as in this patient)
- tachycardia, hypertension.

- violent behavior, suicidal or homicidal ideation, and hallucinations.

Choice A [Marijuana] intoxication is associated with conjunctival injection (red eye), dry (cotton) mouth, euphoria, giddiness, anxiety, disinhibition, intensification of sensory experiences, increased appetite, motor impairment, psychosis & hallucination.

Choice B [Diazepam] and other Benzodiazepine intoxication may include drowsiness, slurred speech, ataxia, horizontal gaze nystagmus, hypotension, coma, respiratory depression, and cardiorespiratory arrest.

Choice C [Cocaine] usually causes mydriasis, hypertension, and tachycardia. The multidirectional nystagmus makes PCP intoxication more likely.

Choice E [Amphetamines] usually cause mydriasis, hypertension, and tachycardia. The multidirectional nystagmus makes PCP intoxication more likely.

90. PSYCHIATRY AND BEHAVIORAL - DOMESTIC PARTNER ABUSE [HEALTH MAINTENANCE]

A woman who leaves an abusive partner has a 70% greater risk of being killed by the abuser in that immediate period after leaving [choice A] compared to staying.

According to the CDC, 1 in 4 women and 1 in 7 men will experience physical violence by their intimate partner at some point during their lifetimes. About 1 in 3 women and nearly 1 in 6 men experience some form of sexual violence during their lifetimes.

91. MUSCULOSKELETAL – RHEUMATOID ARTHRITIS [HEALTH MAINTENANCE]

In patients with Rheumatoid arthritis (RA), early use of disease-modifying antirheumatic drugs (DMARDs), such as Methotrexate [choice A] or Leflunomide have been shown to slow disease progression before irreversible injury occurs and reduce disease activity.

Anti-citrullinated peptide antibodies are specific to the diagnosis of Rheumatoid arthritis.

Use of anti-inflammatory agents, including nonsteroidal anti-inflammatory drugs (NSAIDs) [choice B] and glucocorticoids [choices D and E], are used as adjuncts to DMARD therapy for acute symptoms but do not slow down the progression of the RA.

92. PSYCHIATRY AND BEHAVIORAL – BULIMIA NERVOSA [PHARMACOLOGY]

Fluoxetine [choice D] is the best studied medication for Bulimia nervosa in adults.

It is FDA-approved for this indication and is usually the first line treatment for Bulimia nervosa in adults due to its efficacy and safety profile.

For patients with Bulimia nervosa who do not respond or tolerate Fluoxetine, second line agents include another SSRI [choice C].

Third-line pharmacotherapy include Tricyclic antidepressants [choice E], Trazodone [choice B], MAO inhibitors, or Topiramate.

Choice A [Bupropion] is contraindicated in eating disorders, such as Bulimia nervosa, due to increased seizure risk.

93. GASTROINTESTINAL/NUTRITION – HIRSCHSPRUNG DISEASE [APPLYING FOUNDATIONAL CONCEPTS]

Hirschsprung disease (HD) is caused by congenital absence of ganglion cells in the distal rectum and may extends proximally into the colon [choice C].

It affects the rectum and part of the sigmoid colon in ~80 percent of patients.

Most patients with HD present in the neonatal period with distal intestinal obstruction (eg, meconium ileus, abdominal distention, failure to pass stool, air expelled on digital rectal examination, and bilious emesis).

Plain abdominal radiographs reveal distended loops of bowel and an absence of gas in the rectum (megacolon).

Choice A [Invagination (telescoping) of a part of the intestine into itself] is hallmark of Intussusception, which presents with abdominal pain, palpable mass, and currant jelly stools.

Choice B [Persistence of the vitelline (omphaloenteric) duct] is hallmark of Meckel diverticulum, which presents with painless gastrointestinal bleeding.

Choice D [Narrowing or blockage of the duodenum] is associated with Duodenal atresia, which is associated with a double bubble on imaging.

Choice E [Part of the intestine protrudes through the umbilical opening in the abdominal muscle] is associated with an umbilical hernia, which is characterized by a soft mass either at, slightly above, slightly below, or to one side of the umbilicus.

94. GASTROINTESTINAL/NUTRITION – OBESITY [HEALTH MAINTENANCE]

For most patients with Obesity despite comprehensive lifestyle intervention, an incretin-based therapy (eg, Tirzepatide, Semaglutide) [choice D] is the preferred first-line pharmacotherapy.

Other options include alternative glucagon-like peptide 1 (GLP-1) receptor agonists (eg, Liraglutide), Phentermine-Topiramate, Naltrexone-Bupropion, Orlistat, or single-agent Phentermine.

Candidates for bariatric surgery [choice A] include adults with a BMI ≥35 kg/m^2, or a BMI of 30 - 34.9 kg/m^2 with type 2 diabetes.

Choice C [Phentermine-Topiramate] is alternative therapy, but Topiramate increases the risk for Nephrolithiasis, making Tirzepatide a better option.

95. NEUROLOGY – GUILLAIN-BARRÉ SYNDROME [LABS AND DIAGNOSTIC STUDIES]

Albuminocytological dissociation (elevated CSF protein count with a normal white blood cell count usually <5 cells/mm^3 [choice A] but may be elevated up to 50 cells/mm^3) is the classic CSF finding of Guillain Barré syndrome (GBS).

Hallmark features of GBS include

- progressive and symmetric ascending flaccid muscle weakness (lower motor neuron symptoms)
- absent or depressed deep tendon reflexes.
- sensory symptoms or dysautonomia may also be seen.

Choice B [Increased opening pressure with otherwise normal CSF parameters] is hallmark of Idiopathic intracranial hypertension, which presents with headache, visual changes, papilledema, and/or cranial nerve 6 palsy.

Choice C [Normal glucose, increased protein, increased white cells (predominantly lymphocytes)] is hallmark of Viral meningitis or Encephalitis.

Choice D [Increased IgG and IgG oligoclonal bands] is hallmark of Multiple sclerosis.

Choice E [Decreased glucose, increased protein, increased white cells (predominantly neutrophils)] is hallmark of Tuberculosis or fungal meningitis.

96. MUSCULOSKELETAL – OSTEOPOROSIS [HEALTH MAINTENANCE]

The patient has a normal T score (≥-1.0), so she requires no additional therapy [choice E].
T score compares bone density with the bone density of a young woman.

Osteoporosis: bone density T-score -2.5 or less, in which Bisphosphonates may be indicated [choice C].
Osteopenia: T-score between -1.0 and -2.5.

Choice A [Advise her to switch to low-impact aerobic activities] is incorrect because high-impact exercises reduce Osteoporosis risk.

97. MUSCULOSKELETAL – LEGG-CALVE-PERTHES DISEASE [MOST LIKELY]

The diagnosis of Legg-Calve-Perthes (LCP) Disease [choice D] requires a high index of suspicion as initial radiographs are often negative.
Legg-Calve-Perthes Disease is an idiopathic avascular necrosis of the proximal femoral epiphysis in children, with a peak at 4-8 years.
Patients with LCP may present with insidious onset of a limp (often painless); intermittent knee, hip, thigh, or groin pain; activity related pain, and gait disturbance (eg, antalgic limp or Trendelenburg gait.

Choice A [Juvenile idiopathic arthritis] is usually associated with more than 1 joint involvement. The affected joint is usually warm, swollen, and tender.
Choice B [Septic arthritis] usually presents with pain, swelling, erythema, and warmth over the affected joint. By 5 weeks, radiologic evidence of lytic lesions would most likely be seen.
Choice C [Slipped capital femoral epiphysis] is classically associated with a painful limp and would show evidence of the slipped capital femoral epiphysis on radiographs. This patient has negative radiographs.
Choice E [Developmental dysplasia of the hip] usually presents much earlier in life.

98. GENITOURINARY – CRYPTORCHIDISM [HEALTH MAINTENANCE]

Surgical treatment with orchiopexy [choice C] of congenitally undescended testes is recommended as soon as possible after 4 months of age and definitely should be completed before the child is 2 years old.
Spontaneous descent is rare after 4 months of age. In testes that remain undescended, there is an increased risk for Infertility, Testicular torsion, and Testicular cancer.

Hormonal therapy [choices D and E] have not proven to be efficacious in inducing testicular descent. However, hormonal therapy may be adjunctive to surgical therapy to improve fertility.
Choice A [Surgical referral for orchiectomy] may be indicated for Cryptorchidism detected in adulthood.

99. PSYCHIATRY AND BEHAVIORAL – GENDER DYSPHORIA [PROFESSIONAL PRACTICE]

The initial management of Gender dysphoria should include assessment of safety [choice C], nonjudgmental support, and child psychiatry and psychology referral.
The treatment of gender dysphoria is controversial and so the most important initial step is supporting services.

Gender dysphoria (previously gender identity disorder), according to the Diagnostic and Statistical Manual of Mental Disorders, is defined as a "marked incongruence between their experienced or expressed gender and the one they were assigned at birth."

100. CARDIOLOGY – ATRIAL FIBRILLATION [HEALTH MAINTENANCE].
Factor Xa inhibitors, such as Rivaroxaban [choice C], Apixaban, Edoxaban, or Direct thrombin inhibitors (eg, Dabigatran) are indicated for patients with a CHA_2DS_2VASC score of ≥2 to reduce the incidence of stroke and other arterial events.

This patient has a CHA_2DS_2VASC score of 4:
- 66-year-old (1 point)
- Female (1 point)
- Hypertension (1 point)
- Type 2 Diabetes mellitus (1 point).

Based on her score of 4, her Stroke risk is 4.8% per year and 6.7% risk of stroke, TIA, or systemic embolism.

Patients with a CHA_2DS_2VASC score of 1 may benefit from Aspirin [choice B].

1. A 22-year-old male is found to have the following rhythm on the heart monitor (see photo).

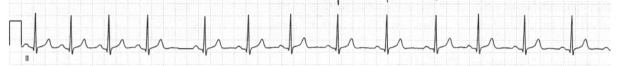

Which of the following is the most likely diagnosis?
a. Sinus arrhythmia
b. Sinus bradycardia
c. Premature atrial complexes
d. First-degree atrioventricular block
e. Mobitz-1 second degree atrioventricular block

Photo credit:
Ewingdo, CC BY-SA 4.0 <https://creativecommons.org/licenses/by-sa/4.0>, via Wikimedia Commons

2. A 38-year-old female is complaining of fatigue, recent easy bruising, and epistaxis 2 days ago that spontaneously resolved. She has no past medical history. She has not noticed any bleeding since this event and is currently asymptomatic. She denies fevers, chills, dyspnea, headaches, or menorrhagia. On examination, lower extremity petechiae are noted, with otherwise normal examination.
- WBC count 8,100/mm^3 (5,000-10,000)
- Hemoglobin 13.4 g/dL (11-15)
- Hematocrit: 39% (36-44)
- Platelet count: 33,000/mm^3 (150,000–450,000)
- PT 11 seconds (11-13)
- aPTT 31 seconds (25-35).

LDH level is normal, and a megakaryocyte is seen on peripheral smear. Which of the following is the first line management of this patient?
a. Splenectomy
b. Intravenous Immunoglobulin
c. Prednisone
d. Platelet infusion
e. Observation and monitoring

3. A 25-year-old male presents to the clinic with polyuria, dizziness, headache, and mild confusion. Physical examination is notable for moist mucous membranes. Initial labs reveal:
- serum sodium 130 mEq/L (135-145)
- serum osmolality 262 mmol/kg (275-295)
- urine sodium 17 mmol/L
- urine osmolality 96 mmol/kg.

Which of the following is the most likely etiology of his presentation?
a. Primary (psychogenic) polydipsia
b. Vomiting
c. Nephrotic syndrome
d. Syndrome of inappropriate ADH secretion
e. Diabetes insipidus (AVP deficiency or resistance)

4. A 54-year-old male presents to the ED after ingesting a substance in a suicide attempt. He has developed flank pain, gross hematuria, and oliguria.
Urinalysis is positive for dumbbell-shaped calcium oxalate crystals.
Laboratory evaluation reveals
- Sodium 137 mEq/L (135-145)
- Potassium 3.7 mEq/L (3.5-5)
- Chloride 96 mEq/L (96-106)
- Serum CO2 7 mEq/L (22-26)

An ABG is performed:
- pH: 7.21 (7.35-7.45)
- PaO2: 96 mm Hg (80-100)
- paCO2: 20 mm Hg (35-45)
- HCO3: 7 mEq/L (22-26)

Which of the following is the most likely acid-base status of this patient?
a. Partially compensated high anion gap metabolic acidosis
b. Partially compensated respiratory acidosis
c. Partially compensated non-anion gap metabolic acidosis
d. Uncompensated non-anion gap metabolic acidosis
e. Uncompensated high anion gap metabolic acidosis

5. A 20-year-old male presents to the emergency department with dyspnea, fever, and lower extremity swelling. Physical examination is notable for fresh needle track marks in the antecubital fossa and a soft holosystolic murmur best head at the left parasternal border in the fourth intercostal space with increased intensity during inspiration. Which of the following is the most likely diagnosis?
a. Mitral regurgitation
b. Tricuspid stenosis
c. Hypertrophic cardiomyopathy
d. Tricuspid regurgitation
e. Mitral stenosis

6. A 2-year-old boy is being evaluated in the pediatric clinic for bilateral eye redness, crusting on his eyelids, right ear pain, and nasal congestion. On examination, T: 98.8°F (37.11°C), BP: 110/68 mmHg, P: 96/min, R: 18 breaths/minute, and SaO2: 99%. There is bilateral conjunctival erythema with minimal purulent discharge. Otoscopic examination reveals a bulging tympanic membrane (TM) in the right ear with fluid behind the TM that is opaque yellow in color. The left tympanic membrane is translucent and grey with a normal light reflex. Which of the following is the most likely etiologic organism for this patient's presentation?
a. Adenovirus
b. Moraxella catarrhalis
c. Nontypeable Haemophilus influenzae
d. Staphylococcus aureus
e. Streptococcus pneumoniae

7. A 22-year-old male presents with headache. He has been experiencing increased thirst, increased trips to the bathroom to urinate, and constant thirst. He has a history of Bipolar disorder that is well controlled. Initial labs reveal:
- Sodium 147 mEq/L (135-145)
- Urine osmolality 202 mOsm/kg (300-900)
- Serum osmolality 304 mOsm/kg (275-295)

After water deprivation:
- Urine osmolality 208 mOsm/kg (300-900)

After Desmopressin (DDAVP) administration:
- Urine osmolality 220 mOsm/kg (300-900)

Which of the following is the most likely etiology of this patient's symptoms and laboratory findings?

a. Dehydration
b. Lithium carbonate
c. Primary (Psychogenic) polydipsia
d. Syndrome of inappropriate ADH
e. Sodium valproate

8. A 48-year-old female with a history of Leiomyoma undergoes an elective hysterectomy. After the procedure, she is given IV fluids and due to large blood loss, she is transfused a total of 4 units packed red blood cells in the ICU. 3 hours after transfusion, she develops breathlessness. Vitals reveal a temperature of 98.8°F (37.1°C), blood pressure 180/94 mmHg (baseline prior to transfusion was 120/70 mmHg), pulse 120/min, respiratory rate 44/min, and SaO2 87% on room air. Physical examination is notable for bilateral rhonchi and a third heart sound. Chest radiographs are obtained (see photo).

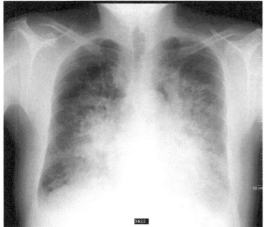

In addition to discontinuing the RBC transfusion and oxygenation, which of the following is the recommended management?

a. IM Epinephrine
b. IV Vancomycin plus Cefepime
c. Endotracheal intubation
d. IV Furosemide
e. Oral Acetaminophen

Photo credit:
Case courtesy of Tomas Jurevicius, Radiopaedia.org, rID: 48089

9. A 20-year-old female at 13 weeks gestation presents to the ED with vaginal bleeding and abdominal cramping since this morning. On the way to the emergency department, she passed large amounts of blood clots and white tissue. Since then, the abdominal cramping and bleeding have significantly improved. Her last prenatal visit 2 weeks ago showed an intrauterine pregnancy. Vitals are normal. Pelvic examination noted a nontender uterus and a closed cervix. Initial labs reveal blood type A negative; hemoglobin 12 g/dL (11.5-13), and a white cell count 6,500 cells/mm^3 (5,000-10,000). Which of the following is recommended at this time?
a. Dilation and evacuation with electric vacuum aspiration
b. Single dose Misoprostol 800 mcg per vagina (four 200 mcg tablets)
c. Anti-D immune globulin 100 mcg (500 international units)
d. IV Ceftriaxone 1 gram plus oral Doxycycline 200 mg IV
e. Mifepristone 200 mg orally followed in 24 hours by Misoprostol 800 micrograms given vaginally (typically given as four 200 microgram tablets)

10. A 6-year-old male is brought to the pediatrician's office by his mother for evaluation of fever. He has been much less active than usual and has been complaining of muscle aches. He recently returned from spending the summer with his grandmother in Vermont. Vitals are temperature of 100.4°F (38.0°C), pulse 95, blood pressure 95/65 mmHg, and respirations 24/min. The following skin lesion is seen (see photo).

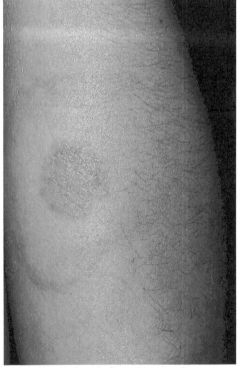

Which of the following is the most appropriate next step in management of this patient?
a. Doxycycline
b. Ceftriaxone
c. Amoxicillin
d. Azithromycin
e. Enzyme immunoassay for IgM and IgG antibodies to *B. burgdorferi*

11. A 35-year-old woman presents with joint stiffness and pain of the hands and wrists for the last two months. Her symptoms are most severe in the morning and improve in the afternoon. She reports an unintentional loss of 15 pounds over the course of 3 months as well as fatigue. On physical examination, there is swelling, warmth, bogginess, and tenderness at the metacarpophalangeal and proximal interphalangeal joints. Which of the following is most specific for the most likely diagnosis?
a. Rheumatoid factor
b. Anti-cyclic citrullinated protein antibodies
c. Anti-Smith antibodies
d. Anti-nuclear antibodies
e. Anti-La

12. A 7-year-old girl presents with fatigue, rash on her extremities, and epistaxis this morning. 6 days ago, she experienced watery diarrhea that became bloody and spontaneously resolved. Vitals reveal a temperature of 98.8°F (37.1°C) and blood pressure 110/70 mmHg. Scattered petechiae on the legs and pale conjunctiva are noted without scleral icterus. Initial labs reveal:
- creatinine 2.1 (0.6-1.2).
- Hemoglobin 8.2 g/dL (10-15)
- Hematocrit 25% (36-44)
- Reticulocyte count 11% (0.5-2.5)
- platelet count 72,400/mm^3 (150,000–450,000)
- PT 12 seconds (11-13)
- aPTT 33 seconds (25-35).

Which of the following is the most likely diagnosis?
a. IgA Vasculitis (Henoch-Schoenlein purpura)
b. thrombotic thrombocytopenic purpura (TTP)
c. Idiopathic thrombocytopenic purpura (ITP)
d. Von Willebrand disease
e. Hemolytic uremic syndrome (HUS)

13. A 20-year-old, G1P1, is complaining of midline lower abdominal pain and fever. She gave birth to a healthy baby boy at 38 weeks gestation via Cesarean section. Vitals reveal a temperature of 101°F (38°C), pulse 114/min, and blood pressure 110/70 mmHg. There is mid abdominal and uterine tenderness with foul-smelling lochia. The surgical site is clean without dehiscence, erythema, or drainage. Initial labs reveal a white cell count of 19,200 cells/mm^3 (5,000-10,000). Which of the following is the most appropriate management of this patient?
a. Dilation and evacuation
b. IV Clindamycin and Gentamicin
c. IV Vancomycin
d. IV Metronidazole and Trimethoprim-sulfamethoxazole
e. IV Cefazolin

14. A 23-year-old female G2P1 presents for routine prenatal care at 13 weeks gestation. She denies any symptoms or any significant past medical history. Her last pregnancy was complicated by Preeclampsia with severe features, requiring immediate Cesarean section at 35 weeks gestation. Vital signs are a blood pressure of 128/84 mmHg and examination reveals a fundal height slightly above the pubic symphysis. Which of the following is recommended in this patient for reduction of the risk of Preeclampsia during this pregnancy?
a. Low-dose Aspirin
b. Magnesium sulfate
c. 17 alpha-hydroxyprogesterone
d. Folic acid
e. Nifedipine

15. A 25-year-old male presents with a 2-week history of increasing fatigue, dyspnea on exertion, fever, and dry cough. He is s/p renal transplant for rapidly progressive Glomerulonephritis. Vitals signs are temperature of 103°F (38.89°C), pulse 104/min, blood pressure 122/72 mmHg, respiratory rate 24/min, and SpO2: 89% on room air. Physical examination is notable for diffuse crackles bilaterally. A chest radiograph is obtained (see photo).

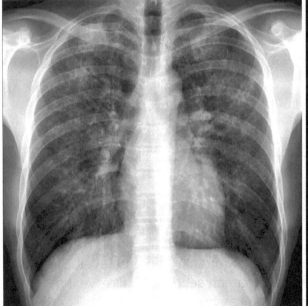 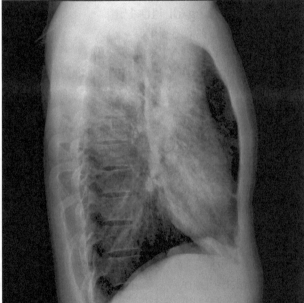

Initial labs are significant for serum lactate dehydrogenase 430 U/L (119-229) and serum 1-3 β-D glucan level 111.8 pg/ml (<6.0). Which of the following is the initial treatment of choice?
a. Doxycycline
b. Trimethoprim-sulfamethoxazole
c. Ceftriaxone plus Azithromycin
d. Isoniazid, Rifampin, Ethambutol, and Streptomycin
e. Ciprofloxacin

Photo credit:
Case courtesy of Andrew Dixon, Radiopaedia.org, rID: 9613

16. A previously healthy 3-year-old boy is brought to the ED for "breathing funny". For 2 days, he had nasal congestion, sneezing, and clear nasal drainage. His parents became concerned when he developed a low-grade fever, hoarseness, a "hacking" cough, and high-pitched noisy breathing worse at night. On physical exam, a deep brassy cough, inspiratory stridor at rest, mild accessory muscle use, and chest retractions are noted. He does not appear anxious, agitated, pale, or fatigued. Which of the following is the most likely etiology?
a. Parvovirus B19
b. Parainfluenza virus
c. Haemophilus influenzae type B
d. Foreign body aspiration
e. Respiratory syncytial virus

17. A 57-year-old man is complaining of intense pruritus after showering, headache, blurred vision, and a burning sensation in his fingers and toes. Physical examination reveals splenomegaly and engorged retinal veins. Laboratory findings include:
- hemoglobin 20 g/dL (12.1-15.1)
- hematocrit 61% (36-48)
- white blood cell count 9,200/mm^3 (5,000-10,000)
- platelet count of 388,000/mm^3 (150,000-450,000)
- Erythropoietin levels 1.3 mIU/mL (2.6-18.5)
Molecular testing revealed the *JAK2* V671F mutation.
Which of the following is the most appropriate initial management of choice?
a. Splenectomy
b. Dabigatran
c. Allogeneic stem cell transplant
d. Phlebotomy
e. Prednisone

18. A 43-year-old patient with a history of generalized seizure disorder develops 10/10 boring epigastric pain radiating to the back. The pain is worse when lying supine and improves slightly with sitting forward. Physical examination reveals epigastric tenderness. Initial lab values reveal
- AST 98 IU/L (8–42)
- ALT 43 IU/L (7–40)
- Amylase 152 IU/L (40-140)
- Lipase 200 IU/L (0-160)
- Serum calcium 7.2 mEq/L (8.5-10)
Which of the following medications is most likely responsible for these findings?
a. Carbamazepine
b. Lamotrigine
c. Valproic acid
d. Phenytoin
e. Topiramate

19. A 34-year-old female presents to the clinic with irritability, anxiety, insomnia, increased appetite, poor concentration at work, and emotional instability. The symptoms occur consistently a couple weeks before onset of her menses and has had a negative impact on her romantic relationship and her position at work. She has missed many days of work, and it frequently causes arguments with her fiancée. Which of the following is the recommended initial management of this patient?
a. Combined Drospirenone/Ethinyl estradiol
b. Leuprolide
c. Bilateral oophorectomy
d. Alprazolam
e. Citalopram

20. A 23-year-old female presents to the clinic with fatigue, especially towards the evening, and difficulty reading for long periods of time due to double vision. She denies any sensory symptoms. Physical examination is notable for bilateral ptosis and 4/5 strength in all 4 extremities. Pupillary reflex is intact, there are no sensory deficits, and deep tendon reflexes are 2+. Which of the following is the primary pathophysiology of her presenting symptoms and signs?
a. Autoantibodies against the postsynaptic acetylcholine receptor
b. Autoantibodies against the presynaptic voltage-gated calcium channels
c. Demyelination of the Schwann cells in the peripheral nervous system
d. Demyelination of the oligodendrocytes in the central nervous system
e. Neuromuscular deficits due to a neurotoxin elaborated by the bacterium *Clostridium botulinum*.

21. A 65-year-old male presents with sudden onset of ataxia, left leg weakness, and soiling of his clothes with urine due to inability to control his bladder. Neurological examination reveals left-sided weakness more pronounced in the left leg than the left arm and gaze deviation to the right. Increased tone with spasticity, hyperextension, plegia, and loss of sensation in the left leg are noted. Which of the following is the most likely diagnosis?
a. Right Middle cerebral artery stroke
b. Left Middle cerebral artery stroke
c. Right Anterior cerebral artery stroke
d. Left Anterior cerebral artery stroke
e. Right Posterior cerebral artery stroke

22. A 27-year-old man presents to his physician with his wife after a referral from a fertility clinic. They have been trying to conceive for the past 15 months without success. He is complaining of decrease in energy. On examination, he is tall, lean in stature, and has long extremities. He has sparse, thin hair in the axillary and pubic areas, decreased muscle mass, and atrophied small, firm testes. Initial labs reveal a serum testosterone of 6.1 nmol/L (11-36). Analysis of his sperm reveals azoospermia. Which of the following would most likely be seen on evaluation of this patient?
a. Reduced luteinizing hormone
b. Elevated follicle-stimulating hormone
c. XO Mocaism on karyotype analysis
d. Elevated 5 alpha-reductase activity
e. Absent gonadotropin releasing hormone

23. A 42-year-old woman presents to her primary care provider complaining of recurrent episodes of moderate dull right upper quadrant discomfort, radiating to the right shoulder blade. The episodes typically last at least 30 minutes, plateauing within 1-2 hours, with an entire attack lasting 2-3 hours. The pain is precipitated with eating fast food meals. She denies fever and chills. She has a history of Obesity and Dyslipidemia. Physical examination is unremarkable. Initial labs reveal:
- WBC count 7,200/mm³ (5,000-10,000)
- Total bilirubin 0.9 mg/dL (up to 1.2)
- ALT 53 U/L (7-55)
- Alkaline phosphatase 61 U/L (44-147)
- GGT 21 IU/L (0-30).

Based on the most likely diagnosis, which of the following is the initial management of choice?
a. ERCP with manometry
b. NPO, IV fluids and rest the pancreas
c. NPO, IV fluids, Metronidazole + Ciprofloxacin + Cholecystectomy when stable
d. NPO, IV fluids Metronidazole + Ciprofloxacin + ERCP when stable
e. Elective cholecystectomy

24. A 24-year-old female is being evaluated by her primary care provider for fatigue. She often craves eating ice chips. On examination, conjunctival pallor and concave shape of the fingernails are noted. A complete blood count with peripheral smear reveals a mean corpuscular volume of 70 fL (80-100) and hypochromia. Which of the following laboratory values is the most useful to test to establish of the most likely etiology?
a. Total serum iron binding capacity
b. Serum iron level
c. Reticulocyte count
d. Serum ferritin level
e. Serum transferrin saturation

25. A 33-year-old male presents to the clinic with constipation and a palpable mass in the neck. Physical examination is notable for decreased bowel sounds and a mass on the left side of the thyroid that moves freely with swallowing.
Initial lab workup is positive for:
- serum TSH 1.4 mIU/L (0.4-4)
- serum parathyroid hormone (iPTH) 432 pg/mL (10–65)
- serum calcium 11.8 mg/dL (8.5-10)
- serum phosphate 2.9 mg/dL (3.4 -4.5)
- serum calcitonin 983 pg/mL (≤185)

Which of the following is the most likely diagnosis?
a. Secondary hyperparathyroidism
b. Multiple endocrine neoplasia I
c. Multiple endocrine neoplasia II (formerly IIA)
d. Multiple endocrine neoplasia III (formerly IIB)
e. Graves' disease

26. A 48-year-old female is being evaluated in the clinic for daytime sleepiness and morning headaches. Her husband complains that she snores loudly, often gasping and choking in her sleep. She has a past medical history of Allergic rhinitis and nasal congestion. She drinks 2 beers nightly and has a 20-pack year smoking history. Her BMI is 36 kg/m². Which of the following clinical features has the strongest association with her presentation?
a. Alcohol use
b. Female gender
c. Obesity
d. Nasal congestion
e. Hypertension

27. A 16-year-old boy presents to his pediatrician. He wants to begin to play football and has begun weightlifting and strength training in preparation. He has type 1 Diabetes mellitus and uses NPH in the morning and evening as well as Insulin aspart prior to meals. His home serum glucose levels range from 80-120 mg/dL. He has not experienced episodes of hypoglycemia. Physical examination is unremarkable. Labs show serum glucose of 75 mg/dL (70-110) and Hemoglobin A1C 6.3%. Which of the following is the most appropriate management of his Diabetes based on his decision to train and play football?
a. Decrease the dosage of the NPH and Insulin aspart
b. Discontinue NPH and initiate regular Insulin on a sliding scale
c. Consume large amounts of carbohydrates after strength training
d. Restrict training sessions to less than 45 minutes
e. Drink orange juice prior to weightlifting

28. A 36-year-old female is complaining of facial redness and "acne" involving her nose, cheeks, forehead, and chin. She is also experiencing flushing of her face with alcohol, prolonged sun exposure, and hot coffee. On examination, there are inflammatory papules and pustules without comedones. Urine beta-hCG is negative. Which of the following is the initial first-line medical management in this patient?
a. Oral Doxycycline
b. Topical Metronidazole
c. Laser and intense pulsed light
d. Oral Isotretinoin
e. Topical Hydrocortisone

29. A 25-year-old male who recently underwent open reduction and internal fixation of a Galeazzi fracture is complaining of sudden onset of dyspnea at rest and exertion, pleuritic chest pain, hemoptysis, and cough. Vitals reveal a temperature of 98.8°F (37.11°C), blood pressure 112/72 mmHg, pulse 118/min, respirations 24/min, and SpO2 94% on room air. The lungs are clear to auscultation and the cardiac examination is within normal limits. Initial labs reveal a serum creatinine of 0.7 mg/dL (0.6-1.2). A chest radiograph is unremarkable. Which of the following is the next recommended step in the evaluation of this patient?
a. D-dimer level
b. Lower extremity venous Ultrasound with Doppler
c. Venography
d. Ventilation-Perfusion scan
e. Helical CT angiography

30. A 65-year-old woman presents with an 8-month history of recurrent low-grade fever, abdominal fullness, and moderately reduced exercise tolerance. Physical examination revealed several palpable cervical and axillary lymph nodes (1-2 cm) that were non-tender and freely mobile, along with palpable splenomegaly.
- leukocyte count 32,000/mm³ (5,000-10,000)
- hemoglobin 9.8 g/dL (12-16)
- platelet count of 145,000/mm³ (150,000-450,000)
- lymphocyte count 26.7 ×10/uL (1–3)
- neutrophil count 1,900/mm³ (2,500- 7,000).

Peripheral smear is performed (see photo)

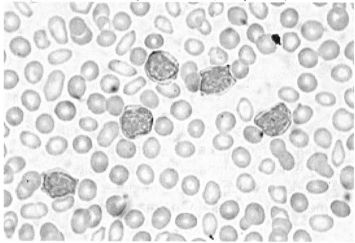

Which one of the following is the most likely cause of his anemia?
a. Acute lymphoblastic leukemia
b. Acute myelogenous leukemia
c. Chronic lymphocytic leukemia
d. Chronic myelogenous leukemia
e. Multiple myeloma

Photo credit:
Ed Uthman, CC BY-SA 2.0 <https://creativecommons.org/licenses/by-sa/2.0>, via Wikimedia Commons

31. A 17-year-old male presents to the ED with severe and acute-onset left abdominal pain and nausea that awoke him from sleep 4 hours ago. The pain is sharp and radiates to his left thigh. Vitals are T: 98.6°F (37.4°C), blood pressure 126/81 mmHg, pulse 119/min, respirations 14/min, and SpO2: 99% on room air. The abdomen is soft, nontender, and nondistended. Scrotal examination reveals an elevated left testicle that is diffusely tender and swollen. Stroking of the patient's inner thigh on the left side does not result in retraction of the left testicle. Which of the following is the most appropriate next step in the management of this patient?
a. IV Ceftriaxone and Azithromycin
b. CT scan of abdomen and pelvis
c. Testicular Doppler ultrasound
d. Observation and IV Morphine
e. Surgical exploration

32. A 21-year-old male presents to the clinic complaining of fatigue, myalgias, weight loss, dizziness, and nausea for 3 months. Vitals reveal a blood pressure of 110/70 mmHg supine and 90/54 mmHg while sitting. Physical examination is notable for patchy hyperpigmentation on the inner surface of his lips and buccal mucosa. A basic metabolic panel reveals:
Na+: 132 mEq/L (135-145)
Cl-: 104 mEq/L (96-106)
K+: 6.0 mEq/L (3.5-5)
CO2: 16 mEq/L (22-26)
Glucose: 64 mg/dL (70-110).
Which of the following is the most likely underlying etiology of this patient's symptoms?
a. Tuberculosis
b. Adrenal hemorrhage
c. Autoimmune adrenalitis
d. Aldosteronoma
e. Bilateral adrenal infarction

33. A 10-year-old male is being evaluated for fever, chills, sore throat, and decreased appetite. He denies cough, runny nose, or sneezing. On examination, there are enlarged tender anterior cervical lymph nodes. There is tonsillar erythema, edema, and white exudates. There is no hepatosplenomegaly. A rapid streptococcal antigen detection test is negative. Which of the following is the recommended next step in the management of this patient?
a. Heterophile antibody test
b. Diphtheria antigen testing
c. Throat culture
d. Administer Penicillin VK
e. Influenza A and B antigen

34. A 60-year-old male presents with worsening vision loss in the left eye. It began as a bright flash of light, followed by small shadowy specks floating in his left visual field. Which of the following would be most associated with the most likely diagnosis?
a. Pain with extraocular movements
b. Vision loss starting in the periphery and then moving centrally
c. Conjunctival erythema
d. Central scotoma
e. Halos around light

35. A 20-year-old female with a history of Anorexia nervosa is being evaluated for bleeding gums, arthralgia, and delayed wound healing. Physical examination is positive for swollen, erythematous, and bleeding gums. Perifollicular hemorrhage, ecchymoses, and coiled hairs are also noted. This patient is most likely deficient in which of the following vitamins?
a. Retinol
b. Cholecalciferol
c. Niacin
d. Ascorbic acid
e. Thiamine

36. A 76-year-old male is brought to the ED from a nursing home via ambulance for a 48-hour history of progressive abdominal cramping, nausea, and several episodes of vomiting. He has a history of chronic constipation. Vitals are stable. Physical examination is notable for diffuse abdominal tenderness to palpation, without rebound tenderness, guarding, or rigidity. Laboratory studies are notable for leukocytosis, and a normal serum lactate. Abdominal radiographs are obtained (see photo).

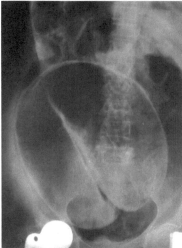

Which of the following is the most likely etiology of his presentation?
a. Functional obstruction of the small bowel
b. Torsion of the sigmoid bowel around its blood supply
c. Mechanical obstruction of the small bowel
d. Telescoping of one part of the bowel into another part of the bowel
e. Inadequate blood supply to the large intestine

Photo credit:
Case courtesy of Wael Nemattalla, Radiopaedia.org, rID: 10633

37. A 7-year-old male presents to the clinic complaining of fatigue and increased bruising. Physical examination is notable for a short stature, café au lait spots on the trunk, extremity petechiae, pallor, and left thumb hypoplasia. Initial labs reveal:
- Hemoglobin: 9.4 g/dL (13.5-17.5)
- Hematocrit: 29% (40-54)
- Platelet count 32,200 cells/mm^3 (150,000-450,000)
- Mean corpuscular volume (MCV): 101 fL (80-100)
- White cell count 4,100/mm^3 (5,000-10,000)
- Reticulocyte count 0.1% (0.5-2.5)

Which of the following is the most likely diagnosis?
a. Sickle cell disease
b. Fanconi anemia
c. Immune thrombotic thrombocytopenia
d. Hemolytic uremic syndrome
e. Neurofibromatosis type 1

38. A 42-year-old woman presents to the clinic with a 4-month history of fatigue, always feeling thirsty, dry eyes, and dyspareunia. She has developed multiple caries that her dentist attributed to dry mouth. Physical examination is notable for bilateral swollen parotid glands, conjunctival erythema, dry oral mucous membranes, and a positive Schirmer test. This patient is at greatest risk for which of the following complications?
a. Acute onset of vision loss
b. Lymphoma
c. Aortic aneurysm
d. Deep vein thrombosis
e. Peritonsillar abscess

39. A 44-year-old woman with no significant medical history presents to the clinic with a 3-month history of gradual onset of weakness. She has difficulty getting out of chairs and raising her arms above her head. She denies muscle pain or stiffness. Physical examination reveals 4/5 muscle strength in the quadriceps and deltoid muscles bilaterally and 5/5 distal muscle strength. There are violaceous skin eruptions on the upper eyelids and midfacial erythema involving the nasolabial folds. Labs reveal increased creatine phosphokinase. Which of the following is the most likely diagnosis?
a. Systemic lupus erythematosus
b. Diffuse systemic sclerosis (Scleroderma)
c. Polymyalgia rheumatica
d. Fibromyalgia
e. Dermatomyositis

40. In evaluating a patient with dysphagia and hoarseness, a palate droop, deviation of the uvula to the right, and loss of the gag reflex is noted. Which of the following would most likely be responsible for these findings?
a. Right Cranial nerve 9 palsy
b. Left Cranial nerve 9 palsy
c. Left Cranial nerve 10 palsy
d. Right cranial nerve 10 palsy
e. Left cranial nerve 12 palsy

41. A 45-year-old male presents to the ED for confusion, disorientation, and restlessness. He has a history of Major depression treated with Escitalopram and GERD treated with Pantoprazole. He was seen in urgent care 48 hours ago and placed on Linezolid for MRSA infection. Vitals reveal a temperature of 39°C (102.2°F), blood pressure 170/94 mmHg, pulse 120/min, and respirations 26/min. He is diaphoretic, tremulous, and shivering. Neurological examination reveals myoclonus more pronounced in the legs, hyperactive bowel sounds, hyperreflexia, and mydriasis. Which of the following is the most likely diagnosis?
a. Neuroleptic malignant syndrome
b. Malignant hyperthermia
c. Serotonin syndrome
d. Alcohol withdrawal
e. Anticholinergic toxicity

42. A 32-year-old male with no past medical history presents to the emergency department with sharp anterior chest pain. The pain worsens when he is supine and with deep inspiration. Vitals reveal a temperature of 100.1°F (37.8°C), blood pressure 118/74 mmHg, pulse 104/min, and respirations 22/min. The rest of the examination is unremarkable. An ECG is obtained (see photo).

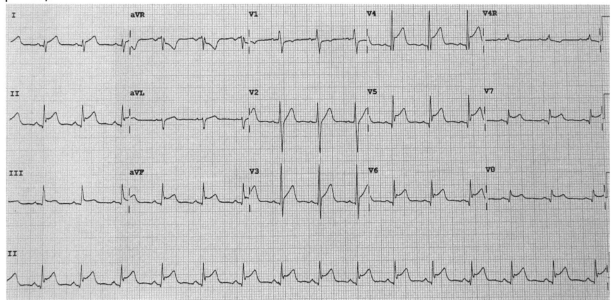

Which of the following is the most appropriate initial management of this patient?
a. Prednisone
b. Naproxen
c. Pericardiocentesis
d. Aspirin and Nitroglycerin
e. Indomethacin and Colchicine

Photo credit:
James Heilman, MD, CC BY-SA 4.0 <https://creativecommons.org/licenses/by-sa/4.0>, via Wikimedia Commons

43. A previously healthy 14-year-old male presents to the emergency department with back pain, abdominal pain, fatigue, and dark urine since last night. 2 days ago, he tested positive for SARS-CoV-2 after experiencing fever, nasal congestion, and cough. Vitals are stable. Scleral icterus and conjunctival pallor are noted. Initial labs are positive for a hemoglobin of 11 g/dL (14-18). Peripheral blood smear reveals Heinz bodies, bite cells, and blister cells. Which of the following is the most likely etiology of his presentation?
a. Oxidative damage to red blood cells
b. Red blood cell cytoskeleton, resulting in a red cell membrane defect
c. Reduction in the synthesis of globin chains
d. Point mutation in the beta globin gene
e. IgM autoantibodies against red blood cell [RBC] antigens

44. A 28-year-old male is brought to the emergency department via ambulance after being picked up from a bar. He has a chronic history of alcohol and Fentanyl misuse. He is noted to have dry vomitus on his shirt and poor dentition. He is producing sputum with a foul putrid odor. Vitals reveal a temperature of 102°F (38.89°C), blood pressure 110/74 mmHg, pulse 118/min, respirations 22/min, and SpO2 93% on room air. There are right-sided crackles. Chest radiographs are obtained (see photo).

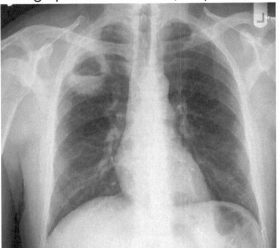 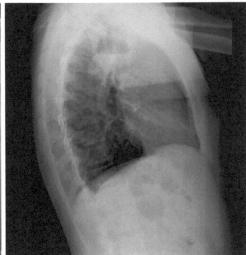

Which of the following is the most likely etiology of his presentation?
a. Extension of infection from parapneumonic sources
b. Aspiration of fluid or endogenous secretions into the lower airways
c. Exposure to contaminated water sources
d. Inhalation of aerosolized droplets
e. Hematogenous spread of pathogenic bacteria

Photo credit
Case courtesy of Abu-Rahmeh Zuhair, Radiopaedia.org, rID: 30554

45. A 24-year-old female presents to the ED for left lower quadrant pain. The pain as sharp, shooting, intermittent, and radiates to her left groin. Physical examination is remarkable for left flank tenderness on palpation.
Urinalysis reveals:
- Red blood cells 12/hpf (<5)
- Nitrites: negative
- Leukocyte esterase: negative
Urine Beta-hCG is negative.
Which of the following is the next best step in management of this patient?
a. KUB (kidneys, ureters, and bladder) plain radiographs
b. Intravenous pyelogram
c. Renal ultrasonography
d. Non-contrast helical CT of the abdomen and pelvis
e. Cystoscopy

46. A 15-year-old boy presents to his pediatrician for right knee pain for 4 weeks. The pain is most noticeable when he climbs stairs, jumps, or squats during soccer practice. He denies any trauma. Physical examination is notable for bony prominence and tenderness with palpation of the right tibial tubercle. The pain is reproduced by extending the knee against resistance. Which of the following is the recommended management of this patient?
a. Knee immobilizer and crutches for weightbearing for 2 weeks
b. Surgical ossicle excision
c. Post activity ice, Ibuprofen, and use of a protective pad
d. Complete avoidance of soccer for 4-6 weeks
e. Triamcinolone injection within the joint space

47. A 65-year-old male presents to the clinic complaining of transient "sticking" of steak and bread, which causes him to have to chew more carefully and eat slower. Over the past few weeks, he has developed regurgitation of saliva and occasional regurgitation or vomiting of undigested food. He denies hoarseness, cough, or weight loss. He has a 20-year history of gastroesophageal reflux disease, for which he takes Nizatidine. Which of the following is the most appropriate next step?
a. Switch to Pantoprazole
b. Esophageal motility studies with barium
c. Esophageal ambulatory pH monitoring
d. Esophagogastroduodenoscopy
e. Esophageal manometry

48. A 3-month-old boy is being evaluated in the clinic for coughing spells, often associated with vomiting after the spells. On examination, he appears healthy until he develops a sustained dry coughing spell, followed by an inspiratory whoop, and perioral cyanosis. His lungs are clear to auscultation. Initial labs reveal lymphocytosis. His 4-year-old sibling has no symptoms and is up to date with his vaccinations. The patient is treated appropriately. Which of the following is the recommended management of his 4-year-old sibling?
a. No management is needed
b. Trimethoprim-sulfamethoxazole if he develops symptoms
c. Azithromycin
d. Administer a DTaP booster
e. Administer Oseltamivir

49. A 29-year-old female comes to the office complaining of cough, runny nose, sneezing, and body aches. At the beginning of the medical interview, she flirts with the provider and asks if he likes her dress with a deep cut plunging neck. When asking about her symptoms, she laughs excessively, lurches forward, and puts her hand on the provider's thigh. When she is told the provider will be back to reassess her after seeing a couple of patients, she pouts her lip, folds her arm, and tells the provider she is "dying" from her viral symptoms. Which of the following is the most likely diagnosis?
a. Illness anxiety disorder
b. Histrionic personality disorder
c. Borderline personality disorder
d. Narcissistic personality disorder
e. Somatic symptom disorder

50. A 62-year-old male is recently diagnosed with Cushing syndrome. He has a recent history of muscular weakness that improves with repeated muscle use. Review of systems is positive for a 30-pack year smoking history. Chest imaging is performed (see photo).

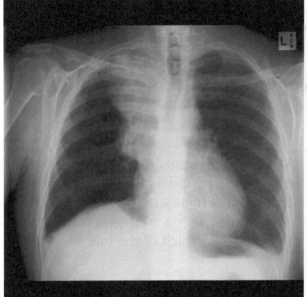 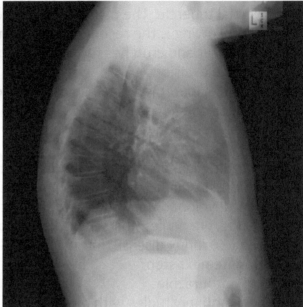

Which of the following is the recommended management?
a. Rifampin, Isoniazid, Pyrazinamide, Ethambutol
b. Surgical excision
c. Broad-spectrum antibiotics and sputum cytology
d. Combination chemotherapy
e. Radiation followed by surgical excision

Photo credit:
Case courtesy of Frank Gaillard, Radiopaedia.org, rID: 10494

51. A 13-year-old boy is evaluated for a palpable mass behind his right nipple. The mass has been gradually increasing in size over the last 3 months. He has no significant past medical history and is not on any medications. Physical examination is notable for mildly tender subareolar rubbery symmetrically shaped masses measuring 3 cm (1.2 in) in the right breast and 2 cm (0.78 in) in the left breast with no skin excess, nipple discharge, nor erythema. His pubic hair is Tanner stage 3 and testicular volume is 9 mL bilaterally (8-10). Which of the following is the best next step for this patient's condition?
a. Brief trial of Tamoxifen for three months
b. Testosterone therapy
c. Serum hCG, estradiol, testosterone, luteinizing hormone (LH), and dehydroepiandrosterone sulfate (DHEAS)
d. Observation and reassurance
e. Ultrasound of the breast tissues

52. A 56-year-old male presents with left-sided weakness, headache, dizziness, and difficulty concentrating. Physical examination reveals vertical nystagmus. The following is seen on imaging.

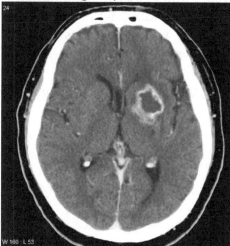

PCR assay of CSF for Epstein-Barr virus (EBV) DNA is positive. Which of the following is a risk factor for this patient's condition?
a. Late-stage HIV infection
b. Radiation exposure
c. Cigarette smoking
d. Multiple sclerosis
e. Diabetes mellitus

Photo credit:
Case courtesy of Frank Gaillard, Radiopaedia.org, rID: 8288

53. A 4-year-old boy presents to the urgent care clinic for a new rash. The rash began on both cheeks 48 hours ago. Since this morning, he has developed a rash on his trunk. He had fever, runny nose, and dry cough 2 days prior to the onset of the facial rash. On physical exam, there is an erythematous rash with circumoral pallor. There is a maculopapular lace-like reticulated rash on both arms. Which of the following is the most likely etiologic agent for his presentation?
a. Human herpesvirus 6
b. Coxsackie virus A16
c. Rubella virus
d. Group A streptococcus
e. Parvovirus B19

54. A 16-year-old girl presents to the clinic with her parents. She is sexually active and is going out of state to complete high school. She is concerned about being compliant with condoms and has trouble remembering to take her iron pills. She is desiring contraception. Which of the following is recommended in this patient?
a. Etonogestrel subdermal implant
b. Estrogen-progestin vaginal ring
c. Transdermal contraceptive patch
d. Combined estrogen-progestin oral contraceptives
e. Depot medroxyprogesterone acetate injection

55. A 34-year-old female presents to the clinic complaining of a small neck mass that she noticed when showering. She denies fatigue, cough, hoarseness, neck pain, or weight loss. She has smoked 1 pack of cigarettes per day since she was 25 years old. Physical examination is notable for a palpable nodule on the left side of the thyroid that is mobile with swallowing. There is no cervical lymphadenopathy. An ultrasound is performed, which confirms a 1.2 cm hyperechoic nodule in the left lobe. Thyroid function labs are drawn:

- Serum TSH: 0.2 mIU/L (0.5-5.0)

Urine beta-hCG is negative and basic metabolic panel is normal. Which of the following is the next best step in management?

a. Fine needle aspiration
b. Levothyroxine
c. Partial thyroidectomy
d. Radioactive iodine
e. Thyroid scintigraphy (Radioactive iodine uptake scan)

56. A 22-year-old male presents to the ED for weakness, malaise, thigh soreness, and dark-colored urine. He has been training excessively for a weightlifting competition. Physical examination is notable for muscle tenderness. An ECG is obtained (see photo).

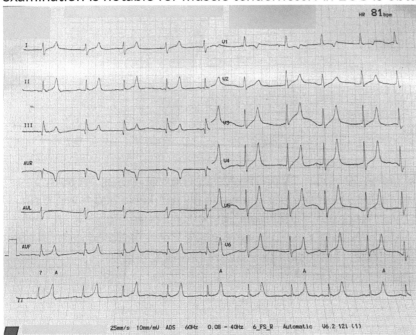

Based on the most likely diagnosis, IV administration of which of the following is the most appropriate next step?

a. Insulin with glucose
b. Sodium bicarbonate
c. Magnesium sulfate
d. Sodium polystyrene sulfonate
e. Calcium gluconate

Photo credit:
Dr. Michael-Joseph F. Agbayani and Dr. Eddieson Gonzales (Manila, Philippines), CC BY 4.0 <https://creativecommons.org/licenses/by/4.0>, via Wikimedia Commons

57. A 13-year-old boy is being evaluated after his mother states he is "out of control". He is resistant to many disciplinary measures she and his father have implemented. He breaks his curfew often, has failed a few classes, and has been suspended from school after physical fights with his classmates and stealing his professor's laptop off of his desk. When the professor confronted him about it, he was hostile, aggressive, and told him "you shouldn't have left it unattended if you didn't want it to be taken." Which of the following is the most likely diagnosis?
a. Narcissistic personality disorder
b. Oppositional defiant disorder
c. Antisocial personality disorder
d. Conduct disorder
e. Intermittent explosive disorder

58. A 50-year-old male presents with increasing fatigue, anorexia, nausea, and decreased urine output. Urinalysis is positive for broad waxy casts and proteinuria. GFR 15 mL/min per 1.73 m². Which of the following is the most common cause?
a. Polycystic kidney disease
b. Hypertension
c. Diabetes mellitus
d. Minimal change disease
e. Rapidly progressive glomerulonephritis

59. A 25-year-old prisoner at a correctional facility returns for an annual Tuberculin skin test (TST) reading. The TST was placed 48 hours ago. He has no significant past medical history denies fever, chills, dyspnea, cough, weight loss. The site of the TST shows 6 mm induration. Which of the following is the most appropriate next step?
a. Isoniazid + Vitamin B6 for 6 months duration
b. Rifampin daily for 4 months (4R)
c. Initiate Rifampin, Isoniazid, Pyrazinamide, Ethambutol
d. No further management at this time; continue routine screening
e. Chest radiograph

60. A 20-year-old female presents to the outpatient department for burning sensation with urination for 3 days. She has been urinating more often but denies any blood in her urine. She denies fever, chills, vaginal discharge, or flank pain. She has been in a monogamous relationship for the past 2 years and uses a Progesterone intrauterine device. Vitals are normal. On physical examination, there is mild tenderness to palpation in the suprapubic area without costovertebral angle tenderness. Urinalysis is positive for trace blood, 10 WBCs/hpf, positive leukocyte esterase and nitrites. Urine beta-hCG is negative. Which of the following is the most appropriate next step in management?
a. Urine culture
b. Nitrofurantoin
c. Doxycycline
d. Ciprofloxacin
e. Cystography

61. A 10-month-old boy presents with worsening constipation, poor feeding, poor ability to suck during feeding, and feeble cry. Physical examination reveals a temperature of 98.8°F, ptosis, poor head control, poor ability to suck, and lethargy. There is diffusely decreased tone, diffuse and symmetric hyporeflexia, and sluggish pupillary response. Which of the following is the most appropriate initial therapy?
a. Equine serum heptavalent immune globulin
b. Plasma exchange therapy
c. Human-derived immune globulin
d. Metronidazole
e. Penicillin G and antitoxin

62. A 35-year-old male is complaining of a 2-day history of nausea, vomiting, malaise, rash, and fever. CBC is notable for peripheral eosinophilia. Physical is notable for a maculopapular rash. Initial labs reveal a serum creatinine of 2.1 mg/dL (0.6-1.2) and BUN 21 mg/dL (7-20). Urinalysis is notable for 3 red cells/hpf (0-5), white cell casts, 1+ proteinuria, and no bacteria or red cell casts. Which of the following is most likely in this patient's recent history?
a. Flare of Systemic lupus erythematosus
b. Pharyngitis
c. Use of Penicillin V potassium
d. Use of Gentamicin
e. Hepatitis C virus

63. A 64-year-old man presents to his primary care physician after noticing blood in his urine, especially towards the end of voiding. He denies dysuria, abdominal pain, urinary frequency, or urgency. Medical history is unremarkable. He has a 20-pack year smoking history. Physical examination is within normal limits. Urinalysis demonstrates a large red blood cell count with normal red blood cell morphology. A cystoscopy is performed, revealing a mass protruding from the bladder wall. Which of the following is the patient's most likely occupation?
a. Coal miner
b. Demolition man of old buildings
c. Rubber manufacturing plant worker
d. Stonecutter
e. Oil refiner

64. A 50-year-old woman presents with intermittent episodes of severe dizziness. During the episodes, she hears "buzzing" sounds in her left ear, gets nauseous, and feels that the "room is spinning", making it difficult for her to walk. The episodes last for minutes up to 3 hours and resolve spontaneously. She also has periodic fluctuation of reduction in hearing "as if I am under water", intense left ear fullness, and head pressure. Vitals are stable. The Weber tests lateralized to the right. Which of the following is the most likely diagnosis?
a. Labyrinthitis
b. Ménière disease
c. Acoustic neuroma (Vestibular schwannoma)
d. Vestibular neuronitis
e. Benign paroxysmal positional vertigo

65. A 38-year-old male presents to the dermatology clinic for a 1-year history of discolored toenails that has become unsightly. Physical examination is notable for thickened yellow discoloration of the nail on the right first toe with involvement of the lunula and the entire width of the nail. Potassium hydroxide (KOH) preparation applied to nail clippings reveal septated hyphae and spores. Fungal culture confirms the most likely diagnosis. Which of the following is the first line therapy for this condition?
a. Oral Fluconazole
b. Oral Terbinafine
c. Oral Griseofulvin
d. Topical Ketoconazole
e. Topical Tree oil

66. A 56-year-old female presents to the emergency department with right wrist pain after a fall from height on an outstretched right wrist. Physical examination is notable for tenderness along the snuffbox and radial side of the right wrist and distal forearm without ecchymosis or soft tissue swelling. Radiographs are obtained. A wrist radiograph is performed.

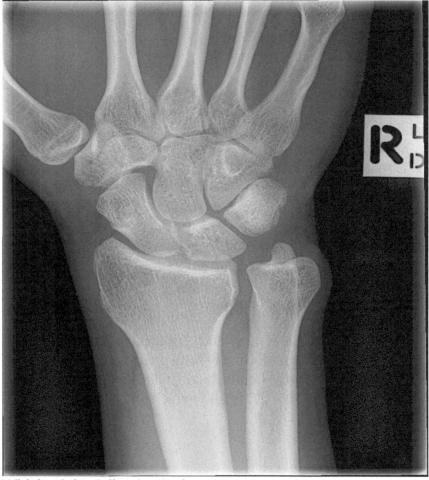

Which of the following is the most appropriate next step?
a. ACE wrap, ice application, and Naproxen
b. Open reduction and internal fixation
c. Ulnar gutter splint
d. Volar (cock up) splint
e. Thumb spica splint

67. A 44-year-old male presents to establish care due to headache, snoring, and tingling sensation in the first 3 fingers of his right hand. Over the last 2 years, he had gained 30 lbs., his voice has gotten deeper, his hat size has increased, and the space between his teeth has widened. On examination, he has coarse facial features, and his skin has moist, soft, doughy feeling. Tinel sign at the wrist is positive. Which of the following is most likely to be associated with his underlying condition?
a. Left ventricular hypertrophy
b. Aortic root dilation
c. Mitral stenosis
d. Mitral valve prolapse
e. Hypotension

68. A 20-year-old male presents to the clinic complaining of pain and swelling to the right index finger. 2 days prior to the swelling, he experienced tingling and burning to the finger. Physical examination is notable for multiple yellowish vesicles, blisters, and ulcers on an erythematous base of the index finger. Which of the following is the first line management of his condition?
a. IV Vancomycin and hospital admission
b. Oral Cephalexin
c. Incision and drainage of the lesions
d. Topical Ivermectin
e. Ibuprofen, clean dry dressing, and hand elevation

69. A 60-year-old male is complaining of generalized weakness, lightheadedness, darkening of the visual fields, and dizziness that occurs with standing. He denies dyspnea, chest pain, palpitations, or diaphoresis. He was recently diagnosed with Postherpetic neuralgia, for which he was placed on Amitriptyline. Which of the following is the most appropriate next step in the evaluation of this patient?
a. Straight leg raise test
b. Blood pressure readings in the supine and standing positions
c. Tilt table testing
d. Transthoracic echocardiography
e. CT scan of the head without contrast

70. A 50-year-old male is placed on Warfarin therapy and Enoxaparin for Deep vein thrombosis. On day 3, the Enoxaparin was discontinued. On day 4, he returns with demarcated ecchymotic patches with central purpuric zones, large hemorrhagic bullae, and some necrotic areas on his trunk and left thigh. Labs reveal an INR of 2.0 (≤1.1). Which of the following is the most likely underlying cause of his presentation?
a. Antithrombin III deficiency
b. Factor V Leiden mutation
c. Protein C deficiency
d. Von Willebrand disease
e. Antiphospholipid syndrome

71. A 70-year-old male presents with an "enlarging mole" on his face. On examination, there is a dome-shaped lesion with central depression (see photo). A biopsy is performed, revealing basophilic palisading cells on histology. Which of the following is the best treatment option in this patient?

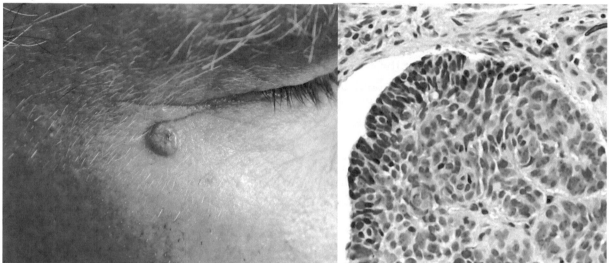

a. Electrodesiccation and curettage
b. Liquid nitrogen cryotherapy
c. Standard excision with 4-5 mm margins and postoperative margin assessment
d. Mohs micrographic surgery
e. Topical imiquimod 5% cream

72. A 62-year-old male presents to his primary care provider for blood pressure management. He has been compliant with Valsartan, Hydrochlorothiazide, and Nifedipine. He has a history of claudication and erectile dysfunction. Vitals reveal a blood pressure of 178/98 mmHg. Which of the following would most likely be seen in this patient?
a. Periumbilical bruit
b. Purple-colored abdominal striae and supraclavicular fat pads
c. Intermittent tachycardia and diaphoresis
d. Pulsatile abdominal mass
e. Systolic murmur radiating to the interscapular area

73. A 21-year-old male is complaining of swelling to his left armpit associated with low-grade fever. He tried to stop his two cats from fighting 3 weeks ago. About one week afterwards, he developed a lesion on his finger. Vitals reveal a temperature of 102°F (38.89°C). There is tender left axillary lymphadenopathy without fluctuance. There is a nontender papule noted at the base of the left middle finger. Which of the following is the first line management?
a. Azithromycin
b. Prednisone
c. Amoxicillin-clavulanic acid
d. Clindamycin
e. Needle aspiration

74. A 40-year-old male is being treated with ABVD therapy (Adriamycin, Bleomycin, Vinblastine, and Dacarbazine) for Hodgkin lymphoma. The clinician mistakenly ordered Vincristine. Prior to infusion of the chemotherapy, the nurse pages the clinician to confirm the medications that were prepared by pharmacy for infusion. The clinician recognizes that the medication should be Vinblastine, discontinues the order for Vincristine, and orders Vinblastine. Which of the following is the most appropriate next step?
a. Inform the patient of the error
b. Let the nurse inform the patient of the error and how it was addressed and corrected
c. No further action needed since the patient is asymptomatic
d. Report the event to Joint commission on Accreditation of Healthcare organizations (JCAHO)
e. Report the event to hospital administration

75. A 60-year-old male presents with substernal chest tightness for 45 minutes. The pain began while he was shoveling snow. He has a past medical history of Hypertension, Dyslipidemia, and Diabetes mellitus. An ECG is obtained (see photo).

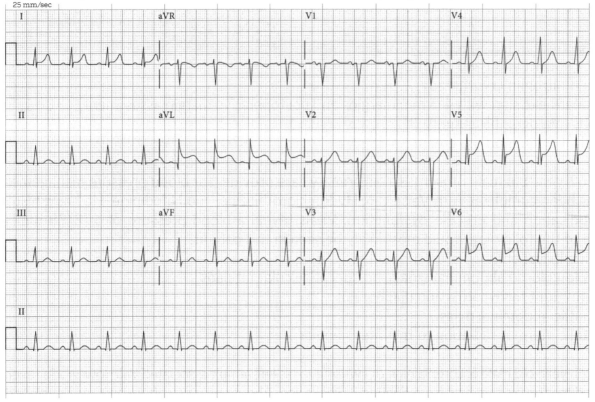

The patient's presentation is most likely due to occlusion of which of the following arteries?
a. Left anterior descending
b. Right coronary artery
c. Left circumflex artery
d. Posterior descending artery
e. Left main coronary artery

Photo credit:
Shutterstock (used with permission)

76. A 46-year-old male presents to the emergency department complaining of epigastric pain, nausea, and vomiting for 48 hours. The pain is worse when supine and relieved with sitting and leaning forward. He has a longstanding history of chronic alcoholism. Physical examination is notable for left upper quadrant tenderness without guarding, rigidity, or rebound tenderness. Labs reveal a serum calcium of 7.2 mg/dL (8.5-10). Which of the following would most likely be seen on physical examination?
a. Radiation of the pain to the left shoulder
b. RLQ pain with palpation of the LLQ
c. Ecchymotic discoloration in the periumbilical region
d. Enlarged left axillary lymph node
e. Retraction of the right iliac fossa

77. A 45-year-old male presents with sudden onset of excruciating right foot pain that woke him out of his sleep. He has recently celebrated his anniversary drinking alcohol at a Brazilian steakhouse. He has a history of stage 3 chronic kidney disease. On examination, the first metatarsophalangeal joint is warm, edematous, erythematous, and tender to palpation. The erythema extends beyond the joint space. Radiographs of the great toe and foot are obtained.

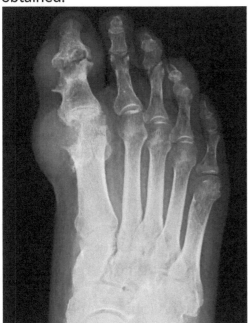

Which of the following medications is most appropriate for the initial management of this patient?
a. Allopurinol
b. Colchicine
c. Prednisone
d. Aspirin
e. Naproxen

Photo credit:
Case courtesy of Naim Qaqish, Radiopaedia.org, rID: 81562

78. A 65-year-old male presents to the clinic with a 3-month history of gradual onset of dyspnea on exertion and nonproductive cough. He denies fever, myalgias, or arthralgias. He has a history of Atrial fibrillation treated with Amiodarone. Physical examination is notable for bibasilar crackles and end-inspiratory "squeaks". Chest radiographs reveal an increase in reticular markings. Pulmonary function testing (PFT) is performed and reveals decrease in 6-minute walking distance. It is thought his symptoms are related to chronic Amiodarone use. Which of the following would most likely be increased on PFTs?
a. Forced expiratory volume in one second/Forced vital capacity (FEV_1/FVC)
b. Residual volume (RV)
c. Total lung capacity (TLC)
d. Forced vital capacity (FVC)
e. Diffusing capacity of carbon monoxide (DLCO)

79. A 60-year-old man presents to the clinic complaining of an episode of painless large-volume bright red blood per rectum. He denies black tarry stool, diarrhea, abdominal pain, nausea, vomiting, fevers, or chills. Vitals are normal. Abdominal examination is soft, nontender, nondistended. Which of the following is the most likely diagnosis?
a. Ischemic colitis
b. Diverticulosis
c. Colorectal cancer
d. Internal hemorrhoids
e. Infectious colitis

80. A 45-year-old male presents to the clinic complaining of moderate dull upper abdominal discomfort that does not radiate. The discomfort is improved with food and antacids but often reoccurs 3-5 hours after a meal and late at night around midnight. Which of the following is the most common complication of this condition?
a. Bleeding
b. Gastric outlet obstruction
c. Perforation
d. Fistulization
e. Penetration

81. An otherwise healthy 2-year-old boy presents to the clinic with his father for persistent left-sided, thick, nasal discharge for 10 days. Vitals are normal. On examination, there is a mucopurulent foul-smelling nasal discharge noted from the left nostril. The right nostril is patent without drainage. He is breathing predominantly through his mouth. There is no pharyngeal or tonsillar erythema, edema, or exudate. Which of the following is the most appropriate next step in the management of this patient?
a. Nasal saline spray
b. CT scan of the sinuses
c. Intranasal Fluticasone propionate
d. Anterior rhinoscopy
e. Oral Amoxicillin-clavulanate

82. A 50-year-old female with chronic alcoholism presents to the emergency department with cough with thick, mucoid, and blood-tinged sputum and fever. A chest radiograph is obtained and reveals an abnormality in the left upper lobe.

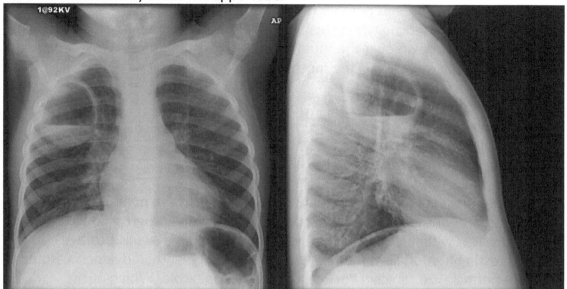

Which of the following is the most likely organism responsible?
a. Pseudomonas aeruginosa
b. Chlamydia pneumoniae
c. Histoplasma capsulatum
d. Klebsiella pneumoniae
e. Mycoplasma pneumoniae

Photo credit:
Case courtesy of Frank Gaillard, Radiopaedia.org, rID: 8288

83. A 6-year-old girl is brought to the ED by her father. She has been having difficulty ambulating for the last 3 days and this morning she refused to bear weight on the right leg. She has a past medical history of Sickle cell disease. Vitals are notable for a low-grade fever. Physical examination reveals an antalgic gait and tenderness over the distal femur. Initial labs reveal an elevated ESR and CRP. Plain radiographs are positive for a periosteal reaction involving the distal femur. Which of the following organisms is most likely responsible?
a. Pseudomonas spp
b. Enterococcus spp.
c. Streptococcus spp.
d. Haemophilus spp.
e. Salmonella spp.

84. Which of the following is decreased during early normal pregnancy?
a. Blood volume
b. Stroke volume
c. Cardiac output
d. Systemic vascular resistance
e. Heart rate

85. A 31-year-old woman presents to the clinic complaining of pain over the lateral aspect of the left wrist, especially when she holds her 5-week-old infant and with gripping objects. She denies trauma, burning, pain, or paresthesias over the dorsum of the hand, wrist, index, and middle fingers. Physical examination is notable for tenderness at the first dorsal compartment. The pain is reproduced when she is asked to bend her thumb across the palm of the hand, bend the fingers down over the thumb, and with bending of the wrist towards the little finger. Which of the following is the most likely diagnosis?
a. Carpal tunnel syndrome
b. Radial sensory nerve entrapment
c. DeQuervain tendinopathy
d. Flexor carpi radialis tenosynovitis
e. Osteoarthritis of the trapeziometacarpal (TMC) joint

86. A 64-year-old male presents to the neurologic clinic for progressive nondisabling intermittent resting tremor of the left hand for 4 years, that has now progressed to the right hand. He has been treated with Levodopa. Neurological examination reveals positive Myerson sign, mild resting tremor, asymmetrical cogwheel rigidity, and bradykinesia. Routine laboratory tests are normal. The clinician decides to initiate Ropinirole. Which of the following describes the primary mechanism of action of this medication?
a. Dopamine receptor agonist
b. Dopamine precursor
c. Selective monoamine oxidase inhibitor
d. Muscarinic (cholinergic) receptor antagonist
e. Catechol-O-methyltransferase inhibitor

87. A 20-year-old male presents to his pediatrician for fever and cough. He experiences 4-6 bulky, foul-smelling stools per day and for the last 5 days, he has been coughing increasing amounts of thick tenacious sputum. He has a history of recurrent pneumonia, chronic sinusitis, and chronic diarrhea. Physical exam is notable for scattered rhonchi in the bilateral lung fields with hepatomegaly. Sweat chloride testing is elevated on 2 separate occasions. Based on his history, sputum culture is most likely to yield which of the following organisms?
a. Pseudomonas aeruginosa
b. Klebsiella pneumoniae
c. Mycobacterium tuberculosis
d. Streptococcus pneumoniae
e. Aspergillus fumigatus

88. A 20-year-old primigravid female presents to the clinic at 12 weeks of gestation to establish care. She recently arrived in the United States from Panama where she never received vaccinations and wants to receive vaccinations to prevent disease in her and her unborn fetus. Which of the following vaccinations is safest in this patient?
a. Intranasal Influenza
b. Inactivated Human papillomavirus (HPV)
c. SARS-CoV-2
d. Measles-Mumps-Rubella (MMR)
e. Varicella (Chickenpox)

89. A 14-year-old male presents with a 3-day history of severe right-sided sore throat, drooling, and change in phonation. He is febrile and ill-appearing. Examination of the oral cavity is positive for tonsillar erythema and exudate. There is a bulge with fullness on the right side of the posterior soft palate and the uvula is displaced to the left. Which of the following is the most appropriate initial management strategy for this patient?
a. Needle aspiration and Amoxicillin-clavulanate
b. Intravenous Dexamethasone
c. Emergent tonsillectomy
d. 24-hour trial of Clindamycin
e. Ibuprofen and gargle with antiseptic mouthwash

90. A 56-year-old male presents to the clinic with a 4-month history of exertional chest discomfort when walking more than 5 blocks, relieved within minutes of cessation of activity. He has a history of Dyslipidemia and a 40-pack year smoking history. Vitals, physical examination, and baseline ECG are unremarkable. An ECG performed during treadmill testing reveals 2-mm ST-segment depression in leads V2, V5, aVL, and II with exercise. Which of the following medications is the first line agent for mortality reduction in this patient?
a. Nitroglycerin
b. Lisinopril
c. Long-acting Diltiazem
d. Ranolazine
e. Metoprolol

91. A 5-year-old boy is being evaluated in the clinic for multiple episodes where he is awakened from sleep crying with sweating, flushed face, and rapid breathing. He sometimes jumps out of bed as if he is running away from an unseen threat. When his parents try to console him, he becomes more agitated. He seems to have no recollection of dreams or episodes. Which of the following is the most likely diagnosis?
a. Sleep terrors
b. Sleepwalking
c. Nightmare disorders
d. Rapid eye movement sleep behavior disorder
e. Confusional arousal state

92. A 28-year-old male presents to his primary care provider complaining of increasing fatigue, constipation, and muscle aches for 3 months. He has a history of Bipolar disorder, GERD, and Asthma, for which he takes Lithium, Pantoprazole, and Albuterol. Physical examination is notable for delayed relaxation of deep tendon reflexes and a puffy face. Which of the following tests would be helpful in establishing the most likely diagnosis in this patient?
a. Urinalysis
b. Thyroid function tests
c. Noncontrast CT scan of the head
d. Single fiber electromyography
e. Complete blood count with peripheral smear

93. A 55-year-old female with a past medical history of Migraine disorder presents with abrupt onset of bilateral frontal headache for 9 hours that began while exercising and did not resolve with Ibuprofen. The headache is more severe than previous headaches. Vital signs are stable, and neurological examination is intact. Non-contrast CT head is normal, but she reports continued pain despite Ketorolac in the emergency department. Which of the following is the next best step in management?
a. Discharge home with outpatient neurology follow up
b. Administer Sumatriptan
c. Consult neurology for intractable headache
d. Perform a Lumbar puncture
e. Perform a Temporal Artery biopsy

94. A 12-year-old female presents to the clinic for unexplained Hypertension. Vital signs reveal a blood pressure of 164/92 mmHg and pulse 90/min. There is a 4/6 systolic ejection murmur best heard at the left upper sternal border and interscapular area. Brachio-femoral pulse delay and decreased femoral pulses are noted. Based on the most likely diagnosis, which of the following would most likely be seen in this patient?
a. Macroorchidism and large ears
b. "Shield" chest with widely spaced nipples
c. Smooth philtrum, thin upper lip, and flat midface
d. Single palmar crease
e. Increased arm span to height ratio

95. A 66-year-old female with no significant past medical history presents with her husband. He reports that she has been increasingly forgetful for the past 6 months, has stopped balancing her checkbook, and recently got lost coming home from the supermarket 2 blocks from their house. Physical examination is unremarkable. A Montreal cognitive assessment is scored 20 out of 30. Laboratory workup is unremarkable. Which of the following classes of medication is the best choice for initial treatment of this patient?
a. Anticholinergic
b. NMDA receptor agonist
c. Dopamine agonist
d. Dopamine antagonist
e. Cholinesterase inhibitor

96. A 21-year-old male is complaining of dizziness while playing tennis. His vitals are stable. Physical examination is notable for a harsh 4/6 systolic murmur heard maximally along the left lower sternal border that does not radiate and increases in intensity with Valsalva maneuver. Which of the following is the first line management of his condition?
a. Isosorbide mononitrate
b. Isolated mitral valve surgery
c. Metoprolol succinate
d. Aortic valve replacement
e. Digoxin

97. Which of the following is most accurate regarding Internal hemorrhoids (IHs)?
a. Symptomatic IHs most commonly present with melena
b. Skin tags are a common associated finding
c. IHs originate below the dentate line
d. Intense pain with defection is hallmark of IHs
e. IHs are generally not palpable on digital rectal examination

98. A 32-year-old female presents with left calf pain and swelling for 3 days. She denies any symptoms or trauma. She uses oral contraception. She drinks occasionally and has a 10 pack-year-smoking history. She works as a mail carrier. Physical examination is positive for an obese woman with left calf swelling, warmth, tenderness, and erythema. Which of the following is most appropriate next step?
a. Venous plethysmography
b. Initiate IV Heparin
c. Warm compresses, leg elevation, Indomethacin
d. Compression ultrasonography (CUS) with Doppler
e. Ankle-brachial index

99. Which of the following instances is considered a HIPAA violation of protected health information (PHI)?
a. Professionals using the names of patients in case reports
b. Discussing diagnosis, workup, and treatment with other healthcare providers
c. Performing imaging and laboratory test and disclosing this information to other providers
d. When referring a patient to another facility or obtaining a consult
e. When calling the pharmacist over the phone to dispense medication to a patient

100. A 55-year-old male presents to the outpatient department. He has a history of Diabetes mellitus, Chronic bronchitis, and Dyslipidemia. He does not remember receiving prior vaccinations. Which of the following vaccines is recommended for this patient to prevent pneumococcal disease?
a. 13-valent pneumococcal conjugate vaccine
b. 20-valent pneumococcal conjugate vaccine
c. Pneumococcal polysaccharide vaccine (PPSV23)
d. 7-valent pneumococcal conjugate vaccine
e. 10-valent pneumococcal conjugate vaccine

END OF EXAM 3

1. CARDIOLOGY - SINUS ARRHYTHMIA [MOST LIKELY]

Sinus arrhythmia [Choice A] is associated with a regularly irregular rhythm, in which the rate increases with inspiration and decreases with expiration (eg, changes with respiration).

There is P-P interval variation of >0.12 seconds.

In respiratory (phasic) Sinus arrhythmia, the heart rate increases with inspiration (due to decreased venous return on the left side with a compensatory increase in the heart rate to maintain cardiac output) and decreases with expiration.

It is a very common benign rhythm and does not usually require intervention.

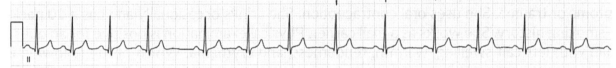

Choice B [Sinus bradycardia] is incorrect as the heart rate is about 79 bpm. The heart rate in Sinus bradycardia is <60 bpm.

Choice C [Premature atrial complexes] are seen on ECG as a P wave that occurs earlier than expected in the cardiac cycle before the next sinus P wave should occur, often with a different morphology from the sinus P wave.

Choice D [First-degree atrioventricular block] is associated with a prolonged PR interval 5 small boxes (≥0.2 seconds).

Choice E (Mobitz-1 second degree atrioventricular block) is associated with progressive lengthening of the PR interval with occasional nonconducted beats.

2. HEMATOLOGY – IMMUNE THROMBOCYTOPENIC PURPURA (ITP) [HEALTH MAINTENANCE]

Close observation and monitoring [choice E] is used in the management of Immune thrombocytopenic purpura (ITP) with minor (skin or mucous membrane bleeding) if the platelet count is ≥30,000/mm^3.

The presence of bleeding, and if present, the site, acuity, and severity determines the management of ITP in adults.

(1) Minor bleeding (platelet count usually < 50,000):
- Glucocorticoids monotherapy first-line therapy [choice C] & preferred, IVIG [choice B], or anti-D.

(2) Severe (critical) bleeding (GI/CNS) + platelets < 30,000:
- Platelet transfusion [choice D] + IVIG + high-dose glucocorticoids.

No bleeding:
- (3) No bleeding + platelet ≥30,000: Observation and monitor the platelet count.
- (4) No bleeding + platelet <20,000-30,000: Glucocorticoids (preferred) or IVIG or anti-D.

3. PSYCHIATRY/BEHAVIORAL MEDICINE – PRIMARY (PSYCHOGENIC) POLYDIPSIA [MOST LIKELY]

Primary polydipsia [choice A] should be suspected in patients with:
Isovolemic hypotonic hyponatremia with dilute urine AND dilute serum:
- **serum osmolality 262 mmol/kg (275-295)**
- **serum sodium 130 mEq/L (135-145)**
- **dilute urine (low urine sodium)**
- **urine osmolality <100 mmol/kg (dilute urine).**

Primary polydipsia (Psychogenic polydipsia) is characterized by a primary increase in water intake.

Choice B [Vomiting] is associated with Hypovolemic hypotonic Hyponatremia but is associated with a concentrated urine (increased urine osmolality), reflecting the kidney's concentration of the urine in response to hypovolemia.

Choice C [Nephrotic syndrome] is not associated with decreased urine osmolality.

Choice D [Syndrome of inappropriate ADH secretion] is associated with an Isovolemic hypotonic hyponatremia but is associated with increased urine osmolality (concentrated urine).

Choice E [Diabetes insipidus (AVP deficiency or resistance)] may develop an Isovolemic Hypertonic hypernatremia if the water intake is less than increased urinary free water loss. The patient's hypotonic Hyponatremia makes this less likely.

4. RENAL – ETHYLENE GLYCOL POISONING/METABOLIC ACIDOSIS [MOST LIKELY]

Ethylene glycol poisoning results in a High anion gap metabolic acidosis [choice A].

Ethylene glycol (antifreeze) poisoning presents with the triad of (1) flank pain, (2) gross hematuria, and (3) oliguria (Acute kidney injury due to tubular damage).

Nausea, vomiting, ataxia, AMS, nystagmus, Kussmaul respirations may also be seen.

UA may reveal envelope- or dumbbell-shaped Ca+ oxalate crystals.

Step 1: look at the pH: 7.21 (decreased) = acidosis.

Step 2: look at CO2 (which is decreased) = metabolic (since the CO2 is in the same direction as the pH).

Step 3: look at the PCO2 to determine compensation for the metabolic acidosis: since the PCO2 moved out of its normal range but the pH is not normal, it reflects partial compensation.

Step 4: Calculate the anion gap $[(137 + 3.7) - (96 + 7)] = [140.7 - 103] = $ AG of 37.7

Choice E [Uncompensated high anion gap metabolic acidosis] would be seen if the PCO2 stayed within its normal range.

Methanol and ethylene glycol poisonings cause dozens of fatal intoxications in the United States annually.

Few conditions other than methanol and ethylene glycol intoxication present with a profound metabolic acidosis (serum bicarbonate <8 mEq/L).

5. CARDIOLOGY – TRICUSPID REGURGITATION [MOST LIKELY]

Tricuspid regurgitation [choice D] is characterized by a holosystolic murmur that is high-pitched, loudest at the left parasternal border in the fourth intercostal space.

The intensity of the murmur increases with increased venous return (eg, during inspiration, exercise, and leg raising) and decreases with decreased venous return (eg, standing position and during the Valsalva maneuver).

The tricuspid valve is the most common valve associated with IV drug use-associated Infective endocarditis (the most likely cause of TR in this patient).

Choice A [Mitral regurgitation] is associated with a soft holosystolic murmur best heard at the apex and would decrease in intensity with inspiration.

Choice B [Tricuspid stenosis] is characterized by an opening snap and low frequency diastolic murmur best heard at the lower left sternal border.

Choice C [Hypertrophic cardiomyopathy] is characterized by a harsh systolic murmur best heard at the lower sternal border.

Choice E [Mitral stenosis] is characterized by a diastolic rumbling murmur best heard at the apex.

6. EENT – OTITIS-CONJUNCTIVITIS SYNDROME [APPLY FUNDAMENTAL CONCEPTS]

The presence of Acute otitis media with purulent conjunctivitis, known as Otitis-conjunctivitis syndrome, is most commonly caused by nontypeable *Haemophilus influenzae* [choice C].

For these patients, antibiotics that cover beta-lactamase producing organisms (eg, high-dose Amoxicillin-clavulanate) is the treatment of choice, as opposed to high-dose Amoxicillin used in the management of isolated Acute otitis media.

Topical ophthalmic antibiotics are not necessary in patients with Otitis-conjunctivitis syndrome.

Other possible bacterial causes include *Moraxella catarrhalis* [choice B] and *Streptococcus pneumoniae* [choice E].

7. ENDOCRINOLOGY – ARGININE VASOPRESSIN RESISTANCE (NEPHROGENIC DIABETES INSIPIDUS) [MOST LIKELY]

Etiologies of Arginine vasopressin resistance (Nephrogenic Diabetes insipidus) include:
- **<u>Medications</u>: Lithium [choice B]**, Amphotericin B, Cidofovir,
- **<u>Electrolyte disorders</u>: eg, Hypercalcemia, Hypokalemia**, and
- Kidney disease, genetic disorders.

Up to 20% of patients on chronic Lithium therapy will develop impaired urinary concentrating ability.

Clinical manifestations of Arginine vasopressin resistance (Nephrogenic Diabetes insipidus) include:
- Polyuria, polydipsia, and nocturia
- <u>Elevation of serum sodium and serum osmolality</u> (dehydration) if water intake is less than urinary free water loss. Hypernatremia + low urine osmolality <300 mOsm/kg is hallmark of DI.
- <u>Decreased urine osmolality</u> <300 mOsm/kg (loss of large-volume diluted urine).
- <u>AVP resistance</u>: The decreased urine osmolality does not change significantly with water deprivation (indicating Nephrogenic DI) nor with administration of DDAVP/ADH (indicating a Nephrogenic cause).

Choice A (Dehydration) is associated with an increased serum sodium and increased serum osmolality; in addition, it is associated with a high urine osmolality (>600 mOsm/kg), reflecting increased renal reabsorption of water to minimize urinary free water loss.

Choice C [Primary (Psychogenic) polydipsia] results in Hyponatremia, decreased serum osmolality, and decreased urine osmolality due to increased free water ingestion. The urine osmolality would increase with water deprivation.

Choice D [Syndrome of inappropriate ADH] causes an Isovolemic hypotonic Hyponatremia.

Choice E [Sodium valproate] may result in Hyponatremia due to Syndrome of inappropriate ADH.

8. CARDIOLOGY/HEMATOLOGY – DECOMPENSATED HEART FAILURE/TRANSFUSION ASSOCIATED CIRCULATORY OVERLOAD [CLINICAL INTERVENTION]

Treatment of TACO is similar to treatment of Cardiogenic pulmonary edema from other causes and includes:
- **discontinuation of the transfusion**
- **fluid mobilization with diuretics, such as Furosemide [choice D]**
- **supplementary oxygen if SaO$_2$ is <90%), and**
- assisted ventilation if indicated (eg, Noninvasive positive pressure ventilation).

TACO should be suspected in patients who develop:
- <u>respiratory distress</u> (dyspnea, orthopnea) or hypertension during or within 12 hours after the end of a transfusion, especially in individuals with underlying heart disease, in the setting of positive fluid balance, and in the ICU.
- hypoxia
- <u>Cardiogenic pulmonary edema</u>: jugular venous distention, pulmonary rales, an S3 gallop, pulmonary edema on chest imaging, and elevated BNP or NT-BNP.

Choice A [IM Epinephrine] can be used in Transfusion-associated anaphylaxis, which can also present with a significant drop in blood pressure (>30 mmHg) but is also associated with respiratory symptoms (eg, respiratory difficulty, wheezing, stridor, angioedema, and pruritus), all of which are absent in this patient.

Choice B [IV Vancomycin plus Cefepime] are used in the management of Transfusion related sepsis, which is characterized by hypotension and fever. This patient is hypertensive and afebrile.

Choice C [Endotracheal intubation] may be required if Noninvasive positive pressure ventilation is ineffective at correcting the hypoxemia in TACO.

Choice E [Acetaminophen] can be used in the management of Febrile nonhemolytic transfusion reaction, which is characterized by fever, chills, headache, & flushing in the absence of other systemic symptoms 1-6 hours after transfusion initiation.

9. REPRODUCTIVE – RH ALLOIMMUNIZATION [HEALTH MAINTENANCE]

For RhD-negative patients experiencing pregnancy loss or induced abortion at ≥12 weeks, RhD immune globulin [choice C] should be given to prevent alloimmunization.
The dosing varies by gestational age.
RhD immune globulin are given to RhD-negative unsensitized women in 3 instances:
- at 28 weeks of gestation
- within 72 hours of delivery of an RhD-positive baby
- during the pregnancy when there is potential missing of blood (eg, spontaneous abortion, pregnancy loss, placenta previa, abruptio placenta, vasa previa).

Because the patient has passed the products of conception with resolving vaginal bleeding and a closed cervix, there is usually no further need for surgical [choice A] or medical management [choices B and E].

Antibiotics [choice D] are not recommended for routine management of first-trimester pregnancy loss without signs of infection.

10. INFECTIOUS DISEASE – LYME DISEASE [PHARMACOLOGY]

In children <8 years of age, Beta lactams, either Amoxicillin [choice C] or Cefuroxime for 14 days, are first line agents for the management of early Lyme disease (erythema migrans).
Doxycycline [choice A] is the first line for nonpregnant adults, children >8 years of age, or children <8 years of age who cannot take a Beta lactam.

Choice B [Ceftriaxone] can be used for patients with acute neurological changes or carditis.
Choice D [Azithromycin] and other Macrolides are an alternative for patients with early Lyme disease who cannot take Doxycycline, Amoxicillin, or Cefuroxime.
Choice E [Enzyme immunoassay for IgM and IgG antibodies to *B. burgdorferi*] is neither necessary or recommended in early Lyme disease (Erythema migrans) as it is frequently negative, and the results do not change management.

11. MUSCULOSKELETAL/RHEUMATOLOGY – RHEUMATOID ARTHRITIS [LABS AND DIAGNOSTIC STUDIES]

Measurement of anti-citrullinated peptide antibodies (ACPA) [choice B] is useful in suspected Rheumatoid arthritis because of the relatively high specificity for RA of ACPA (>90% specificity; 70-75% sensitivity).
The sensitivities of ACPA and RF are similar, but ACPA positivity is more specific.
ACPA has greater specificity than RF for early Rheumatoid arthritis.

Rheumatoid factor (RF) [choice A] is sensitive but not specific for Rheumatoid arthritis. A positive RF can be seen in conditions, such as Infective endocarditis and Juvenile idiopathic arthritis.
Rheumatoid arthritis classically presents with pain, stiffness, and/or swelling of certain joints [eg, metacarpophalangeal (MCP) joints, proximal interphalangeal (PIP) joints], often with systemic symptoms (eg, fever, fatigue, etc.).

Choice C [Anti-Smith antibodies] are specific for Systemic lupus erythematosus.
Choice D [Anti-nuclear antibodies] can be seen in various autoimmune diseases, so it lacks significant specificity.
Choice E [Anti-La] antibodies are seen with Sjögren's syndrome.

12. RENAL – HEMOLYTIC UREMIC SYNDROME [HISTORY AND PHYSICAL EXAMINATION]

The diagnosis of Hemolytic uremic syndrome (HUS) [choice E] is based on the classic triad of:
- **microangiopathic hemolytic anemia**
- **thrombocytopenia, and**
- **acute kidney injury.**

Shiga toxin-producing Escherichia coli (STEC) HUS is responsible for >90% of pediatric HUS cases.
In children, HUS is often preceded by a prodromal illness with abdominal pain, vomiting, and diarrhea (that may have become bloody).

Choice A [IgA Vasculitis (Henoch-Schoenlein purpura)] is associated with purpura on the lower extremities, joint pain, abdominal pain, and hematuria, especially after a viral infection. The purpura is due to vasculitis not thrombocytopenia or coagulopathy. The patient has thrombocytopenia, making HSP less likely.

Choice B [Thrombotic thrombocytopenic purpura (TTP)] is more common in adults and present with the pentad of microangiopathic hemolytic anemia, thrombocytopenia, and acute kidney injury.

Choice C [Idiopathic thrombocytopenic purpura (ITP)] presents with an isolated thrombocytopenia without anemia or hemolysis.

Choice D [Von Willebrand disease] presents with a mucocutaneous bleeding without anemia or hemolysis. The aPTT may be normal or prolonged.

13. REPRODUCTIVE – ENDOMETRITIS [PHARMACOLOGY]

Because postpartum Endometritis is often polymicrobial first line IV regimen for postpartum Endometritis includes coverage for gram-positive, gram-negative, and anaerobic organisms, including:

- **IV Clindamycin 900 mg every eight hours plus IV Gentamicin [choice B]** 5 mg/kg every 24 hours (preferred) **or** 1.5 mg/kg every eight hours (without a loading dose). This regimen resolves the infection in up to 97% of cases.
- If the patient is colonized with GBS: either [1] add Ampicillin to the above regimen or [2] use **Ampicillin-Sulbactam instead.**

In patients who do not respond to IV Clindamycin plus Gentamicin within 24-48 hours, options include adding:

- Ampicillin or
- Vancomycin [choice C] in Penicillin-allergic patients.

Cesarean section is the most important predisposing factor for the development of postpartum Endometritis, which presents with:

- fever and tachycardia
- midline lower abdominal pain
- tachycardia that parallels the rise in temperature
- uterine tenderness
- purulent vaginal discharge or foul-smelling lochia.

Choice E [IV Cefazolin] is used in prevention of Endometritis, not for the treatment of Endometritis. Antibiotic prophylaxis within 60 minutes prior to making the skin incision is significantly reduces the incidence of post cesarean Endometritis, for both planned and intrapartum procedures.

14. REPRODUCTIVE – PREECLAMPSIA [HEALTH MAINTENANCE]

Patients at increased risk for developing Preeclampsia are given Low-dose Aspirin [choice A] prophylaxis, around the 12th or 13th week of gestation and ideally prior to 16 weeks of gestation and continued daily until delivery.

Low-dose Aspirin prophylaxis is associated with ≥10% reduction in the overall incidence of Preeclampsia and its complications.

Although its exact mechanism of action is unknown, it is thought Aspirin may prevent platelet aggregation & help prevent placental ischemia.

Choice B [Magnesium sulfate] can be used to prevent Eclampsia in patients with Preeclampsia with severe features. Magnesium sulfate is also used for neuroprotection to pregnancies <32 weeks of gestation (protects against motor dysfunction & cerebral palsy).

Choice C [17 alpha-hydroxyprogesterone] can be used with or without cerclage for Cervical insufficiency.

Choice D [Folic acid] is used in pregnant women to reduce the incidence of neural tube defects.

Choice E [Nifedipine] may be used in women who are pregnant with Hypertension. This patient is not hypertensive.

15. INFECTIOUS DISEASE – PNEUMOCYSTIS PNEUMONIA (PCP) [PHARMACOLOGY]

Trimethoprim-sulfamethoxazole (TMP/SMX) [choice B] is the first line treatment and prophylaxis for *Pneumocystis* pneumonia (PCP).

TMP-SMX is the most effective regimen for PCP.

Adjunctive corticosteroids are used in some patients with severe hypoxemia (eg, SpO2 <92% on room air or PaO2 <70 mmHg).

PCP most commonly occurs in those with immunocompromised states [eg, HIV (AIDS-defining illness), solid organ transplant recipients (this patient is post kidney transplant), HIV, malignancy (especially hematologic malignancies), individuals with cancer, chemotherapy, and those receiving glucocorticoid therapy.

PCP presents in these patients with fever, dry cough, dyspnea, and hypoxia.

The most common radiographic features of PCP are diffuse, bilateral, interstitial infiltrates (as seen in this radiograph).

Choice A [Doxycycline] is first line for Community-acquired Pneumonia treated as an outpatient.

Choice C [Ceftriaxone plus Azithromycin] is first line for Community-acquired Pneumonia treated as an inpatient.

Choice D [Isoniazid, Rifampin, Ethambutol, and Streptomycin] is used as first line for active Tuberculosis infection.

Choice E [Ciprofloxacin] is not a respiratory Fluoroquinolone and is not used for PCP.

16. PULMONOLOGY – CROUP [APPLYING FOUNDATIONAL CONCEPTS]

Parainfluenza viruses [choice B], especially type 1, are the most common cause of Laryngotracheobronchitis (Croup).

Parainfluenza virus causes inflammation of the upper airway edema, and infiltration of inflammatory cells this causes narrowing of subglottic airway, resulting in hoarseness, stridor, barking cough (hallmark), and increased work of breathing.

It is a self-limited disease most commonly seen in children <5 years of age.

Other causes include influenza A and B, measles, adenovirus, and respiratory syncytial virus (RSV).

Respiratory syncytial virus [choice E] and influenza virus account for 1%-10% of cases. RSV is the most common cause of Acute bronchiolitis, which presents with lower respiratory symptoms (eg, wheezing).

Choice A [Parvovirus B19] is associated with Erythema infectiosum, which presents with a facial "slapped cheek" rash, followed by a lace-like reticular rash on the extremities.

Choice C [Haemophilus influenzae type B] is associated with Acute epiglottitis, which is not associated with a barking cough. Drooling, dyspnea, and dysphagia are hallmark of Croup.

Choice D [Foreign body aspiration] may be associated with inspiratory stridor and hoarseness and is often associated with a history of choking episode, monophonic focal wheezing, and is not associated with the prodromal viral symptoms.

17. HEMATOLOGY – POLYCYTHEMIA VERA [CLINICAL INTERVENTION]

Periodic phlebotomy [choice D] until hematocrit <45% + low-dose Aspirin to reduce vasomotor symptoms and to prevent thrombosis is the first line treatment for Polycythemia vera (PV) in low-risk patients (<60 years & no thrombosis).

Phlebotomy is the quickest way to reduce red blood cell mass in patients with PV.

Pegylated interferon may be given in some patients to reduce the need for phlebotomy.

For high-risk patients (≥60 years old and/or prior thrombosis) treatment includes a cytoreductive agent (eg, Hydroxyurea) plus low-dose Aspirin.

Polycythemia vera (PV) is a myeloproliferative neoplasm characterized by excessive, clonal proliferation of red cells (increased red cell mass), often a result of a JAK2 mutation.

PV may present with vasomotor symptoms such as pruritus, erythromelalgia (burning pain in feet or hands), headache, abdominal pain/fullness from splenomegaly, and increased thromboembolic events.

18. NEUROLOGY – SEIZURE DISORDER [PHARMACOLOGY]

Adverse effects of Valproic acid [choice C] adverse effects include pancreatitis, hepatotoxicity, and teratogenicity.

Medication-induced Pancreatitis is uncommon, but accumulation of a toxic metabolite is thought to be the cause of Valproic acid-induced Pancreatitis.

Choice A [Carbamazepine] adverse effects include diplopia, ataxia, Stevens-Johnson syndrome, agranulocytosis, Aplastic anemia, hepatotoxicity, SIADH, and teratogenicity.

Choice B [Lamotrigine] adverse effects include Stevens-Johnson syndrome.

Choice D [Phenytoin] is associated with gingival hyperplasia, hirsutism, nystagmus, ataxia, diplopia, sedation/CNS depression, SLE-like syndrome, osteopenia, megaloblastic anemia (decreased folate absorption), and teratogenicity.

Choice E [Topiramate] adverse effects include weight loss, sedation, and Nephrolithiasis.

19. PSYCHIATRY/BEHAVIORAL MEDICINE – PREMENSTRUAL DYSPHORIC DISORDER [PHARMACOLOGY]

Selective serotonin reuptake inhibitors (SSRIs), such as Citalopram [choice E] are the first-line treatment for women with moderate to severe Premenstrual symptoms and Premenstrual dysphoric disorder (PMDD), especially for depressive and anxious symptoms.

SSRIs can be administered as a continuous daily therapy, luteal phase-only treatment (starting on cycle day 14), or symptom-onset therapy.

Compared to combined estrogen-progestin oral contraceptive (COC), SSRIs are more effective at treating depressive and anxious symptoms (this patient experiences anxiety).

In patients where contraception is the patient's main priority, a combined estrogen-progestin oral contraceptive (COC) containing Drospirenone [choice A] is an alternative to SSRIs. However, SSRIs are more effective at managing depression and symptoms of anxiety.

Choice B [Leuprolide], a GnRH agonist, is an alternative for PMDD that is refractory to first line options (SSRIs or COCs).

Choice C [Bilateral oophorectomy] is an invasive treatment for PMDD.

Choice D [Alprazolam] and other Benzodiazepines are not recommended in the management of PMDD as the risk and potential for misuse outweigh benefits of their effects.

20. NEUROLOGY – MYASTHENIA GRAVIS [APPLYING FOUNDATIONAL CONCEPTS]

Myasthenia gravis (MG) is an autoimmune disorder of the neuromuscular junction most commonly due to autoantibodies directed against the postsynaptic nicotinic acetylcholine receptor (AChR) [choice A].

Myasthenia gravis (MG) is characterized by
- fluctuating weakness involving ocular (diplopia, ptosis), bulbar, limb, and/or respiratory muscles that WORSENS with repeated muscle use,
- Pure motor involvement: lack of autonomic and sensory symptoms and signs
- Normal deep tendon reflexes (DTRs)
- No pupillary involvement

Choice B [Autoantibodies against the presynaptic voltage-gated calcium channels] is the hallmark pathophysiology of Lambert-Eaton myasthenic syndrome.

Choice C [Demyelination of the Schwann cells in the peripheral nervous system] is the hallmark pathophysiology of Guillain-Barre syndrome.

Choice D [Demyelination of the oligodendrocytes in the central nervous system] is the hallmark pathophysiology of Multiple sclerosis.

Choice E [Neuromuscular deficits due to a neurotoxin elaborated by the bacterium *Clostridium botulinum*] is hallmark of Botulism.

21. NEUROLOGY – ANTERIOR CEREBRAL ARTERY STROKE [MOST LIKELY]

Key features of a right Anterior cerebral artery stroke [choice C] include:
- **Contralateral hemiparesis, with motor weakness in the lower extremity/leg > arm/hand/face (left side in this patient);** the face may be spared in some
- **Sensory changes in the same distribution as above**
- **Urinary incontinence** (due to the involvement of the medial paracentral gyrus)
- **Cognitive impairment** may be seen if the lesion is very proximal (involving the prefrontal cortex). Disinhibited behavior in some

ACA territory infarcts are less common because if the A1 segment is occluded there is often enough collateral flow via the contralateral A1 segment to supply the distal ACA territory.

Choice A [Right Middle cerebral artery stroke] usually presents with left-sided motor and sensory deficits greater in the upper extremity/face > lower extremity.

Choice B [Left Middle cerebral artery stroke] usually presents with right-sided motor and sensory deficits greater in the upper extremity/face > lower extremity.

Choice D [Left Anterior cerebral artery stroke] usually presents with contralateral (right-sided) deficits in lower extremities > arm/hand/face.

Choice E [Right Posterior cerebral artery stroke] presents with contralateral homonymous hemianopsia (may spare the macula); alexia without agraphia (if dominant hemisphere - left PCA); visual hallucinations, sensory loss, coma, limb ataxia, nystagmus, cerebellar signs, nausea, vomiting & drop attacks.

22. ENDOCRINOLOGY/REPRODUCTIVE – PRIMARY HYPOGONADISM/KLINEFELTER SYNDROME [APPLY FUNDAMENTAL CONCEPTS]

Primary hypogonadism (Hypergonadotropic hypogonadism) should be expected in patients with
- **elevated serum LH &/or FSH [choice B] as a pituitary response to testicular atrophy and low testosterone.**
- **below normal serum testosterone and/or sperm count**

In patients with Primary hypogonadism (Hypergonadotropic hypogonadism), Karyotype analysis should be performed to look for Klinefelter syndrome (Karyotype 47, XXY).

Klinefelter syndrome should be suspected in men with:
- infertility
- signs of androgen deficiency (gynecomastia, female hair distribution, small firm testes, sexual dysfunction, decreased energy and libido, Osteoporosis)
- long extremities, tall stature.

Choice A (Reduced luteinizing hormone) is hallmark of Secondary hypogonadism (hypogonadotropic hypogonadism).

Choice C [XO Mocaism on karyotype analysis] is hallmark of Turner syndrome in women.

Choice D [Elevated 5 alpha-reductase activity] in men is often associated with Benign prostatic hypertrophy and premature male pattern baldness.

Choice E [Absent gonadotropin releasing hormone] is incorrect as it is often elevated in Primary hypogonadism as a hypothalamic response to low serum testosterone.

23. GASTROINTESTINAL/NUTRITION – CHOLELITHIASIS [CLINICAL INTERVENTION]

Elective cholecystectomy [choice E] is the management of choice for isolated Biliary colic associated with Cholelithiasis without complications and gallstones on imaging.

Expectant management is an alternative in patients who wish to avoid surgery.

Biliary colic due to uncomplicated gallstone disease usually presents with biliary colic with normal physical examination and labs (eg, complete blood count, aminotransferases, bilirubin, alkaline phosphatase, amylase, and lipase).

Choice B [NPO, IV fluids and rest the pancreas] is the management of Acute pancreatitis.

Choice C [NPO, IV fluids, Metronidazole + Ciprofloxacin + Cholecystectomy when stable] is hallmark of Acute cholecystitis which is associated with the triad of fever, RUQ pain, and leukocytosis. This patient is afebrile with a normal white cell count.

Choice D [NPO, IV fluids Metronidazole + Ciprofloxacin + ERCP when stable] is the management Acute cholangitis.

24. HEMATOLOGY – IRON DEFICIENCY ANEMIA [LABS AND DIAGNOSTIC STUDIES]

Ferritin [choice D] is the most useful test in an iron studies panel to establish the diagnosis of Iron deficiency anemia (IDA) as Iron deficiency is the only cause of a low Ferritin.

The first occurrence in IDA is
- [1] a depletion of iron stores (ferritin) without anemia, followed by
- [2] anemia with a normal red blood cell size (normal MCV/normocytic anemia), followed by
- [3] anemia with reduced red blood cell size (low MCV/microcytic anemia.

Pica, pagophagia, and koilonychia are hallmark features of IDA.

Otherwise, serum iron [choice B] and total iron binding capacity (TIBC) [choice A] can be used to determine the transferrin saturation (TSAT) [choice E].

25. ENDOCRINOLOGY – MULTIPLE ENDOCRINE NEOPLASIA [MOST LIKELY]
The hallmarks of Multiple endocrine Multiple endocrine neoplasia II (formerly IIA) [choice C] include:
- **[1] Medullary thyroid cancer (MTC), often with an elevated calcitonin**
- **[2] Pheochromocytoma**
- **[3] Primary parathyroid hyperplasia** (increased iPTH, increased calcium, decreased phosphate).

Almost all patients will develop Medullary thyroid carcinoma.

Choice A [Secondary hyperparathyroidism] is associated with Hypocalcemia, increased PTH, and increased serum phosphate, often in the setting of Chronic kidney disease.
Choice B [Multiple endocrine neoplasia I] is characterized by the "3 Ps": Parathyroid tumors, Pituitary tumors (eg, Prolactinomas), and Pancreatic tumors (eg, Gastrinoma).
Choice D [Multiple endocrine neoplasia III (formerly IIB)] is characterized by Medullary thyroid carcinoma and Pheochromocytoma but not Hyperparathyroidism. Patients often have a Marfanoid habitus and may develop mucosal neuromas.
Choice E [Graves' disease] is associated with a Primary hyperthyroid profile, which would result in a decreased TSH. A normal TSH makes this diagnosis less likely.

26. PULMONOLOGY – OBSTRUCTIVE SLEEP APNEA [HEALTH MAINTENANCE]
The major risk factors for Obstructive sleep apnea (OSA) in adults are obesity [choice C], male gender, and advancing age. Increased neck circumference is a strong risk factor.
~40–60% of cases of OSA are attributable to excess weight.
Obesity predisposes to OSA because upper airway fat narrows the airway and obesity decreases chest wall compliance lung volumes.
Weight loss can dramatically reduce the severity of OSA.

Ingestion of alcohol [choice A] or sedatives before sleeping or nasal obstruction of any type [choice D], may precipitate or worsen OSA.

27. ENDOCRINOLOGY – TYPE 1 DIABETES MELLITUS [HEALTH MAINTENANCE]
To reduce the risk of exercise-induced Hyperglycemia, patients with type 1 diabetes this patient should reduce his insulin dosages [choice A] and adjust as necessary.
Measures to reduce early post-exercise hypoglycemia include:
- reducing insulin dose,
- interspersing brief episodes of intense exercise (which tends to raise plasma glucose concentrations), or
- adding carbohydrate ingestion (eg, 1 g/kg/h),

Choice B [Discontinue NPH and initiate regular Insulin on a sliding scale] may result in the development of Diabetic ketoacidosis.
Choice D [Restrict training sessions to less than 45 minutes] is not necessary.

28. DERMATOLOGY – ROSACEA [PHARMACOLOGY]

First-line therapies in mild to moderate Rosacea include topical Metronidazole [choice B], topical Azelaic acid, or topical Ivermectin.

Although the exact mechanism of Metronidazole is unknown, its effects are thought to result from its anti-inflammatory, antimicrobial, and/or antioxidant properties.

Topical Metronidazole is most effective for the treatment of inflammatory papules and pustules but also results in some improvement of facial erythema.

Choice A [Oral Doxycycline] and other systemic Tetracyclines are options for the management of Rosacea with inadequate response to one or more topical therapies.

Choice C [Laser and intense pulsed light] is a second-line option for the management of Rosacea for the management of the vascular findings of Rosacea, particularly telangiectasis.

Choice D [Oral Isotretinoin] is an option for Rosacea that fails to respond to topical therapies and oral antibiotics.

Choice E [Topical Hydrocortisone] is not a first-line agent for Rosacea, and prolonged used on the face can lead to thinning of the skin and telangiectasias.

29. PULMONOLOGY – PULMONARY EMBOLISM [LABS AND DIAGNOSTIC STUDIES]

For most patients with suspected PE, CTPA (chest CT angiogram with contrast) [choice E], is the first-choice diagnostic imaging modality because it is sensitive and specific for the diagnosis of PE. His Wells score is 7.

Many experts believe that a subset of patients in the intermediate risk category (eg, those in the upper zone of the intermediate range [eg, Wells score 4 to 6 or Modified Geneva sore 8 to 10]) should undergo imaging based upon the higher probability of PE in these patients since the sensitivity of D-dimer is not as good.

Choice A [D-dimer levels] can be used in patients with moderate risk, but an elevated D dimer may also be observed in malignancy (this patient has Hodgkin lymphoma), pregnancy, following trauma, and surgery.

Choice B [Venous Doppler ultrasound] is most useful to diagnose PE in patients suspected of having a PE when imaging (CTPA, V/Q scan) is negative, contraindicated, or indeterminate.

Choice C [Venography] would not be the most appropriate next step as it is invasive.

Choice E [Ventilation-Perfusion scan] can be used to make the diagnosis of PE when CTPA is contraindicated or inconclusive, or when additional testing is required.

30. HEMATOLOGY – CHRONIC LYMPHOCYTIC LEUKEMIA (CLL) [MOST LIKELY]

Smudge cells are most often associated with abnormally fragile lymphocytes in disorders such as Chronic lymphocytic leukemia (CLL) [choice C].

Smudge cells are remnants of cells that lack any identifiable cytoplasmic membrane or nuclear structure. It is a lab artifact.

Most patients are initially asymptomatic but may painless lymphadenopathy.

The classic findings of CLL on peripheral smear include marked lymphocytosis (morphologically mature-appearing small lymphocytes) and smudge cells.

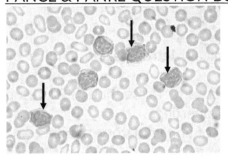

31. GENITOURINARY – TESTICULAR TORSION [CLINICAL INTERVENTION]

Early surgical consultation for orchiopexy [choice E] is recommended in patients with a high probability (high TWIST score) of Testicular torsion without need for Ultrasound (eg, nausea, vomiting, testicular swelling, high-riding testis, absent cremasteric reflex).

A color Doppler ultrasound of the scrotum [choice C] should be obtained if history and clinical findings are equivocal for a Testicular torsion.

Choice A [IV Ceftriaxone and Azithromycin] can be used in the management of Acute epididymitis.

Choice B [CT scan of abdomen and pelvis] is not the imaging used to establish the diagnosis of Testicular torsion. When imaging is needed, a color Doppler ultrasound of the scrotum is recommended.

Choice D [Observation and IV Morphine] is inappropriate as delay in performing Orchiopexy reduces the chance of viability of the affected testis.

32. ENDOCRINOLOGY – PRIMARY ADRENAL INSUFFICIENCY [APPLYING FUNDAMENTAL CONCEPTS]

Autoimmune adrenalitis [choice C] is the most common cause of Primary adrenal insufficiency (AI), accounting for 70-90% of cases of Primary AI.

The remaining causes include infectious diseases [choice A], replacement by metastatic cancer or lymphoma, adrenal hemorrhage or infarction [choices B and E], or medications.

Choice D [Aldosteronoma] is associated with Primary hyperaldosteronism, which is characterized by the triad of Hypertension, Hypokalemia, and Metabolic alkalosis.

33. EENT – STREPTOCOCCAL PHARYNGITIS [LABS AND DIAGNOSTICS]

Follow-up testing with the criterion standard Throat culture [choice C] is recommended in children and adolescents with an exudative pharyngitis with negative RADT testing because RADT may miss as many as 30% of cases of GAS pharyngitis.

Failure to adequately treat children and adolescents with GAS increases the risk of Acute rheumatic fever (ARF) and suppurative complications.

Confirmation of negative RADT with Throat culture is not necessary in adults because the risk of ARF is low.

The diagnosis of GAS pharyngitis is supported by a positive throat culture, Rapid antigen detection test (RADT), or molecular assay for GAS.

Microbiologic confirmation of GAS in the pharynx before initiation of antibiotic therapy [choice D] prevents unnecessary administration of antibiotics in children with viral pharyngitis, the most common cause of pharyngitis in children.

Choice A [Heterophile antibody test] is helpful in the diagnosis of Infectious mononucleosis.
Choice B [Diphtheria antigen testing] may be used if Respiratory Diphtheria is suspected (eg, grey-white pseudomembranes).
Choice E (Influenza A and B antigen) can be ordered in patients with viral symptoms consistent with Influenza.

34. EENT – RETINAL DETACHMENT [HISTORY AND PHYSICAL EXAMINATION]

Retinal detachment should be suspected in patients who develop sudden onset if unilateral
- **progressive or fixed visual field loss, often starting in the periphery and then moving centrally ("curtain coming down") over the visual field [choice B].**
- **photopsia (flashes of light) in their vision and floaters (moving spots in the visual field)**
- evidence of detachment on funduscopic examination.

Ocular erythema [choice C] and pain with eye movements (ophthalmoplegia) [choice A] suggests an alternative diagnosis, such as Anterior uveitis (Iritis).
Choice D [Central scotoma] can be seen with Optic neuritis, which is associated with eye pain and ophthalmoplegia.
Choice E [Halos around light] can be associated with Acute angle closure glaucoma, which is associated with ocular pain and peripheral vision loss often described as tunnel vision.

35. GASTROINTESTINAL/NUTRITION – VITAMIN C DEFICIENCY [MOST LIKELY]

Because inadequate consumption of vitamin C (Ascorbic acid) [choice D] leads to impaired hydroxylation of collagen, Scurvy results in the 4 "Hs": Hemorrhage, Hyperkeratosis, and Hematologic abnormalities:
- **gingivitis: swollen/bleeding gums**
- **coarse corkscrew (coiled) hair with perifollicular hemorrhage**
- bruising, petechiae, hemarthrosis, anemia, and poor wound healing

Choice A [Retinol], or Vitamin A deficiency, presents with night blindness and Bitot spots.
Choice B [Cholecalciferol], or Vitamin D deficiency, presents with Osteomalacia in adults and Rickets in children.
Choice C [Niacin], or Vitamin B3 deficiency, presents with Pellagra: diarrhea, dermatitis, and dementia.
Choice E (Thiamine), or Vitamin B1 deficiency, presents with [1] dry Beri Beri (peripheral neuropathy), [2] wet Beri Beri (dilated cardiomyopathy), [3] Wernicke's encephalopathy, &/or [4] Korsakoff syndrome.

36. GASTROINTESTINAL/NUTRITION – VOLVULUS [APPLYING FOUNDATIONAL CONCEPTS]

A Sigmoid volvulus occurs when a portion of the intestine twists around its blood supply [choice B].
Patients often present with signs of obstruction (eg, nausea, vomiting, abdominal pain, distention), especially in patients with a history of constipation.

The classic radiograph findings of a Sigmoid volvulus is the presence of a U-shaped, distended sigmoid colon with no haustra (often described as the "coffee bean" or "bent inner tube" sign) arising from the pelvis up towards the right upper quadrant.

Choice A [Functional obstruction of the small bowel] describes a Paralytic ileus, which is characterized by dilated loops of small bowel without a transition zone.

Choice C [Mechanical obstruction of the small bowel] describes a Small bowel obstruction, which is characterized by a step ladder appearance.

Choice D [Telescoping of one part of the bowel into another part of the bowel] is hallmark of Intussusception.

Choice E [Inadequate blood supply to the large intestine] is hallmark of Ischemic colitis, which is characterized by segmental bowel wall thickening with a classic thumbprinting appearance.

37. HEMATOLOGY – APLASTIC ANEMIA/FANCONI ANEMIA [MOST LIKELY]

Fanconi anemia (FA) [choice B] is a rare inherited bone marrow failure syndrome characterized by pancytopenia (Aplastic anemia), predisposition to malignancy, and characteristic physical abnormalities/congenital malformations.

Children with Fanconi anemia have characteristic congenital abnormalities, including short stature, thumb hypoplasia, café au lait spots, and heart defects.

Choice A [Sickle cell disease] is not associated with Aplastic anemia, unless in the setting of Parvovirus B19 infection. It is not associated with the congenital findings.

Choice C [Immune thrombotic thrombocytopenia] presents with an isolated thrombocytopenia.

Choice D [Hemolytic uremic syndrome] is associated with the triad of (1) hemolytic anemia, (2) thrombocytopenia, and (3) Acute kidney injury.

Choice E [Neurofibromatosis type 1] is characterized by café au lait macules >5 mm, Lisch nodules on the iris, axillary and inguinal freckling, Neurofibromas, optic glioma, and Pheochromocytoma.

38. MUSCULOSKELETAL/RHEUMATOLOGY – SJÖGREN'S SYNDROME [HEALTH MAINTENANCE]

Lymphoma [choice B] is one of the most serious complications of Sjögren's syndrome, occurring in up to 5-10% of patients.

Rarely, malignant transformation of B lymphocytes in the focal lymphocytic infiltrates of the exocrine glands result in non-Hodgkin lymphoma.

Patients with Sjögren's syndrome may also have a higher risk of head and neck cancers.

Sjögren's syndrome is a chronic systemic autoimmune disorder characterized by diminished lacrimal and salivary gland function, resulting in dry eyes dry mouth, dyspareunia (vulvovaginal dryness), and parotid gland enlargement.

Choice A [vision loss] is a classic complication of Giant cell arteritis.

39. MUSCULOSKELETAL/RHEUMATOLOGY – DERMATOMYOSITIS [MOST LIKELY]

Key features of Dermatomyositis [choice E] include
- **Heliotrope eruption: erythematous to violaceous eruption on the periorbital skin and eyelids**

- **Gottron sign** raised violaceous macules, patches, or papules on the extensor surfaces of the hands, elbows, knees, or ankles.
- **Facial erythema** that can mimic the malar erythema seen in Systemic lupus erythematosus (SLE) but involves the nasolabial folds, unlike SLE, which spares the nasolabial folds.
- **Muscle weakness:** objective weakness on examination involving the proximal muscles of the hip and shoulder girdles.
- Elevated muscle enzymes.

Choice A [Systemic lupus erythematosus] is associated with a malar rash that spares the nasolabial folds and is not associated with increased muscle enzymes.

Choice B [Diffuse systemic sclerosis (Scleroderma)] can present with skin thickening, sclerodactyly, calcinosis cutis, Raynaud phenomena, and esophageal disorders.

Choice C [Polymyalgia rheumatica] is associated joint achiness and stiffness (which this patient denies), no objective muscle weakness on examination, and normal muscle enzymes.

Choice D [Fibromyalgia] is characterized by widespread muscle pain, fatigue, cognitive disturbances, sleep disturbances, and point tenderness in at least 11 out of 18 trigger points.

40. NEUROLOGY – CRANIAL X PALSY [HISTORY AND PHYSICAL EXAMINATION]

This patient most likely has a left Cranial nerve X (10) palsy [choice C] due to deviation of the uvula to the contralateral side (right).

Cranial nerve X (10) palsies:

- palate droop
- dysphagia
- **deviation of the uvula away from the side of the lesion** (towards the strong side)
- **loss of gag reflex** (the sensory component of this reflex is mostly via CN IX).

A hoarse voice can indicate Vagus nerve injury.

Choice A [Right Cranial nerve 9 palsy] is associated with difficulty swallowing and absent gag reflex, but it not associated with hoarseness.

Choice B [Left Cranial nerve 9 palsy] is associated with difficulty swallowing and absent gag reflex, but it not associated with hoarseness.

Choice D [Right cranial nerve 10 palsy] would be associated with deviation of the uvula to the contralateral side (left).

Choice E [Left cranial nerve 12 palsy] is associated with deviation of the tongue toward the side of the lesion and muscle atrophy that may be visible on examination.

41. PSYCHIATRY/BEHAVIORAL MEDICINE – SEROTONIN SYNDROME/DELIRIUM [MOST LIKELY]

Serotonin syndrome [choice C] is characterized by

- **neuromuscular hyperreactivity** eg, tremor, hyperreflexia, myoclonus
- **serotonergic effects on GI system:** diarrhea, hyperactive bowel sounds
- **altered mental status:** eg, agitation, confusion
- **autonomic instability:** eg, hyperthermia, hypertension, tachycardia
- **diaphoresis, mydriasis**

Interactions with serotonergic medications, such as SSRIs and MAO inhibitors (eg, Linezolid is an antibiotic with MAOI properties), can induce Serotonin syndrome with concomitant use.

Choice A [Neuroleptic malignant syndrome] and SS share similar symptoms (eg, autonomic instability, altered mental status but NMS occurs slower (days to weeks), has sluggish responses (hyporeflexia, lead pipe rigidity), and occurs with the use of dopamine receptor antagonist medications (eg, antipsychotics).

Choice B [Malignant hyperthermia] occurs in the setting of depolarizing muscle relaxant use (eg, Succinylcholine) and presents with tachycardia, hyperthermia, acidosis, and rigor mortis-like muscle rigidity.

Choice C [Alcohol withdrawal] and other sedative hypnotic withdrawal lack the neuromuscular activation signs (eg, tremor, hyperreflexia and clonus that are greater in the lower extremities, ocular clonus).

Choice D [Anticholinergic toxicity] can present similar, but patients are usually hot and dry as opposed to diaphoretic, have decreased bowel sounds (as opposed to increased), and lack the neuromuscular activation signs (eg, tremor, hyperreflexia and clonus that are greater in the lower extremities, ocular clonus).

42. CARDIOLOGY – ACUTE PERICARDITIS [PHARMACOLOGY]

Combination therapy with a Nonsteroidal anti-inflammatory drug (NSAID) plus Colchicine [choice E] is preferred rather than an NSAID alone for most patients with acute idiopathic or viral Pericarditis.

The addition of Colchicine decreases pain, symptom length, complications, and recurrence rate.

Acute pericarditis should be suspected in patients with the **Ps of Pericarditis**:

- **P**leuritic chest pain
- **P**ositional chest pain (worse when supine; improves with sitting up)
- **P**ericardial friction rub
- **P**R depression and diffuse ST elevation in the same leads as PR depression
- **P**yrosis (may be febrile)
- **P**ericardial effusion

Choice A [Prednisone] or other glucocorticoids are usually reserved for severe or refractory cases, if NSAIDs/ASA or Colchicine is contraindicated (eg, kidney disease), in connective tissue disease, autoreactivity, uremia, SLE, or pregnancy.

Choice B [Naproxen] and other NSAIDs can be used for Acute pericarditis but combination therapy is preferred due to reduce recurrence rates.

Choice C [Pericardiocentesis] can be performed if Pericardial tamponade is suspected (eg, hypotension, distended neck veins, muffled heart sounds, also known as Beck's triad).

Choice D [Aspirin and Nitroglycerin] may be used in the setting of Acute coronary artery syndrome.

43. HEMATOLOGY – G6PD DEFICIENCY [APPLYING FOUNDATIONAL CONCEPTS]

Glucose-6-phosphate dehydrogenase (G6PD) deficiency results in oxidative injury during times of oxidative stress (eg, infection, medications, food such as Fava/broad beans, etc.) [choice A].

G6PD deficiency is an X-linked recessive inherited disorder (most commonly seen in males) caused by a genetic defect in the red blood cell enzyme G6PD, which normally generates NADPH to protects RBCs from oxidative damage.

G6PD deficiency can result in episodic hemolytic anemia during oxidative stress.

There is usually no hemolysis in the steady state.

Choice B [Red blood cell cytoskeleton, resulting in a red cell membrane defect] is hallmark of Hereditary spherocytosis.

Choice C [Reduction in the synthesis of globin chains] is hallmark of Thalassemia.

Choice D [Point mutation in the beta globin gene] results in Sickle cell disease.

Choice E [IgM autoantibodies against red blood cell [RBC] antigens] results in Cold agglutinin disease.

44. PULMONOLOGY – ASPIRATION PNEUMONIA [HISTORY AND PHYSICAL]

Aspiration of fluid or endogenous secretions into the lower airways [choice B] is a cause of Aspiration pneumonia when normal protective mechanisms of the airway are compromised.
Infections can be caused by oral bacteria (eg, anaerobic or aerobic bacteria).
Risk factors for Aspiration include chronic drug or alcohol use (loss of normal gag reflex), dysphagia from neurologic deficits, and poor dental hygiene. This patient has both substance use and periodontal disease.
Radiographs of Aspiration pneumonia may reveal a right lobe infiltrate or cavitary lesion (lung abscess), as seen in this patient.

Choice A [Extension of infection from parapneumonic sources] is not a cause of Aspiration pneumonia.

Choice C [Exposure to contaminated water sources] is the mode of transmission of *Legionella pneumoniae*.

Choice D [Inhalation of aerosolized droplets] is the mode of transmission of *Mycobacteria tuberculosis*.

Choice E [Hematogenous spread of pathogenic bacteria] is not a cause of Aspiration pneumonia.

45. GENITOURINARY – NEPHROLITHIASIS [LABS AND DIAGNOSTIC STUDIES]

Non-contrast helical CT [choice D] is the most sensitive modality to detect renal or ureteral stones.
CT can also detect ureteral stones and small stones (eg, <5 mm), which may not be detected by ultrasonography.
Nephrolithiasis is associated with renal colic or flank pain and gross or microscopic hematuria.

Choice A [KUB (kidneys, ureters, and bladder) plain radiographs] is not the first line imaging modality as it can miss radiolucent and small stones.

Choice B [Intravenous pyelogram] is not the initial imaging of choice for suspected Nephrolithiasis.

Choice C [Renal ultrasound] can be used to diagnose Nephrolithiasis in younger children and in pregnant women to avoid radiation. Her beta-hCG is negative.

Choice E [Cystoscopy] is used in the workup of suspected Bladder carcinoma.

46. MUSCULOSKELETAL/RHEUMATOLOGY – OSGOOD-SCHLATTER DISEASE [CLINICAL INTERVENTION]

Conservative (nonsurgical) management is the mainstay of treatment of Osgood-Schlatter disease includes control of pain and swelling (ice, brief use of NSAIDs) [choice C], continuation of activity, physical therapy to strengthen the quadriceps, and improve the flexibility of the hamstrings, and use of a protective pad over the tibial tubercle.

Patients may continue activity as tolerated as long as the pain is tolerated and resolves within 24 hours (activity may need to be modified).

Symptoms usually subside once the growth plate is ossified, often within 6-19 months. Osgood-Schlatter disease most commonly occurs during growth spurts (ages 9-14 years). Physical examination is notable for tenderness and bony prominence of the tibial tubercle near the patellar tendon insertion.

Crutches are rarely needed and knee immobilizers [choice A] are contraindicated as casting can result in atrophy of the hamstring and quadriceps muscles.

Surgical management [choice B] is reserved for patients who fail to respond to conservative measures; if necessary, it is usually performed after closure of the proximal tibial growth plate (which is often the time that the symptoms improve or resolve in most).

Complete avoidance of sports activity [choice D] is neither necessary nor recommended. Inactivity may result in deconditioning.

Glucocorticoid injections [choice E] are generally not recommended due to various associated complications.

47. GASTROINTESTINAL/NUTRITION – GASTROESOPHAGEAL REFLUX DISEASE [LABS AND DIAGNOSTIC STUDIES]

Upper endoscopy [choice D] can be used to detect esophageal complications of GERD (eg, Barrett's metaplasia, Erosive esophagitis, stricture, or Esophageal adenocarcinoma) in patients with alarm symptoms.

Although upper endoscopy is not required to make a diagnosis of uncomplicated GERD but should be performed in patients with alarm features:

- new onset of dyspepsia in patient ≥60 years
- Evidence of gastrointestinal bleeding (hematemesis, melena, hematochezia, occult blood in stool)
- Iron deficiency anemia
- Dysphagia, odynophagia
- Unexplained weight loss.

Choice A [Switch to Pantoprazole] may be used in patients with uncomplicated GERD or persistent GERD.

Choice B [Esophageal motility studies with barium] is not first line to evaluated GERD with alarm features.

Choice C [Esophageal ambulatory pH monitoring] may be used in the diagnosis of classic GERD symptoms not responsive to appropriate treatment.

Choice E [Esophageal manometry] may be used to exclude an esophageal motility disorder in patients with suspected GERD with chest pain and/or dysphagia and a normal upper endoscopy.

48. PULMONOLOGY – PERTUSSIS [HEALTH MAINTENANCE]

It is recommended that all household and close contacts of a person with Pertussis receive postexposure antibiotics, such as Macrolides (eg, Azithromycin, Erythromycin) [choice C], regardless of their vaccination status.

Trimethoprim-sulfamethoxazole is an alternative.

Young, healthy adults who have been fully vaccinated (including with a booster dose within five years) may still develop an infection during an outbreak.

Postexposure prophylaxis is most effective when started within 21 days of the onset of symptoms in the index patient.

Pertussis should be suspected in patients with paroxysms of coughing, followed by an inspiratory whoop, and post tussive vomiting.

Pertussis occurs in 3 stages:
- [1] catarrhal stage symptoms similar to an upper respiratory infection; lasts 1-2 weeks.
- [2] paroxysmal stage characterized by paroxysms of coughing, an inspiratory whoop, and posttussive vomiting or cyanosis; lasts 2-8 weeks.
- [3] convalescent stage: resolution of cough; subsides over several weeks to months.

49. PSYCHIATRY/BEHAVIORAL MEDICINE – HISTRIONIC PERSONALITY DISORDER [HISTORY AND PHYSICAL]

Histrionic personality disorder [choice B] is characterized by excessive emotionality and attention seeking, behaviors characterized by:
- inappropriate sexually seduction, flirtatious, and provocative behavior
- attention seeking: needs to be the center of attention
- resorts to child-like behavior when they are not the center of attention
- displays rapidly shifting and shallow expression of emotions.
- consistently uses physical appearance to draw attention to self.

Choice A [Illness anxiety disorder] is a preoccupation of having contracted an illness despite little to no symptoms of that illness.

Choice C [Borderline personality disorder] is associated with black-and white thinking, intense reactions, fear of abandonment, and mood swings.

Choice D [Narcissistic personality disorder] is characterized by grandiosity, need for attention and admiration, superficial interpersonal relationships, and a lack of empathy.

Choice E [Somatic symptom disorder] is a preoccupation of at least 1 symptom over a long period of time.

50. PULMONOLOGY – SMALL CELL LUNG CANCER [CLINICAL INTERVENTION]

Combination chemotherapy (eg, either Cisplatin or Carboplatin plus Etoposide) [choice D] or concurrent chemoradiotherapy is often the standard of treatment of Small cell lung cancer (SCLC) to slow growth and increase survival.

SCLC is a highly aggressive disease characterized by its rapid doubling time, early development of metastatic disease [eg, Cushing syndrome, Lambert-Eaton syndrome, SVC syndrome], and dramatic response to first-line chemotherapy and radiation. This patient was diagnosed with Cushing syndrome and has weakness improved with repeated use, consistent with Lambert-Eaton syndrome.

In general, surgical resection is *not* routinely recommended because even patients with Limited disease-SCLC often have occult micro metastases.

SCLC is often seen as a central lesion on imaging.

Choice A [Rifampin, Isoniazid, Pyrazinamide, Ethambutol] is used in the management of Tuberculosis, which usually appears as a consolidation or miliary pattern on imaging.

Choice B [Surgical excision] is the treatment of choice for clinical stage I and II Non-small cell lung cancer [NSCLC] for individuals who can tolerate surgery.

Choice C [Broad-spectrum antibiotics and sputum cytology] may be indicated for infectious Pneumonia.

Choice E [Radiation followed by surgical excision] is incorrect as SCLC is not usually amenable to surgery.

51. REPRODUCTIVE – GYNECOMASTIA [HEALTH MAINTENANCE]

Observation and reassurance alone [choice D] that is it a benign physiologic process is a reasonable approach for most adolescent boys with pubertal gynecomastia.

Pubertal gynecomastia is thought to be caused by a faster elevation in estradiol than the rise of testosterone, resulting in an imbalance that normally regresses with time as testosterone increases.

It typically develops between ages 10 and 12 years, with a peak prevalence between ages 13 and 14 years, followed by regression in 80% within six months to two years.

Features of typical pubertal Gynecomastia include a **palpable rubbery or firm mass of tissue,** often >2 cm, with 4 classic characteristics:
- [1] centrally located (usually underlying the nipple and extending from the nipples),
- [2] symmetrical in shape,
- [3] bilateral in most, and
- [4] often tender to palpation in the early phase (first 6 months).

Choice A [Brief trial of Tamoxifen for three months] may be used in some adolescent boys with severe breast enlargement identified as glandular tissue with significant tenderness or embarrassment.

Choice B [Testosterone therapy] may be indicated in men with hypogonadism detected by laboratory evaluation. This patient has no features suggestive of hypogonadism.

Laboratory evaluation [choice C] is generally not necessary for adolescents with clinical features typical of pubertal gynecomastia. Laboratory evaluation may be indicated [1] in prepubertal males without any other secondary sexual characteristics (eg, increased testicular volume, pubic hair) or [2] if gynecomastia persists >2 years or if >17 years of age.

Choice E [Ultrasound of the breast tissues] is not indicated unless there is suspicion for malignancy or infection.

52. INFECTIOUS DISEASE – CNS LYMPHOMA [HISTORY AND PHYSICAL EXAMINATION]

Aside from increasing age, immunosuppression, especially those infected with the human immunodeficiency virus (HIV) [choice A] or organ transplant recipients, is the most important risk for the development of Primary CNS lymphoma (PCNSL).

Epstein-Barr virus (EBV) plays a significant part in the pathogenesis of PCNSL in this population.

Primary CNS lymphoma (PCNSL) is second to CNS Toxoplasmosis as a cause of a brain mass lesion in patients with advanced HIV.

The classic finding of PSCNL on imaging, as with Toxoplasmosis, is a ring-enhancing lesion.

53. INFECTIOUS DISEASE – ERYTHEMA INFECTIOSUM [HISTORY AND PHYSICAL]

Classic presentations of Parvovirus B19 infections [choice E] include:

- **Fifth disease/Erythema infectiosum in children**: facial rash with a slapped cheek appearance, followed by a lace-like reticular rash on the trunk or extremities.
- **Arthropathy** in older children and adults, especially women
- Transient Aplastic crisis in individuals with hemoglobinopathies (Sickle cell, Thalassemia), and G6PD deficiency, or
- Pure red blood cell aplasia in immunocompromised individuals.

Choice A [Human herpesvirus 6] is associated with Roseola infantum, which is characterized by a rash that starts on the trunk and then spreads to the face. It is usually seen in children <2 years of age.

Choice B [Coxsackie virus A16] is associated with Hand foot and mouth disease, characterized by painful oral lesions on the tongue and buccal mucosa, followed by a rash on the hands, feet, buttock, and extremities.

Choice C [Rubella virus] classically presents with a maculopapular facial rash associated with low-grade fever, swollen glands (suboccipital and posterior cervical), joint pain and non-exudative conjunctivitis.

Choice D [Group A streptococcus] causes Scarlet fever, which also associated with facial erythema and circumoral pallor, but Scarlet fever is also associated with diffuse erythema that blanches with pressure, papular elevations with a rough "sandpaper" quality, and a strawberry tongue.

54. REPRODUCTIVE – CONTRACEPTION [PHARMACOLOGY]

Long-acting, reversible contraceptives, such as the subdermal progestin implant [choice A] and intrauterine devices (IUDs) Levonorgestrel or Copper are first-line contraception options for adolescents.

Benefits of Etonogestrel implant include:

- Etonogestrel implant is the most effective form of any contraceptive method, with an average failure rate of 0.05%.
- Lasts 3 years
- Does not impact endogenous estradiol levels and thus does not induce significant bone loss (unlike Depot Medroxyprogesterone acetate/DMPA).

Choice B [Estrogen-progestin vaginal ring] may be an issue in adolescent when compliance may be an issue (she expresses compliance issues).

Choice C [Transdermal contraceptive patch] is not one of the first line options in adolescents.

Choice D [Combined estrogen-progestin oral contraceptives] is an alternative but with issues of compliance IUDs or implants are a more effective option and reduces the need for constant compliance.

Choice E [Depot medroxyprogesterone acetate injection] lasts for 3 months (she is going away to school and can be used for no more than 2 years due to increased bone loss and Osteoporosis risk.

55. ENDOCRINOLOGY – THYROID NODULE [LABS AND DIAGNOSTIC STUDIES]

In patients with a thyroid nodule with a subnormal TSH concentration (suggesting subclinical or overt hyperthyroidism), Thyroid scintigraphy [choice E] should be performed to rule out a hyperfunctioning nodule (Thyroid adenoma).

Autonomous thyroid nodule may suppress TSH production (Primary hyperthyroidism) and is characterized by a hot nodule (focal increased uptake) on Thyroid scintigraphy.

Because hyperfunctioning nodules are rarely cancerous, a hyperfunctioning nodule on thyroid scintigraphy does not require FNA.

Choice A [Fine needle aspiration] are indicated for large thyroid nodules (>1.5 cm), suspicious nodules on physical examination, suspicious nodules on ultrasound, or suspicious nodules on scintigraphy. A hyperechoic nodule <1.5 cm is most likely benign.
Choice B [Levothyroxine] is not indicated in the diagnosis of a thyroid nodule.
Choice D [Partial thyroidectomy] is not the most appropriate next step in the evaluation and management of a suspected benign thyroid nodule.
Choice E (Radioactive iodine) is a therapeutic option for the management of Hyperthyroidism once the diagnosis and etiology has been established.

56. RENAL – HYPERKALEMIA [CLINICAL INTERVENTION]
Calcium gluconate [choice E] or Calcium chloride is the first step in the management of severe Hyperkalemia (eg, serum potassium >6.5 mEq/L, ECG changes).
Calcium directly antagonizes the membrane actions of hyperkalemia and stabilizes the cardiac membranes, allowing time for potassium lowering therapy to take their effect.

After administration of Calcium gluconate, the next step is administration of Insulin [choice B] to rapidly lower the serum potassium concentration by driving potassium into the cells, primarily by enhancing the activity of the Na-K-ATPase pump in skeletal muscle. Glucose is coadministered with insulin to prevent the development of hypoglycemia.

Choice B [Sodium bicarbonate] is used as an antidote for ECG changes associated with Tricyclic antidepressant toxicity.
Choice C [Magnesium sulfate] is used in the management of severe Hypomagnesemia and Torsades de pointes.
Choice D [Sodium polystyrene sulfonate] is not commonly used in the management of Hyperkalemia, and if it is used, it is done to slowly lower potassium if other GI cation exchangers are not available.

57. PSYCHIATRY/BEHAVIORAL MEDICINE – CONDUCT DISORDER [MOST LIKELY]
Conduct disorder [choice D] is characterized by consistent aggressive and disobedient behavior that violates the basic rights of others or violates age-appropriate society norms.
Key features may include:
- threats of harm to people and animals
- property loss or damage, deceitfulness or theft, and serious rule violations
- lack of remorse or guilt, callousness/lack of empathy.

Choice A [Narcissistic personality disorder] is also associated with lack of empathy but is associated with a grandiose attitude.
Choice B [Oppositional defiant disorder] is associated with increased irritability and anger but is not classically associated with aggression towards people or animals, or destruction of property.
Choice C [Antisocial personality disorder] presents with behaviors similar to Conduct disorder but requires the patient to be ≥18 years of age.
Choice E [Intermittent explosive disorder] may also be associated with aggression towards others. However, aggression in intermittent explosive disorder is often not premeditated or to achieve a specific benefit, as seen with Conduct disorder.

58. RENAL – END STAGE RENAL DISEASE/CHRONIC KIDNEY DISEASE [HEALTH MAINTENANCE]

Diabetes mellitus [choice C] is the most common cause of End stage renal disease in the United states.

Hypertension [choice B] is the second most common cause.

Diabetes and high blood pressure account for 3 out of 4 cases of ESRD in the US.

Broad waxy casts seen on Urinalysis is associated with End stage renal disease and reflect dilated collecting ducts.

59. INFECTIOUS DISEASE – TUBERCULOSIS [HEALTH MAINTENANCE]

Because a negative Tuberculin skin test (TST) is considered negative if <10 mm (eg, living in group settings, such as prisons, nursing homes, and homeless shelters), the patient should continue routine screening without any further intervention [choice D].

A repeat TST or perform an Interferon-gamma release assay (IGRA) can be considered if the patient is considered at high risk of developing an active TB infection.

Choice A [Isoniazid + Vitamin B6 for 6 months duration] and choice B [Rifampin daily for 4 months (4R)] are treatment options for Latent TB infection: [1] a positive PPD, [2] chest imaging with no evidence of an active infection, and [3] no symptoms of an active infection.

Choice C [Initiate Rifampin, Isoniazid, Pyrazinamide, Ethambutol] is the treatment of choice for an active Tuberculosis infection.

Choice E [Chest radiograph] is the most appropriate next step in patients with a positive screening test [eg, TST or an Interferon-gamma release assay (IGRA)].

60. GENITOURINARY – ACUTE CYSTITIS [PHARMACOLOGY]

First line antibiotic treatment for Acute uncomplicated cystitis includes Nitrofurantoin [choice B], Fosfomycin, or Trimethoprim-sulfamethoxazole.

Symptoms of acute uncomplicated Cystitis in women include dysuria, increased urinary frequency, urinary urgency, and suprapubic discomfort.

Acute cystitis is considered uncomplicated if the patient is female, immunocompetent, premenopausal, and not pregnant.

She has no symptoms or signs consistent with Acute pyelonephritis, such as flank pain, costovertebral angle tenderness, and she has no symptoms of systemic illness (eg, fever, rigors).

The diagnosis of uncomplicated Acute cystitis is mainly clinical, and additional workup (eg, urine culture [choice A] or cystography [choice E) are not required unless the patient fails initial treatment.

Choice C [Doxycycline] is used in the management of Urethritis caused by Chlamydia trachomatis. The presence of suprapubic tenderness and nitrites on UA is more suggestive of Acute cystitis.

Choice D [Ciprofloxacin] and other Fluoroquinolones are usually reserved for cases when first line agents cannot be used.

61. INFECTIOUS DISEASE – BOTULISM [CLINICAL INTERVENTION]

Infant botulism (<1 year of age) is treated with human-derived intravenous Botulism immune globulin [choice C] (BIG-IV or BabyBIG).

BIG-IV should be administered as early as in the course of illness as possible.

Equine serum heptavalent BAT [choice A] is used to treat non-infant botulism >1 years of age.
Antibiotics [choice E] are **not** recommended for types of botulism other than wound botulism.
With infant botulism lysis of intraluminal *C. botulinum* with antibiotics may release additional toxin, worsening the condition.

62. RENAL – ACUTE INTERSTITIAL NEPHRITIS [HISTORY AND PHYSICAL EXAMINATION]
Medications are the most common cause of Acute interstitial nephritis (AIN), with common offenders including:
- **Penicillins [choice C], Cephalosporins, and Fluoroquinolones**
- NSAIDs, including selective COX-2 inhibitors
- Proton pump inhibitors
- Rifampin
- Allopurinol
- Diuretics (especially sulfonamides).

Patients with AIN may present with rash, fever, eosinophilia, and nonspecific symptoms. Other causes of AIN include infection and autoimmune causes [choice A].

Choice B [Pharyngitis] may proceed postinfectious Glomerulonephritis, which is associated with dysmorphic RBCs and red cell casts.
Choice D [Use of Gentamicin] is associated with epithelial cell and muddy brown casts.
Choice E [Hepatitis C virus] is associated with Membranous nephropathy.

63. GENITOURINARY – BLADDER CANCER [HEALTH MAINTENANCE]
In addition to smoking, risk factors for Bladder cancer include industrial exposure: eg, rubber industry workers [choice C], leather workers, aniline dyes in paint/pigment exposure, auto or metal workers, beauticians, and exposure to textile & electrical, carpets, plastics, & industrial chemicals.

Choice A [Coal miner] increases the risk for Coal worker's pneumoconiosis.
Choice B [Demolition man of old buildings] increases the risk for Asbestosis and Mesothelioma.
Choice D [Stonecutter] increases the risk for Silicosis.
Choice E [Oil refiner] increases exposure to Benzene, which can increase the risk for blood-related cancers (eg, Leukemia, Lymphoma).

64. EENT – MÉNIÈRE DISEASE [MOST LIKELY]
Ménière disease [choice B] is characterized by:
- **≥2 spontaneous episodes of vertigo, each lasting 20 minutes to 12 hours**
- **sensorineural hearing loss**: audiometry will reveal low- to mid-frequency hearing loss in the affected ear
- **fluctuating aural symptoms (reduced or distorted hearing, tinnitus, or fullness)** in the affected ear
- symptoms not better accounted for by another vestibular diagnosis.

Choice A [Labyrinthitis] is associated with continuous vertigo and hearing loss.
Choice C [Acoustic neuroma (Vestibular schwannoma)] presents with progressive asymmetric sensorineural hearing loss. Although patients may experience imbalance and disequilibrium, true vertigo is not common.
Choice D [Vestibular neuronitis] is associated with continuous vertigo without hearing loss.
Choice E [Benign paroxysmal positional vertigo] is associated with episodic vertigo, usually lasting seconds but no more than a minute and is exacerbated by changes in head position. BPPV is not associated with hearing loss.

65. DERMATOLOGY – ONYCHOMYCOSIS [PHARMACOLOGY]

Oral Terbinafine [choice B] is the first-line oral agent for mild to moderate dermatophyte onychomycosis.
Oral Itraconazole is an alternative in patients who do not respond to or cannot tolerate Itraconazole.
First-line topical therapies include Eficonazole, Tavaborole, Amorolfine, and Ciclopirox.

Topical antifungal agents developed for cutaneous fungal infections [choice D] generally are poorly effective for Onychomycosis because of poor penetration of the nail plate.

Choice A [Oral Fluconazole] is not the first line treatment of Onychomycosis.
Choice C [Oral Griseofulvin] is first line agent for Tinea capitis.
Choice E [Topical Tree oil] may be helpful but lack scientific evidence of benefit.

66. MUSCULOSKELETAL/RHEUMATOLOGY – SCAPHOID FRACTURE [CLINICAL INTERVENTION]

The preferred immobilization technique for a confirmed or suspected (anatomic snuffbox tenderness) Scaphoid fracture is a Thumb spica splint or cast [choice E] until a definitive imaging study can be performed, even if the initial radiographs are negative (as in this case).
If the initial radiographs are negative, options for repeat imaging include:
  • MRI (most accurate) or
  • immobilization and repeat imaging with a bone scan (after 3-5 days) or
  • Plain radiographs (after 7-10 days).
Because the blood supply is distal to proximal, these fractures have a high risk on nonunion or malunion.

Choice A [ACE wrap, ice application, and Naproxen] is insufficient as the thumb should be immobilized if there is anatomical snuffbox tenderness.
Choice B [Open reduction and internal fixation] is not the initial management as the thumb should be immobilized for stabilization and follow-up with orthopedic surgery to determine the best approach for further management.
Choice D [Ulnar gutter splint] can be used in the management of a Boxer fracture.
Choice E [Volar (cock up) splint] is an alternative to Thumb spica splint but Thumb spica splint is preferred.

67. ENDOCRINOLOGY – ACROMEGALY [APPLY FUNDAMENTAL CONCEPTS]

Cardiovascular manifestations of Acromegaly include
  • **Left ventricular hypertrophy [choice A]**

- **Hypertension**
- **Cardiomyopathy (often associated with diastolic dysfunction and arrhythmias).**

All of these manifestations may progress to the development of Heart failure.

Acromegaly, a clinical syndrome due to excess of growth hormone, is almost always a result of a pituitary adenoma (somatotroph adenoma).
Other manifestations of Acromegaly include:

- Increase growth of the hands, feet, and head
- Doughy moist handshake
- Increased spacing between the teeth
- Deepening of the voice
- Sleep apnea
- Carpal tunnel syndrome.

Choice B [Aortic root dilation] may be seen with smoking, Marfan syndrome, and other inflammatory disorders.
Choice C [Mitral stenosis] is almost always caused by Rheumatic fever.
Choice D [Mitral valve prolapse] can be seen with collagen diseases, such as Marfan syndrome and Ehlers-Danlos syndrome.
Choice E [Hypotension] is unlikely in Acromegaly as it is classically associated with Hypertension.

68. DERMATOLOGY – HERPETIC WHITLOW [CLINICAL INTERVENTION]
The management of primary Herpetic whitlow is conservative (rest, elevation, and anti-inflammatory agents) [choice E].
A dry dressing is used to cover the digit to prevent transmission of the infection.
If detected early, oral antiviral agents can hasten resolution of symptoms.

Herpetic whitlow is characterized by a single vesicle or a cluster of vesicles.
The vesicles progress into shallow ulcers that form crusts that eventually leave behind a healed epidermis.

Choice A [IV Vancomycin and hospital admission] are not indicated in the management of uncomplicated Herpetic whitlow.
Choice B [Oral Cephalexin] is not usually indicated in the management of Herpetic whitlow unless a secondary bacterial infection is suspected.
Surgery [choice C] is contraindicated because it will only spread the infection and may result in secondary bacterial infection. The lesions should not be incised and drained.
Choice D [Topical Ivermectin] can be used in the management of Rosacea.

69. CARDIOLOGY – ORTHOSTATIC HYPOTENSION [HISTORY AND PHYSICAL]
Orthostatic hypotension is diagnosed by comparing blood pressure readings in the supine and standing positions [choice B].
Orthostatic hypotension is defined as a reduction of

- systolic blood pressure reduction of ≥20 mmHg &/or
- diastolic blood pressure reduction of ≥10 mmHg.

Orthostatic hypotension is a common adverse effects of Tricyclic antidepressants, such as Amitriptyline, due to alpha adrenergic blockade, resulting in vasodilation.

Choice A [Straight leg raise test] is used in the diagnosis of Sciatica.

Choice C [Tilt table testing] can be used in the evaluation of Orthostatic hypotension when it is suspected in patients with negative orthostatic blood pressure evaluation.

Choice D [Transthoracic echocardiography] may be used in the workup of Cardiogenic syncope.

Choice E [CT scan of the head without contrast] can be used to rule out CNS causes if suspected.

70. DERMATOLOGY/HEMATOLOGY - WARFARIN INDUCED SKIN NECROSIS/PROTEIN C DEFICIENCY [APPLYING FUNDAMENTAL CONCEPTS]

Preexisting protein C deficiency [choice C] is the most common predisposing factor for the development of Warfarin-induced skin necrosis.

This is because although Warfarin's anticoagulant effect is to inhibit Vitamin K dependent clotting factors II, VII, IX and X, its inhibition of the vitamin K dependent anticoagulant proteins C & S occur more rapidly initially (due to their shorter half-lives, resulting in an acquired transient protein C deficiency).

Therefore, there is a greater imbalance and tendency towards thrombosis during the first few days of initiation of Warfarin therapy, which is why patients are often bridged with Heparin. Lesions appear in the absence of Heparin because the early effect of Warfarin is procoagulant.

Warfarin induced skin necrosis is a very rare adverse effect of Warfarin use and estimated at 0.01% to 0.1% of patients on Warfarin.

Other less common predisposing factors include Protein S deficiency, Factor V Leiden mutation [choice B], Antithrombin III deficiency [choice A], and Antiphospholipid syndrome [choice E].

Choice D [Von Willebrand disease] may present with mucocutaneous bleeding (eg, epistaxis, menorrhagia, bleeding gums, petechiae, and purpura without necrosis).

71. DERMATOLOGY – BASAL CELL CARCINOMA [CLINICAL INTERVENTION]

Mohs micrographic surgery [choice D] is the first line management for nodular Basal cell carcinoma on cosmetically sensitive areas (like facial involvement), difficult cases, high-risk cases, or recurrent disease.

Mohs micrographic surgery has a cure rate of up to 99% (best long-term rates) and has tissue sparing benefit.

Choice A [Electrodesiccation and curettage] is used most commonly for non-facial Basal cell carcinoma with low risk of recurrence.

Choice B [Liquid nitrogen cryotherapy] is the most commonly used treatment for localized Actinic keratosis.

Choice C [Standard excision with 4-5 mm margins and postoperative margin assessment] may be used for tumors with either low or high risk of tumor recurrence (eg, primary nodular BCCs <20 mm on low-risk areas of the trunk or extremities).

Choice E [Topical imiquimod] can be used for the management of superficial BCCs at low-risk sites, patients who prefer not to have surgery, or if there is a concern for poor wound healing after surgery.

72. CARDIOLOGY – RENOVASCULAR HYPERTENSION/SECONDARY HYPERTENSION [HISTORY AND PHYSICAL]

An abdominal bruit or flank bruit [choice A] is highly specific for Renovascular hypertension (99%), with a sensitivity of ~40%; however, it may be absent in many patients.

Renovascular hypertension is the most common potentially correctable causes of Secondary hypertension, representing 4% of the 5% of the causes of Secondary Hypertension. 95% of Hypertension is idiopathic (Essential hypertension).

Renal artery stenosis may present in patients with other manifestations of atherosclerosis, such as Peripheral arterial disease (as seen in this patient) and Coronary artery disease.

Choice B [Abdominal striae and supraclavicular fat pads] are hallmark of Cushing syndrome, a less common cause of Secondary Hypertension.

Choice C [Intermittent tachycardia and diaphoresis] are hallmark of Pheochromocytoma, a less common cause of Secondary Hypertension.

Choice D [Pulsatile abdominal mass] are hallmark of Abdominal aortic aneurysm.

Choice E [Systolic murmur radiating to the interscapular area] are hallmark of Coarctation of the aorta.

73. INFECTIOUS DISEASE – CAT SCRATCH DISEASE [PHARMACOLOGY]

Azithromycin [choice A] is the first line regimen for Lymphadenitis associated with Cat scratch disease [CSD] due to *Bartonella henselae*.

Alternative agents include Clarithromycin, Rifampin, or Trimethoprim-sulfamethoxazole.

CSD often begins with a nontender cutaneous lesion at the site of inoculation, followed by enlarged tender lymph nodes around 2 weeks afterwards.

Choice B [Prednisone] and other corticosteroids can be used adjunctively in patients with CSD neuroretinitis.

Choice E [Needle aspiration] may be indicated in severe or persistent suppurative lymph nodes. There is no fluctuance seen in this patient.

74. HEMATOLOGY – HODGKIN LYMPHOMA [PROFESSIONAL PRACTICE]

Near-miss events, where no actual harm comes to the patient as the error occur in the process of medical care detected and corrected before a patient is harmed, should be reported to hospital administration [choice E].

Near miss events represent an opportunity to improve patient safety, address patient expectations regarding disclosure of medical errors, and allow the opportunity for meaningful changes in policy and practice.

Fatal errors can occur, often due to name similarity, when patients are given vincristine at a vinblastine dose.

Choice A [Inform the patient of the error] is not required if the patient is not aware of the near miss since the patient. Any medical error that has an impact on the care of the patient, it should be disclosed as soon as possible.

Disclosing the near miss may be troubling to some patients. However, if the patient is aware of the near miss, disclosure is recommended as it will decrease anxiety and improve trust. However, any medical error that impacts patient care or causes harm to a patient should be promptly disclosed.

It is not required that the near miss be reported to JCAHO.

75. CARDIOLOGY – LATERAL WALL MYOCARDIAL INFARCTION [APPLICATION OF BASIC CONCEPTS]

A lateral wall Myocardial infarction usually represents occlusion of the circumflex [choice C] or diagonal branch of the left anterior descending artery.

The ECG shows ST elevation in aVL, V5, and V6, consistent with a lateral infarction.

Lateral STEMI (ST-Elevation Myocardial Infarction)

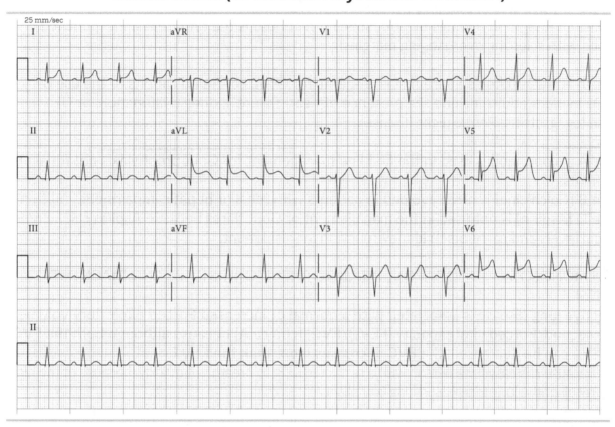

Choice A [Left anterior descending] is associated with ST elevations in the anterior leads (V1, V2, V3, &/or V4).

Choice B [Right coronary artery] is associated with an inferior wall MI.

Choice E [Left main coronary artery] is associated with anterolateral wall MI.

76. GASTROINTESTINAL/NUTRITION – ACUTE PANCREATITIS [HISTORY AND PHYSICAL EXAMINATION]

In 3% of patients with Acute pancreatitis, ecchymotic discoloration may be observed in the periumbilical region (Cullen's sign) [choice C] or around the flank (Grey Turner sign).

After gallstones, alcohol use is the second most common cause of Acute pancreatitis.

Acute pancreatitis presents with severe upper abdominal pain often radiating to the back, nausea, vomiting, and abdominal tenderness to palpation.

Choice A [Radiation of the pain to the left shoulder] describes Kehr sign, which is indicative of a ruptured spleen or ruptured Ectopic pregnancy.

Choice B [RLQ pain with palpation of the LLQ] describes Rovsing sign, which is indicative of Acute appendicitis.

Choice D [Enlarged left axillary lymph node] describes Irish sign, which is usually indicative of metastases from a GI malignancy.

Choice E [Retraction of the right iliac fossa] describes Dance's signs, which is usually indicative of Intussusception.

77. MUSCULOSKELETAL/RHEUMATOLOGY – GOUT [PHARMACOLOGY]

Glucocorticoids [choice C], either oral or intraarticular, are often the preferred treatment of Gout in patients with Chronic kidney disease as the other options (NSAIDs and Colchicine) are generally avoided in patients with kidney dysfunction.

The classic radiograph findings of Gout seen in the photo is the rat bite lesions (punched erosions with sclerotic overhanging margins).

Although NSAIDs [choice E] are first line agents for Gout, contraindications to the use of NSAIDs in older adults include the presence of heart failure, kidney dysfunction, or GI disease (eg, gastritis, Peptic ulcer disease).

Choice A [Allopurinol] is used in the first line management for Gout prophylaxis not for acute Gout flares.

Choice B [Colchicine] is often avoided in patients with renal or hepatic impairment.

Choice D [Aspirin] is not used in the management of Gout flares because Aspirin can increase uric acid levels and can worsen kidney function in this patient.

78. PULMONOLOGY – AMIODARONE INDUCED PNEUMONITIS [LABS AND DIAGNOSTIC STUDIES]

Restrictive lung disease is associated with a normal or increased Forced expiratory volume in one second/Forced vital capacity (FEV_1/FVC) [choice A] because although both the FVC and FEV1 can be decreased, the FVC decreases more than the FEV1.

This is because it is easy for a person with a restricted lung to breath out quickly, because of the high elastic recoil of the lung (decreased lung compliance).

Amiodarone-induced pulmonary toxicity is often associated with a restrictive pattern (reduced forced vital capacity and total lung capacity) and a reduction in diffusing capacity (DLCO).

79. GASTROINTESTINAL/NUTRITION – DIVERTICULOSIS [MOST LIKELY]

Diverticulosis [choice B] is the most common cause of acute Lower GI bleed/LGIB (60%).

Although left-sided diverticula are more common, right-sided diverticular are more prone to cause bleeding.

Inflammatory (colitis) is the second most common cause — Inflammatory bowel disease (Crohn, Ulcerative colitis , Ischemic colitis, infectious); Meckel diverticulum.

Other causes include benign anorectal disease: Hemorrhoids [choice D], Anal fissure, Fistula-in-ano.

Neoplastic polyps or neoplasms of the small intestine, colon, rectum, and anus.

Vascular: angiodysplasia, ischemic, radiation-induced, AV malformations, coagulopathies

80. GASTROINTESTINAL/NUTRITION – PEPTIC ULCER DISEASE [HISTORY AND PHYSICAL EXAMINATION]

Acute upper gastrointestinal hemorrhage [choice A] is the most common complication of Peptic ulcer disease.

Peptic ulcer disease is the most common cause of an Upper gastrointestinal bleed. Classic presentation of bleeding from a Peptic ulcer may include nausea, hematemesis (red blood or coffee-ground emesis), or melena (black, tarry stool).

81. EENT – NASAL FOREIGN BODY [HISTORY AND PHYSICAL]

In most patients, the first step is visualization of a nasal foreign body (FB) during physical examination (eg, Anterior rhinoscopy) [choice D].

The presence of foul-smelling unilateral discharge distinguishes nasal FB from other causes of **bilateral** nasal discharge (eg, URI, sinusitis, or allergic rhinitis).

Fiberoptic nasopharyngoscope is an alternative for direct visualization of a nasal FB.

All patients with nasal discharge should undergo a meticulous examination of the nasal cavity to rule out foreign body before instituting treatment for other conditions (eg, antibiotics for sinusitis [choice E] or allergy medications for allergic rhinitis [choices A and C]).

Clues for potential nasal FB include:
- history of nasal FB insertion (often asymptomatic)
- mucopurulent nasal discharge
- malodorous discharge
- epistaxis
- nasal obstruction (may result in mouth breathing).

Choice B [CT scan of the sinuses] is not usually necessary in the workup of a nasal FB. It is also not commonly indicated for Acute Sinusitis unless there is suspicion for complications.

82. PULMONOLOGY – KLEBSIELLA PNEUMONIA/CAP [HISTORY AND PHYSICAL]

In addition to the symptoms of other causes of Bacterial pneumonia (eg, cough, pleuritic chest pain, fever, sputum production, crackles on examination, increased WBC), *Klebsiella pneumoniae* [choice D] is also associated with significant inflammation and necrosis of the surrounding tissue, which results in
- **[1] thick, mucoid, and blood-tinged sputum ("currant jelly") sputum and**
- **[2] cavitary lung disease or a lobar infiltrate may be seen** (this patient has a cavitary infiltrate).

However, *K. pneumoniae* is also associated with marked inflammation and necrosis that can lead to thick, mucoid, and blood-tinged sputum, referred to as "currant jelly" sputum
K. pneumoniae most often occurs in alcoholics and patients with diabetes, severe chronic obstructive pulmonary disease, or hospitalized patients.

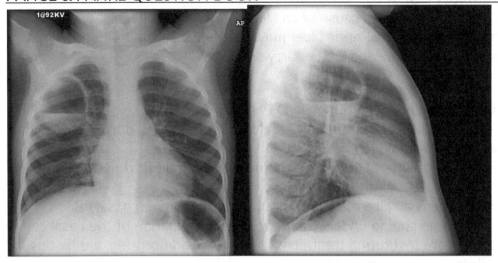

Choice A [Pseudomonas aeruginosa] classically causes a lobar consolidation and thick green sputum production.

Choice B [Chlamydia pneumoniae] is a cause of atypical pneumonia, commonly associated with mild pulmonary symptoms, extrapulmonary symptoms (eg, pharyngitis, laryngitis, and sinusitis), and a chest radiograph pattern of unilateral alveolar infiltrates or bronchopneumonia.

Choice C [Histoplasma capsulatum] is associated with living or travel to endemic areas in the Mississippi and Ohio river valleys. Chest radiograph findings are similar to bronchopneumonia or may reveal hilar or mediastinal lymphadenopathy.

Choice E [Mycoplasma pneumoniae] is a cause of atypical pneumonia, commonly associated with mild pulmonary symptoms, extrapulmonary symptoms [eg, hemolysis, central nervous system (CNS) disease, dermatitis, carditis, joint disease, and gastrointestinal disease], and a chest radiograph pattern of unilateral alveolar infiltrates or bronchopneumonia.

Photo credit:
Case courtesy of Frank Gaillard, Radiopaedia.org, rID: 8288

83. MUSCULOSKELETAL/RHEUMATOLOGY – OSTEOMYELITIS [MOST LIKELY]

In children with SCD, the most common organism responsible for osteomyelitis is nontyphoidal Salmonella spp. [choice E].

The majority of Salmonella infections in Sickle cell patients involve bones (especially long bones) and joints and occur most frequently in early childhood.

Functional asplenia due to Sickle cell disease, in addition to reticuloendothelial system dysfunction, suppress clearance of Salmonella and other encapsulated organisms from the blood stream.

84. REPRODUCTIVE – EARLY PREGNANCY [HISTORY AND PHYSICAL]

During early pregnancy, systemic vascular resistance (peripheral vasodilation) [choice D] decreases, which is compensated for by the increased stroke volume & cardiac output.

During pregnancy, the following parameters increase:
- Blood volume (10-15% as early as 6 weeks), cardiac output, stroke volume, RBC mass.
- Increased tidal volume to meet the increased oxygen demand. Hypercoagulable state.
- Heart rate increases 10–15 bpm; increased intensity of S1, exaggerated splitting of S2.

The following parameters decrease during pregnancy:
- Functional residual capacity by 20%, decreased exercise capacity for some.
- Hemoglobin
- Systemic vascular resistance
- Blood pressure decreases in the second trimester (decreases of 5-7 mmHg of both SBP & DBP). Blood pressure normalizes in the third trimester.
- Decreased GI motility (may lead to GERD).

85. MUSCULOSKELETAL/RHEUMATOLOGY – DEQUERVAIN TENDINOPATHY [MOST LIKELY]

DeQuervain tendinopathy [choice C] should be suspected when there is
- **pain, tenderness, and/or enlargement over the radial styloid at the first dorsal compartment (radial side of the wrist)**
- **positive Finkelstein test**: pain at the radial styloid with active or passive stretch of the thumb tendons in thumb flexion.

DeQuervain tendinopathy is tendon entrapment affecting the dorsal compartment of the wrist [affects the abductor pollicis longus (APL) and extensor pollicis brevis (EPB) tendons].
It is most commonly seen in women ages 30-50 years and also seen in women ~4-6 weeks after delivery.

Choice A [Carpal tunnel syndrome] results from median nerve entrapment, characterized by pain, paresthesias, and numbness to the thumb, index finger, middle finger, and the radial side of the ring finger.
Choice B [Radial sensory nerve entrapment] causes burning pain and paresthesias over the dorsum of the hand, wrist, thumb, index, and middle fingers (which this patient denies).
Choice D [Flexor carpi radialis tenosynovitis] is a condition characterized by pain over the volar radial wrist caused by inflammation of the FCR tendon sheath.
Choice E [Osteoarthritis of the trapeziometacarpal (TMC) joint] causes pain and tenderness at the thumb joint distal to the radial styloid.

86. NEUROLOGY – PARKINSON DISEASE [PHARMACOLOGY]

The 3 nonergot Dopamine receptor agonists [choice A] used in the management of Parkinson disease are Ropinirole, Pramipexole, and Rotigotine.
Parkinson disease results from progressive degeneration of dopamine-producing neurons in the substantia nigra of the midbrain.
This results in relative dopamine depletion (which has a depressive effect at the neuromuscular junction) compared to acetylcholine (which has an excitatory effect at the NM junction), resulting in the classic triad of tremor, rigidity, and bradykinesia.

Choice B [Dopamine precursor] describes the mechanism of action of Levodopa.
Choice C [Selective monoamine oxidase inhibitor] describes the mechanism of action of Selegiline and Rasagiline.
Choice D [Muscarinic (cholinergic) receptor antagonist] describes the mechanism of action of Benztropine and Trihexyphenidyl.
Choice E [Catechol-O-methyltransferase inhibitor] describes the mechanism of action of Tolcapone.

87. PULMONOLOGY – CYSTIC FIBROSIS [HISTORY AND PHYSICAL]
Patients with Cystic fibrosis (CF) are predisposed to colonization with Pseudomonas aeruginosa [choice A] and is often isolated from respiratory secretions of most adults with CF.
This predisposition to *P. aeruginosa* infection may be in part because of impaired clearance directly induced by a defect in CFTR.

All of the other choices listed can be isolated in CF but not as common as *P. aeruginosa*.

88. REPRODUCTIVE – COVID 19-SARS-COV-2 [HEALTH MAINTENANCE]
COVID-19 vaccination [choice C] is recommended regardless of pregnancy or breastfeeding status, in agreement with major medical organizations and public health authorities.
This recommendation is based on data showing vaccine safety and efficacy in pregnant people and data that pregnancy is associated with an increased risk of severe infection.

Other vaccines safe in pregnancy include:
- Meningococcal
- Tetanus (eg, Td, Tdap)
- Hepatitis B
- Inactivated influenza
- Rabies
- Diphtheria

Vaccines contraindicated in pregnancy include:
- BCG
- Intranasal influenza [choice A]
- Live vaccines: Varicella (Chickenpox), MMR, Polio, BCG [choices D and E]
- Inactivated HPV vaccine [choice B]
- Yellow fever (in most)
- Smallpox.

89. EENT – PERITONSILLAR ABSCESS [CLINICAL INTERVENTION]
The initial management of Peritonsillar abscess (PTA) includes:
- **surgical drainage**: eg, needle aspiration [choice A], which is often preferred, or incision and drainage
- **antibiotic therapy** with gram positive (Group A streptococcus and *Staphylococcus aureus*) and respiratory anaerobic coverage (eg, Amoxicillin clavulanate)
- **supportive care**: adequate hydration and analgesia and monitoring for complications.

Drainage procedures, in combination with antimicrobial therapy and supportive management (eg, hydration), results in resolution in >90% of cases of PTA.
Hallmark physical examination findings of a PTA include:
- an enlarged and fluctuant tonsil with deviation of the uvula to the opposite side &/or
- fullness or bulging of the posterior soft palate near the tonsil with palpable fluctuance.

Choice B [Intravenous Dexamethasone] and the role of other glucocorticoids is controversial in the management of PTA as evidence regarding the benefits of glucocorticoids in the management of PTA is inconsistent.

Tonsillectomy [choice C] is usually reserved for patients who fail to respond to drainage, PTA with complications (eg impending airway obstruction), prior episodes of PTA, or recurrent severe pharyngitis.

Choice D [24-hour trial of antibiotics only] can be used in some patients with Peritonsillar cellulitis or very mild abscesses but in most cases surgical drainage (any of the 3 procedures) is indicated for large PTA.

Choice E [NSAIDs and gargle with antiseptic mouthwash] may be part of supportive therapy for some but is not the mainstay of treatment.

90. CARDIOLOGY – CHRONIC CORONARY SYNDROME/STABLE ANGINA PECTORIS [PHARMACOLOGY]

Beta blockers, such as Metoprolol [choice E], are first-line therapy for Chronic coronary syndrome (Stable angina pectoris) because they:

- are the most effective antianginal and anti-ischemic agents
- reduce anginal episodes by decreasing cardiac work (reducing contractility) and by causing coronary peripheral vasodilatation
- improve exercise tolerance, especially in those individuals with other indications for beta-blocker therapy (eg, recent acute myocardial infarction, heart failure with reduced ejection fraction)
- blunt exercise-induced elevations in heart rate and blood pressure and control exertionally and emotionally induced angina.
- improve survival in certain subgroups of patients with stable coronary disease [patients with Myocardial infarction or Heart failure with reduced ejection fraction (systolic dysfunction)].

Choice A [Nitroglycerin] is used for acute symptom control of Chronic coronary syndrome. It does not have significant mortality benefit in CCS.

Choice B [Lisinopril], other Angiotensin-converting enzyme (ACE) inhibitors, and Angiotensin receptor blockers (ARBs) are used in a subset of patients with CCS (eg, those with decreased LV ejection fraction <40%, Chronic kidney disease, Hypertension, Diabetes mellitus). However, in the absence of these conditions, it is not certain if ACE inhibitors or ARBs have a cardioprotective or vascular protection effect outside of their benefits of Hypertension reduction.

Choice C [Long-acting Diltiazem] and other Calcium channel blockers (eg, long-acting Verapamil, Amlodipine, or Felodipine) are alternatives to Beta blockers as monotherapy but do not have mortality benefit. Short-acting dihydropyridines (eg, Nifedipine) are usually avoided unless used in conjunction with a Beta blocker and are avoided if there is systolic dysfunction.

Choice D [Ranolazine] is a late sodium channel blocker than can be added as a third line agent, for persistent symptoms of CCS.

91. PSYCHIATRY/BEHAVIORAL MEDICINE – SLEEP TERRORS [MOST LIKELY]

Sleep terrors [choice A] is associated with

- **abrupt, terrifying arousal (wakening from sleep) with panicky screams or crying accompanied by**

- **fear and signs of autonomic arousal (eg, tachycardia, sweating, flushed face, rapid breathing, agitation, and inconsolable** (may become more agitated when consoled).
- **amnesia for the event (no recollection).**

Parasomnias are disturbing or strange behaviors or experiences during sleep.
A sleep terror usually lasts from seconds to a few minutes, but it may last longer.
Most children outgrow sleep terrors by their teenage years.

Choice B [Sleepwalking] is characterized by toddler sits up and crawls around the bed or walks up quietly to stand by the bed of the parents.
Choice C [Nightmare disorders] are associated with dream recollections and full alertness generally returns immediately waking.
Choice D [Rapid eye movement sleep behavior disorder] is characterized by aggressive motor behavior as part of dream enactment, resulting from loss of muscle atonia during REM sleep and often leading to injury.
Choice E [Confusional arousal] is not associated with autonomic arousal (eg, sweating, flushed face, etc.).

92. PSYCHIATRY/BEHAVIORAL MEDICINE – LITHIUM [PHARMACOLOGY]
Thyroid function tests [choice B] should be performed in patients on Lithium therapy as Hypothyroidism is common in Lithium-treated patients.
The Hypothyroidism is often subclinical but may become overt.
Lithium may cause Hypothyroidism through a number of mechanisms:
- increased iodine content in the thyroid gland,
- reduction of the thyroid gland's ability to produce T4 and T3,
- blockage of the release of thyroid hormone from the thyroid gland, and
- alteration of the structure of thyroglobulin.

Symptoms of Hypothyroidism include fatigue, constipation, delayed and decreased deep tendon reflexes.

93. NEUROLOGY – SUBARACHNOID HEMORRHAGE [LABS AND DIAGNOSTIC STUDIES]
Lumbar puncture [choice D] is often required to exclude a Subarachnoid hemorrhage (SAH) for most patients with a normal head CT if there is a high suspicion.
This is because although Head CT is the initial test of choice, its sensitivity is highest within the first 6 hours after SAH and then declines. In addition, the sensitivity of head CT may be decreased with low-volume bleeds.

Subarachnoid hemorrhage (SAH) should be suspected in patients with:
- Sudden-onset severe headache, often described as "the worst headache of my life"
- increased intracranial pressure: nausea, vomiting
- meningismus: neck stiffness, positive Brudzinski &/or Kernig signs
- may be associated with brief loss of consciousness, seizures.

Choice A [Discharge home with outpatient neurology follow up] is incorrect because a life-threatening SAH should be ruled out.

Choice B [Administer Sumatriptan] can be given for Migraine headache. This patient has bilateral headache (Migraine is usually unilateral) and is worse than previous headaches (worse headache of their life), making a Migraine headache unlikely.

Choice C [Consult neurology for intractable headache] can be done after confirmation of SAH.

Choice E [Perform a Temporal Artery biopsy] is used in the diagnosis of Giant cell (Temporal) arteritis.

94. CARDIOLOGY – COARCTATION OF THE AORTA [HISTORY AND PHYSICAL]

Coarctation has an increased association with Turner syndrome, which can present with a webbed neck and widely spaced nipples [choice B].

~5-15% of girls with Coarctation of the Aorta have Turner syndrome.

Coarctation of the aorta is associated with upper extremity hypertension, lower extremity hypotension, and brachio-femoral delay.

Choice A [Macroorchidism and large ears] are hallmark of Fragile X syndrome.

Choice C [Smooth philtrum, thin upper lip, and flat midface] can be seen with Fetal alcohol syndrome.

Choice D [Single palmar crease] can be seen with Trisomy 21 (Down syndrome).

Choice E [Increased arm span to height ratio] can be seen with Marfan syndrome.

95. NEUROLOGY – ALZHEIMER DISEASE [PHARMACOLOGY]

Cholinesterase inhibitors [choice E], such as Donepezil Galantamine, and Rivastigmine, are first-line agents for patients with newly diagnosed Alzheimer disease (AD) dementia (mild to moderate severity with a Mini-Mental State examination 10-26).

AD is associated decreased cortical acetylcholine; cholinesterase inhibitors increase cortical cholinergic function.

In patients with moderate to advanced dementia (eg, MMSE ≤18), adding the NMDA antagonist Memantine to a cholinesterase inhibitor or as monotherapy is recommended.

Choice A [Anticholinergic] medications can be used in the management of Parkinson disease.

Choice B [NMDA receptor agonist] is incorrect because Memantine is an NMDA antagonist.

Choice C [Dopamine agonist] is used in the management of Parkinson disease.

Choice D [Dopamine antagonist] is used in the management of Schizophrenia.

96. CARDIOLOGY – HYPERTROPHIC CARDIOMYOPATHY [CLINICAL INTERVENTION]

For most patients with Hypertrophic cardiomyopathy (HCM), initial therapy with a Beta blocker are first line agents, such as nonvasodilating Beta blockers Nadolol or Metoprolol succinate [choice C].

Beta blockers decrease heart rate, improve ventricular filling and relieve symptomatic HCM.

Alternative medications include Nondihydropyridine Calcium channel blockers [eg, Verapamil (extended release), Diltiazem], Disopyramide, or myosin inhibitors.

Septal reduction options include Surgical myectomy or Alcohol septal ablation.

Choice A [Isosorbide mononitrate] is often avoided in HCM as it may worsen with left ventricular outflow obstruction in HCM.

Choice B [Isolated mitral valve surgery] has been shown to have little to no benefit in the management of HCM. Mitral valve surgery without concomitant septal myectomy is not recommended as management of LVOT obstruction.

Choice D [Aortic valve replacement] is used in the management of Aortic stenosis (AS). The murmur of AS decreases in intensity with Valsalva, often radiates to the carotids, and is maximally heard at the right upper sternal border.

Choice E [Digoxin] is often avoided in HCM as it may worsen with left ventricular outflow obstruction in HCM.

97. GASTROINTESTINAL/NUTRITION – INTERNAL HEMORRHOIDS [HISTORY AND PHYSICAL EXAMINATION]

Internal hemorrhoids are generally not palpable on digital examination in the absence of thrombosis [choice E], unless prolapsed.

Anoscopy can be used to evaluate the anal canal for Internal hemorrhoids not detected on digital rectal examination.

Internal hemorrhoids
- are often asymptomatic
- associated with hematochezia (painless bright red blood per rectum), leakage of stool, intermittent pruritus
- originate above the dentate line
- often not painful.

98. CARDIOLOGY – DEEP VEIN THROMBOSIS [LABS AND DIAGNOSTIC STUDIES]

Compression ultrasonography [choice D] with Doppler is the diagnostic test of choice in patients with suspected DVT.

The presence of noncompressibility of a deep vein establishes the diagnosis of DVT.

DVT should be suspected in patients with unilateral calf pain, swelling, erythema, and tenderness, especially with risk factors (eg, combined oral contraception and smoking in this patient).

Choice A [Venous plethysmography] can be used to assess for degree of venous outflow obstruction, reflux, and efficiency of the venous calf pumps.

Choice B [Initiate IV Heparin] can be done if Compression ultrasonography is positive.

Choice C [Warm compresses, leg elevation, Indomethacin] can be used in the management of Superficial thrombophlebitis.

Choice E [Ankle-brachial index] is used to make the diagnosis of Peripheral arterial disease.

99. PROFESSIONAL PRACTICE

Professionals should not use the names of patients in case reports [choice A].

Anything that can identify a patient is not permitted.

All of the other information can be shared in the other choices listed.

100. PULMONARY – PNEUMOCOCCAL VACCINE [HEALTH MAINTENANCE]

In patients ages 19-64 with underlying medical condition, options for Pneumococcal vaccine include:

- **Administer one dose of 20-valent pneumococcal conjugate vaccine (PCV20) [choice B] OR**
- One dose of PCV15, followed by one dose of PPSV23 [choice C] at least 1 year later.

The minimum interval (8 weeks) can be considered in adults with an immunocompromising condition, cochlear implant, or cerebrospinal fluid leak.

1. A 10-year-old boy is being evaluated for abrupt onset of nonrhythmic, involuntary movements. About 5 weeks ago, he had sore throat, migratory joint pain associated with swelling, high-grade fever, and a nonpruritic rash involving his trunk. Physical examination is notable for a harsh diastolic murmur. ECG reveals diffuse ST elevations and PR depressions in the precordial leads. Which of the following is considered a minor criterion for the most likely diagnosis?
a. Arthritis
b. Erythema marginatum
c. Carditis
d. Sydenham chorea
e. High-grade fever (≥38.5°F)

2. A 10-year-old boy is being evaluated in the clinic for an intensely pruritic rash that is worse at night. His brother has a similar rash. On examination, there are multiple small erythematous papules and excoriations noted on the periumbilical skin, extensor aspects of the elbows, sides and webs of the fingers, and waist. Based on the most likely diagnosis, which of the following is the preferred initial management of this condition?
a. Topical Lindane
b. Clotrimazole cream
c. Topical Permethrin
d. Topical Hydrocortisone
e. Oral Prednisone

3. A 40-year-old female presents to the clinic with leg discomfort, heaviness, and aching that improves with rest and leg elevation. The pain is not association with exercise. Chronic venous insufficiency is suspected. Which of the following physical examination findings is most supportive of this diagnosis?
a. Dependent pitting edema
b. Dependent rubor
c. Lateral malleolar ulcer
d. Thin shiny skin with loss of hair
e. 1+ posterior tibialis and dorsalis pedis pulses

4. A 7-year-old boy is brought to the emergency department for crampy abdominal pain and dyspnea. He was eating an orange and a peanut butter sandwich at school when he felt itching in his mouth, followed by vomiting. Vitals reveal a blood pressure of 78/40 mmHg, pulse 120/min, respirations 32/min, and SaO2: 88% on room air. He is in moderate distress. There is tonsillar erythema, periorbital edema, and multiple raised wheals on his trunk and extremities. There is stridor, scattered wheezing, fair aerations, and minimal retractions. No angioedema is noted. Which of the following is the most important next step in the management of this patient?
a. Albuterol
b. Epinephrine
c. Methylprednisolone
d. Cetirizine
e. Diphenhydramine

5. A 55-year-old male presents to the clinic for a routine well visit. He has a 30-pack year smoking history but quit 5 years ago. He drinks 2 beers daily. He underwent a colonoscopy at 50, which was negative. Which of the following should be performed in this patient?
a. Colonoscopy
b. Chest radiography
c. Low-dose CT of the chest
d. Abdominal ultrasonography
e. Pulmonary function testing

6. A 50-year-old man is brought to the emergency room for altered mental status. His wife endorses he has been slow to respond and has been walking unsteady. He has a longstanding history of chronic alcohol use. On physical examination, jaundice, erythematous palms, and jerking movements of the outstretched hands when bent upward at the wrist are noted. Which of the following would most likely be seen on physical examination?
a. Shifting dullness
b. Ecchymosis to the flank
c. Papilledema
d. Palpable nontender gallbladder
e. Tenderness in the right upper quadrant with deep palpation

7. A 22-year-old male presents with recurrent episodes of Acute bronchitis. He complains of cough most days of the week associated with production of thick, tenacious sputum and occasional hemoptysis. On physical examination, there are rales and wheezing heard throughout both lung fields. A Chest radiograph shows atelectasis. A CT scan of the chest is performed (see photo).

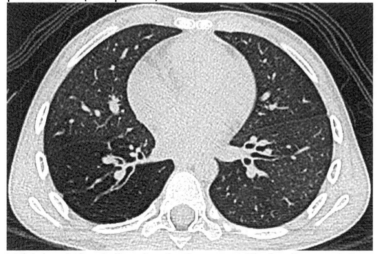

Which of the following is the most likely diagnosis?
a. Asthma
b. Chronic bronchitis
c. Tuberculosis
d. Bronchiectasis
e. Pulmonary embolism

Photo credit:
Case courtesy of Tee Yu Jin, Radiopaedia.org, rID: 71538

8. A 46-year-old woman was evaluated for intermittent episodes of palpitations, diaphoresis, and headaches. She is found to have a blood pressure of 156/110 mmHg. Her 24-hour urine metanephrines and VMA are elevated. Abdominal CT reveals a 5.1 cm right adrenal mass. Which of the following is the most appropriate next step in the management of the patient?
a. Right adrenalectomy
b. Initiate Phenoxybenzamine
c. Initiate Metoprolol
d. No pharmacologic intervention required
e. Initiate Lisinopril

9. A 27-year-old man is complaining of a 6-month history of weight gain, muscle weakness, and generalized fatigue. He has a 5-pack year smoking history and does not take any medications. His blood pressure is 158/98 mmHg. Abdominal obesity, abdominal stretch marks, and thin extremities are noted. Labs reveal:
Serum glucose 298 mg/dL (70-110)
24-hour urinary cortisol 488 µg (<300)
Late night salivary cortisol 385 ng/dL (29-101 ng/dL)
Serum adrenocorticotropin-releasing hormone 1.7 pg/mL (>5).
Which of the following is the most appropriate next step in the evaluation of this patient?
a. CT chest
b. CT abdomen and pelvis
c. Low dose dexamethasone suppression test
d. High dose dexamethasone suppression test
e. MRI pituitary

10. A 44-year-old man is brought to the emergency department due to altered mental status and lethargy. He has a history of Type 2 Diabetes mellitus. Vitals are blood pressure 140/70 mmHg, pulse 120/min, and temperature 98.8°F (37.11°C). He is drowsy with dry mucous membranes. Labs reveal:
Sodium 152 mEq/L (135-145)
Potassium: 5.5 mEq/L (3.5-5)
Chloride: 122 mEq/L (96-106)
Bicarbonate: 20 mEq/L (22-26)
Blood urea nitrogen: 51 mg/dL (7-20)
Creatinine: 1.5 mg/dL (0.6-1.2)
Glucose 1,234 mg/dL (70-110)
Serum ketones: negative
ECG reveals Atrial flutter.
Which of the following represents the most important initial intervention for this patient?
a. Metoprolol
b. Insulin bolus followed by continuous infusion
c. IV Potassium chloride
d. IV Calcium gluconate
e. IV 0.9% sodium chloride

11. A 53-year-old woman presents to the clinic due to increased shortness of breath with exertion. Physical examination is notable for reddish-brown hyperpigmentation of the skin and increased liver span without tenderness. Initial labs are notable for
- Sodium 140 mEq/L (135-145)
- Potassium 4.6 mEq/L (3.5-5)
- AST 199 U/L (8-48)
- ALT 137 U/L (7-55)
- Random blood glucose of 154 mg/dL (70-110).

An echocardiogram shows impaired diastolic relaxation of the ventricles and marked dilation of the atria. Which of the following is the most likely diagnosis?
a. Sarcoidosis
b. Wilson disease
c. Hereditary hemochromatosis
d. Nonalcoholic fatty liver disease
e. Primary Adrenal insufficiency

12. A 27-year-old female presents for follow-up for chronic aching in the head, arm, chest, abdomen, back, and buttocks. She also experiences fatigue, mild cognitive disturbance, and nonrestorative sleep. Examination is positive for multiple sites of tenderness with 5/5 muscle strength. ESR is 8 mm/hr (0-15). She has tried increased physical activity and exercise. Which of the following is the best next step in the management of this patient's symptoms?
a. Low-dose Prednisone
b. High-dose Prednisone
c. Amitriptyline
d. Indomethacin
e. Tramadol

13. A 36-year-old male is complaining of bouts of severe right-sided periorbital and temporal headaches lasting from 15 minutes up to 3 hours before spontaneously resolving. The bouts occur more frequently at night. During the headaches, he paces about or sits and rocks back and forth. Triggers include alcohol intake, sexual activity, and glare. Which of the following is the most likely associated symptom or sign?
a. Miosis and conjunctival erythema of the right eye
b. Vision loss
c. Photophobia and nausea
d. Papilledema and right cranial nerve IV palsy
e. Reproduction of the pain with stroking the right side of the face at trigger zones

14. A 15-year-old girl is being evaluated after a school nurse noted truncal asymmetry. Adams forward bend test shows left thoracic (rib) prominence. Radiographs reveal a Cobb angle of 13 degrees. Which of the following is the best next step in management of this patient?
a. Magnetic resonance imaging (MRI) of the spine
b. Orthopedic referral for surgery
c. Observation with follow up every 6-9 months
d. Repeat of radiographs every 12 months
e. Back bracing

15. A 57-year-old female presents with diffuse pain, swelling, and tenderness to the left distal forearm, wrist, and hand. Radiographs are obtained (see photo).

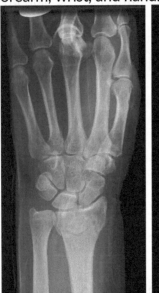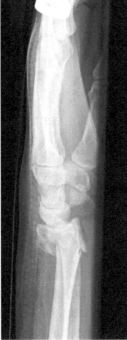

Which of the following is the most common mechanism of injury?
a. Fall forward landing on the back of their wrist with their hand flexed or bent in toward their body
b. Direct blow to the anterior or posterior aspect of the wrist and hand
c. Falling on an outstretched hand with a pronated forearm in wrist extension
d. Punching a stationary object with a clenched fist
e. Compression load driving the scaphoid or lunate into the distal radius

Photo credit:
Case courtesy of Frank Gaillard, Radiopaedia.org, rID: 12382

16. An 11-year-old male is brought for evaluation. His twin brother awoke from sleep when he heard the patient making grunting sounds and was smacking his lips, which lasted for no more than a minute. Afterwards, he sat up in bed and stared at his hands, making gripping movements. When his twin asked the patient what was wrong or what he was doing, he did not answer "as if he was in a trance." He seemed to be confused for 2 to 3 minutes and did not recall the event happening. There was no associated urinary or bowel incontinence. Which of the following is the most likely diagnosis?
a. Myoclonic seizure
b. Absence seizure
c. Focal seizure with impaired awareness
d. Tonic–clonic seizure
e. Atonic seizure

17. A 15-year-old girl is complaining of lower abdominal pain and dizziness. She denies fever, vaginal discharge, or dysuria. She feels nauseous and has missed her last menstrual period, which usually occurs every 28 days. Her mother asserts her pain is most likely due to appendicitis and that her daughter is a virgin. Vitals are only notable for tachycardia with a normal physical examination. Her mother would like for a CT scan of the abdomen and pelvis to be performed. Which of the following is the most appropriate initial step in the management of this patient?
a. Perform MRI of the abdomen and pelvis
b. Obtain a quantitative serum hCG test
c. Perform a rapid Ultrasound at the bedside
d. Obtain a urine hCG test
e. Perform a CT scan of the abdomen and pelvis

18. A 25-year-old male is admitted for Infective endocarditis treated with IV Vancomycin and Gentamicin. On hospital day 6, he is experiencing decreased urine output. Initial labs reveal:
- serum creatinine 2.2 mg/dL (0.6-1.2)
- BUN 28 mg/dL (6-20)
- urine specific gravity of 1.040
- urine sodium 55 mEq/L.
- urine specific gravity 1.010
- urine osmolality 400 mOsm/kg H2O (500-850)

Which of the following casts would most likely be seen on microscopic examination of the urine?
a. Broad waxy casts
b. Red cell casts
c. White cell casts
d. Epithelial cell casts
e. Fatty casts

19. A 50-year-old male is brought to the emergency department via ambulance after a witnessed syncopal episode without head trauma. He was recently treated with lobectomy for Lung adenocarcinoma and is currently undergoing postoperative adjuvant chemotherapy. Vitals reveals a blood pressure 72/48 mmHg, pulse 120/min, respirations 23/min, and oxygen saturation 89% on room air. He is diaphoretic, ill-appearing, and clammy with distended neck veins. Bedside echocardiogram shows a dilated right ventricle, new right ventricular strain, and early systolic notching of the pulsed wave Doppler waveform in the right ventricular outflow tract. Which of the following is the most appropriate next step in management of this patient?
a. IV Alteplase
b. CT head
c. CT angiogram chest
d. D-dimer
e. IV Heparin

20. A 20-year-old female presents with 4-day history of vaginal discharge. She denies dysuria, urgency, or frequency. She is sexually active with 2 partners. Physical examination revealed a mucopurulent exudate in the endocervical canal and endocervical bleeding from gentle passage of an endocervical swab through the cervical os. Point of care testing on the discharge reveals gram-negative intracellular diplococci. Which of the following medications is first line management?
a. Nitrofurantoin
b. Doxycycline
c. Ceftriaxone
d. Metronidazole
e. Penicillin G

21. A 60-year-old male is complaining of progressive dyspnea on exertion and dry cough. He has worked in construction since he was a teenager including demolition, renovation, and repair of old buildings. Physical examination is notable for crackles without wheezing. PFTs reveal a normal FEV1/FVC and decreased residual volume (RV). Chest radiographs are obtained (see photo).

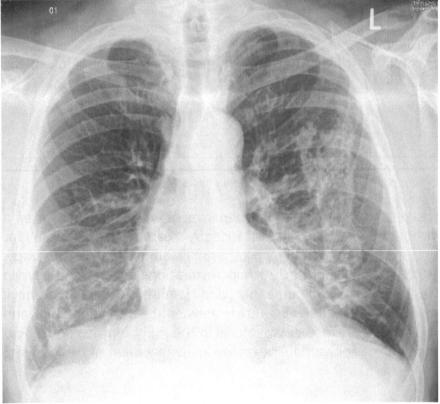

This patient is at greatest for the development of which of the following?
a. Caplan syndrome
b. Mesothelioma
c. Lofgren syndrome
d. Emphysema
e. Bronchiectasis

Photo credit
Case courtesy of Roberto Schubert, Radiopaedia.org, rID: 17322

22. A 26-year-old female with no significant medical history presents to the emergency department for dizziness, heart racing, and a pounding sensation in her chest. She is not on any medications. Vitals are temperature 98.6°F (37°C), blood pressure 128/82 mmHg, pulse 150/min, and respirations 20/min. Physical examination is unremarkable. An ECG is performed (see photo).

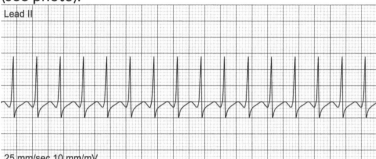

Which of the following is the most appropriate next step in management?
a. IV Adenosine
b. Synchronized (direct current) cardioversion
c. IV Amiodarone
d. Carotid massage
e. IV Esmolol

Photo credit:
Shutterstock (used with permission)

23. A 22-year-old female at 15 weeks gestation is complaining of urgency, frequency, and dysuria. Physical examination is notable for suprapubic tenderness. Urinalysis is positive for pyuria and positive leukocyte esterase. Which of the following is the first line management?
a. Ciprofloxacin
b. Trimethoprim-sulfamethoxazole
c. Cephalexin
d. Doxycycline
e. Clindamycin

24. A 52-year-old female presents to the clinic for headache, dizziness, and blurred vision. She occasionally experiences a painful burning of the hands accompanied by erythema. Labs reveal:
- Hemoglobin: 15 g/dL (12-16)
- Hematocrit: 45% (36-48)
- Platelets 537,000/mm^3 (150,000-450,000)
- White cell count 9,200/mm^3 (5,000-10,000)

Which of the mutations would most likely be present in this patient?
a. CALR
b. BCR-ABL
c. MPL
d. t(15;17)
e. JAK 2

25. A 16-year-old boy is being evaluated in the emergency department complaining of mild headache, dizziness, and nausea after a head on collision while playing football. There was no witnessed loss of consciousness, but he was "dazed" shortly after impact. Vitals are stable and physical examination is within normal limits with normal gait and neurological examination. Glasgow coma scale score is 15. His parents are inquiring when he can return to play football. Which of the following is the best recommendation for this patient?
a. Complete bed rest until full resolution of symptoms
b. Physical rest for 24-48 hours followed by a gradual progressive return to normal activity
c. He can immediately return to playing football
d. Perform gradually increasing activities for the next 48 hours
e. He should not return to football for this season

26. A 20-year-old female presents to establish care. She denies any symptoms currently, but experiences occasional fatigue. Initial labs reveal:
  • Hemoglobin: 9.2 g/dL (11-16)
  • Hematocrit: 28% (36-46)
  • Mean corpuscular volume (MCV): 74 fL (80-100)
  • Ferritin: 148 ng/mL (13-150)
A peripheral smear shows the following (see photo).

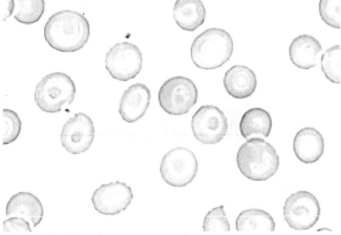

Hemoglobin electrophoresis:
  • Hemoglobin A: 97% (96-98%)
  • Hemoglobin A2: 2.5% (2-3.3%)
  • Hemoglobin F: 0.5% (<1%).
Which of the following is the most likely diagnosis?
a. Hemochromatosis
b. Beta thalassemia minor
c. Alpha thalassemia intermedia
d. Alpha thalassemia trait
e. Iron deficiency anemia

27. A 44-year-old male is brought to the ED by his wife due to a seizure. Prior to the event, he complained of headache, fever, and nausea. Her husband appeared confused. On examination, he cannot clearly answer questions. A facial nerve palsy and right hemiparesis are noted. Head CT shows no evidence of a hemorrhage, or a space-occupying lesion. MRI of the brain shows temporal lobe enhancement. A lumbar puncture is performed, and cerebral spinal fluid analysis shows:

- normal opening pressure
- lymphocytic pleocytosis
- normal glucose
- elevated protein.

Which of the following is the most common likely etiologic agent?

a. *Neisseria meningitidis*

b. *Streptococcus pneumoniae*

c. Enterovirus

d. Herpes Simplex Virus

e. *Cryptococcus neoformans*

28. A 41-year-old primigravid woman presents to the clinic to establish prenatal care. Her last menstrual period was 12 weeks ago. She is concerned because she has felt pelvic pressure and had some vaginal spotting. Vital signs are normal. Physical examination shows fundal height midway between the pubis and the umbilicus. A transvaginal ultrasound is performed (see photo).

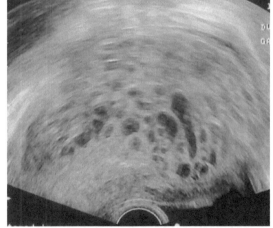

Serum quantitative hCG is 223,000 IU/L. Which of the following is the best next step in management of this patient?

a. Suction aspiration and sharp curettage

b. Repeat ultrasound in 1 week

c. Administer Methotrexate

d. Observation and serial B-hCG levels

e. Diagnostic laparoscopy

Photo credit:
Mikael Häggström. When using this image in external works, it may be cited as:Häggström, Mikael (2014). "Medical gallery of Mikael Häggström 2014". WikiJournal of Medicine 1 (2). DOI:10.15347/wjm/2014.008. ISSN 2002-4436. Public Domain.orBy Mikael Häggström, used with permission., CC0, via Wikimedia Commons

29. A neonate is being evaluated because his mother is concerned his lips turn blue when he is nursing or cries. He was born via spontaneous vaginal delivery, but his mother did not undergo routine prenatal care. Physical examination is notable for a harsh systolic ejection murmur. A chest radiograph is performed (see photo).

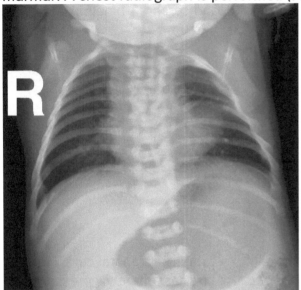

Which of the following is the most likely diagnosis?
a. Transposition of the great vessels
b. Atrial septal defect
c. Tetralogy of Fallot
d. Coarctation of the aorta
e. Hypoplastic left heart syndrome

Photo credit:
Case courtesy of Mohammed Alshammari, Radiopaedia.org, rID: 16268

30. A 20-year-old male with no past medical history presents to the clinic for an annual well visit. He is on a basketball team and does not drink or smoke. He denies chest pain, shortness of breath, or dizziness. Vitals are blood pressure 128/72 mmHg, P: 44 bpm, SpO2: 99% room air. The following is seen on ECG (see photo).

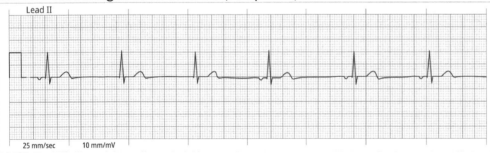

Which of the following is the most appropriate next step in management of this patient?
a. Atropine
b. No further management is needed
c. Transcutaneous pacing
d. Epinephrine
e. Permanent pacemaker placement

31. A 26-year-old male presents to the urgent care department complaining of acute onset of pain and vision loss in his eyes. He describes the vision loss as central with paracentral scotomas in the visual fields and decreased color saturation. He has a history of Tuberculosis, for which he is treated with multidrug therapy. Physical examination is notable for pain with eye movements and a relative afferent pupillary defect noted on the swinging light test of the left eye. Which of the following medications is most likely responsible for these findings?
a. Ethambutol
b. Rifampin
c. Streptomycin
d. Isoniazid
e. Pyrazinamide

32. A 25-year-old tall, thin male with a 2 pack-year smoking history presents to the emergency department complaining of 9/10 right-sided pleuritic chest pain and dyspnea. He has a past medical history of Asthma. Vitals are blood pressure 130/80 mmHg, pulse: 120/min, and respirations 20/min. Lung examination reveals decreased breath sounds, tympany to percussion, and unequal respiratory expansion on the right side. A chest radiograph is obtained:

Which of the following is the most appropriate management strategy for this patient?
a. Supplemental oxygen and observation
b. Needle decompression followed by chest tube thoracostomy
c. Needle thoracentesis
d. Chest tube thoracostomy
e. Video-assisted thoracoscopic surgery (VATS)

33. A 25-year-old woman presents to her primary care physician with progressive fatigue, increasing anxiety, and weight loss despite a good appetite. Vitals reveal a blood pressure 160/94 mmHg and pulse 112/min. Bilateral exophthalmos, lid retraction, diaphoresis, and brisk reflexes are noted. Based on the most likely diagnosis, which of the following antibodies would most likely be present?
a. Triiodothyronine
b. Thyroid peroxidase
c. Thyroglobulin
d. TSH receptor blocking
e. Thyrotropin receptor

34. A 32-year-old female presents to the ED after collapsing at home. Her husband said she had been complaining of fever and URI symptoms for the last 2 days. She has a history of Sarcoidosis for which she completed treatment with Prednisone 1 month ago. Vitals reveal temperature 103°F (39.4°C), blood pressure 88/52 mmHg, pulse 124/min, and respirations 12/min. Initial labs reveal:
- sodium 129 mEq/L (135-145)
- potassium 5.8 mEq/L (3.5-5)
- blood urea nitrogen 33 mg/dL (7-20)
- creatinine 2.1 mg/dL (0.6-1.2)
- glucose 54 mg/dL (70-110)
- white blood cell count 22,000 (5,000-10,000).

Which of the following is the most appropriate next step in the management?
a. Perform an ACTH (Cosyntropin) stimulation test and obtain cortisol levels
b. 0.9% normal saline
c. 5% dextrose in 0.9% normal saline and IV Hydrocortisone
d. IV Hydrocortisone and IV Levothyroxine
e. 5% dextrose in water and Hydrocortisone

35. A 22-year-old male is complaining of severe right eye pain, tearing, blurred vision, and discomfort in bright light for 48 hours. He also reports foreign body sensation in the right eye. He admits to sleeping in and using his daily-wear soft contact lenses for extended periods. On examination, he has difficulty keeping the right eye open and the conjunctiva is injected. Slit lamp examination is positive for a staining epithelial defect with an underlying yellow hazy infiltrate spreading into the stroma without a hypopyon. Which of the following is the most appropriate next step?
a. Initiate ophthalmic Prednisolone
b. Apply an eye patch to the right eye for comfort
c. Irrigate the eye with Lactated ringers or normal saline
d. Immediate referral to an ophthalmologist
e. Initiate Moxifloxacin, discharge the patient, and inform the patient to use glasses until the symptoms resolve

36. A 5-month-old girl is brought to the clinic because she has had a fever and tugging her right ear. She also has had nasal congestion for the past 3 days. She is up to date on her vaccinations. Vitals are temperature 102.2°F (39°C) and pulse is 125/min. Examination of her right ear shows a bulging, diffusely erythematous tympanic membrane. There is reduced mobility with insufflation. The left ear is unremarkable and there is no mastoid tenderness. Which of the following is the best next step in management of this patient?
a. High-dose Amoxicillin
b. Observation with a scheduled follow up appointment in 48-72 hours
c. High-dose Amoxicillin with clavulanate
d. Tympanocentesis with culture
e. Cefdinir

37. A 14-year-old male presents to an outpatient clinic in December for persistent rhinorrhea and nasal stuffiness. Examination of the nasal and oral mucosa reveals pale bluish hue and edema of the turbinate, clear rhinorrhea, and cobblestoning of the posterior pharynx. Which of the following is the most likely etiology of his presentation?
a. Nontypeable *Haemophilus influenzae*
b. Environmental allergen
c. Rhinovirus
d. Cold and dry air exposure
e. Streptococcus pneumoniae

38. A 20-year-old male is being evaluated for agitation, paranoia, unexplained weight loss, and absenteeism at work. Vitals are blood pressure of 146/92 mmHg, pulse 112 bpm, and respirations 32/minute. During examination, psychomotor agitation, restlessness, tremor, diaphoresis, and easy distractibility are noted. His pupils are dilated and reactive to light, with intact extraocular movements. His speech is loud and pressured. Which of the following is the most likely diagnosis?
a. Alcohol withdrawal syndrome
b. Cocaine use disorder
c. Bipolar disorder with manic episode
d. Phencyclidine intoxication
e. Heroin withdrawal

39. A 25-year-old G2P0100 at 14 weeks of gestation presents for routine testing. She has a history of 2 pregnancy loss related to painless cervical dilation at 22 weeks and 20 weeks of gestation 3 and 5 years ago respectively. A transvaginal ultrasound is performed at this visit reveals a viable singleton gestation and cervical length of 32 mm. Which of the following is the most appropriate management?
a. IM progesterone
b. Cervical cerclage
c. Observation and serial cervical length monitoring
d. Vaginal progesterone
e. IV Betamethasone

40. A 24-year-old male presents to the clinic for chronic low back pain. The pain is worse at night but improved as the day progresses and when he goes to the gym. Physical examination reveals a stooped posture, limited spinal mobility, and decreased chest wall expansion. Pulmonary function test reveals
- Vital capacity: 68% predicted (80-120%)
- FEV1/FVC: 97% predicted (>70%)

The following is seen on lumbar radiographs (see photo).

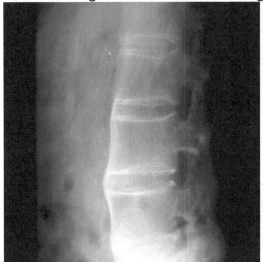 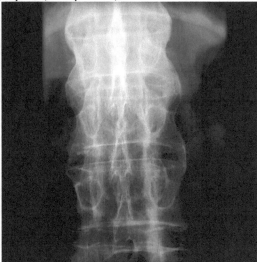

Which of the following is the most common extraarticular manifestation of this condition?
a. Anterior uveitis
b. Aortic regurgitation
c. Osteoporosis
d. Inflammatory bowel disease
e. Psoriasis

Photo credit:
Case courtesy of Frank Gaillard, Radiopaedia.org, rID: 7163

41. A 25-year-old male presents with injuries after his legs were pinned under a metal beam during a construction accident. Vital signs are stable. The legs are swollen, tender, and bruised. Laboratory results are as follows:
Sodium 142 mEq/L (135-145)
Potassium 5.3 mEq/L (3.5-5)
Creatinine 2.1 mg/dL (0.6-1.2)
Calcium 7.3 mg/dL (8.5-10)
Creatine kinase, serum 79,000 U/L (39-308)
Which of the following is the most appropriate initial therapy for this patient?
a. Emergent hemodialysis
b. IV Sodium bicarbonate
c. IV 0.9% sodium chloride solution
d. Intravenous Furosemide
e. IV 0.45% sodium chloride solution with 5% dextrose

42. A 25-year-old female presents to the clinic after noticing a breast lump. She denies nipple discharge. Physical examination is positive for a 3-cm ovoid, firm, nontender, mobile, rubbery mass in the lower inner quadrant of the right breast. There is no axillary lymphadenopathy. Which of the following is the most likely diagnosis?
a. Fibrocystic changes
b. Intraductal papilloma
c. Infiltrative ductal carcinoma
d. Fibroadenoma
e. Galactocele

43. A 5-year-old boy from Columbia is to undergo an umbilical hernia repair. Preoperative labs were only significant for an elevated eosinophil count. Shortly after induction of anesthesia, a large worm is seen wriggling out of his mouth. Which complication is most likely to occur in this patient?
a. Pleuritis
b. Pericarditis
c. Pneumonitis
d. Lymphadenitis
e. Myocarditis

44. A 21-year-old male presents to the emergency department with fever, chills, malaise, and dyspnea. Vitals reveal a temperature of 103°F (39.44°C), blood pressure 112/66 mmHg, and pulse 116/min. There are multiple pink macular lesions on the palm of his left hand, small puncture wounds, fresh scarring at the antecubital fossae, and a holosystolic murmur that is best heard at the left lower sternal border accentuated with inspiration. Blood cultures are obtained. Which of the following is the first line therapy?
a. Penicillin G plus Gentamicin
b. Amphotericin B
c. Vancomycin
d. Nafcillin
e. Clindamycin

45. A 10-year-old boy presents with swelling around his eyes and scrotal region. Associated symptoms include dark brown urine with a foamy appearance and malaise. Labs are positive for serum creatinine 2.5 mg/dL (0.6-1.2) and BUN 34 mg/dL (7-20). Urinalysis findings include specific gravity 1.020 and protein 1+. Microscopic examination of the urine reveals erythrocyte 10+ with dysmorphic red cells, and leukocytes 1+. Which of the following is most likely in this child's recent history?
a. Diarrheal illness
b. Protracted vomiting
c. Recent Antibiotic use
d. Impetigo
e. Recent allergies

46. A 39-year-old male develops a painful rash preceded by a 3-day history of myalgia, conjunctivitis, sore throat, and fever. He has a history of Gout for which he takes Allopurinol. On examination, there are erythematous macules, bullae, desquamation, sloughing off of the skin, and skin tenderness to palpation of the skin involving the entire trunk and both arms in their entirety. Some of the lesions are annular with purpuric centers. There are painful ulcerations in the mucous membranes in the mouth. Which of the following is the most likely diagnosis?
a. Bullous pemphigoid
b. Erythema multiforme major
c. Staphylococcal scalded skin syndrome
d. Stevens-Johnson syndrome
e. Toxic epidermal necrolysis

47. A 75-year-old male presents with decreased urine output for 72 hours and lower abdominal distention. He has a history of Benign prostatic hypertrophy but is not on any medications. On examination, dullness to percussion in the pelvis and lower abdomen is noted. Bladder scan reveals a postvoid residual of 200 mL. Initial labs reveal:
BUN: 19 mg/dL (7-20)
Creatinine 1.9 mg/dL (0.6-1.2)
Renal ultrasonography is performed (see photo).

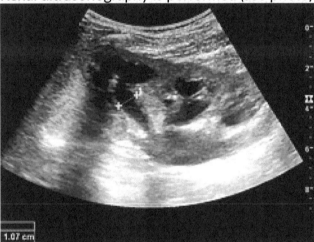

Which of the following is the recommended next step?
a. Suprapubic catheterization
b. Foley catheter placement
c. IV Normal saline
d. Initiate Finasteride
e. Emergent hemodialysis

Photo credit
Kristoffer Lindskov Hansen, Michael Bachmann Nielsen and Caroline Ewertsen, CC BY 4.0 <https://creativecommons.org/licenses/by/4.0>, via Wikimedia Commons

48. The presence of which of the following laboratory findings is most consistent with multiple gestation?
a. Decreased beta-hCG
b. Increased maternal serum alpha-fetoprotein
c. Increased serum pregnancy-associated plasma protein-A
d. Low unconjugated estriol
e. Increased maternal serum glucose

49. A 79-year-old male is admitted to the hospital for Pneumonia. On examination, he is noted to have a pressure ulcer on his sacrum. He stays in bed most hours of the day and often, his grandson, who is his caretaker, often forgets to feed him or change his diapers. Physical examination is notable for caked feces on his skin, dry mucous membranes, and ligature marks on his wrists. When the patient is informed that social work is to be involved in the case, he states he does not want social work to call his son. Which of the following is the most appropriate action?
a. No further intervention is indicated
b. Notify adult protective services
c. Psychiatry evaluation for determination of capacity
d. Educate the patient on signs to look out for elder abuse
e. Call the son to discuss and explain the physical findings

50. A 47-year-old male presents to the clinic with a 3-month history of dyspnea on exertion and fatigue. On examination, 2+ pitting pedal edema and a rise in jugular venous pressure with inspiration are noted. Transthoracic echocardiogram is performed and reveals an ejection fraction of 62% (55-60), impaired diastolic relaxation, speckling, and biatrial enlargement. Which of the following is likely the etiology?
a. Previous treatment with Doxorubicin
b. Autosomal dominant mutation of genes that encode for cardiac cell sarcomere proteins
c. Coxsackie virus infection
d. Chronic inflammation of the pericardium
e. Amyloid deposition into the cardiac tissue

51. A 20-year-old male presents to the dermatology clinic with a worsening rash. On examination, there are well-circumscribed erythematous flat-topped plaques with thick silver-white scales. Which of the following nail findings would most likely be seen?
a. Concave shaped nails
b. Few to multiple tiny pits distributed over the nail plate
c. Banded longitudinal brown to black pigmentation of the nail
d. Convex curving of the nails
e. Transverse grooves of the nail plate

52. A 50-year-old male presents to the clinic to establish care. He has a family history of coronary artery disease. Initial labs reveal:
- Total cholesterol 235 mg/dL
- LDL 148 mg/dL
- Triglycerides 180 mg/dL.
He is prescribed the first-line agent to reduce his cardiovascular risk. Which of the following is the most significant adverse effect of this medication?
a. Generalized pruritus
b. Myopathy
c. Impaired hearing
d. Cutaneous flushing
e. Erectile dysfunction

53. A 35-year-old male is complaining of intermittent burning retrosternal chest discomfort, which is aggravated by drinking coffee, alcohol, eating fatty foods, and reclining after dinner. His symptoms are sometimes accompanied by a "sour" taste in his mouth. The episodes occur on average 3 times a week. He denies dysphagia, odynophagia, weight loss, vomiting, or melena. An ECG reveals normal sinus rhythm. Hemoglobin is 13.5 g/dL (13.2-16.6). Which of the following is the most appropriate next step in the management of this patient?
a. Upper GI series (Barium esophagram)
b. Ambulatory 24-hour esophageal pH monitoring
c. Upper endoscopy
d. Famotidine
e. Pantoprazole

54. A 40-year-old female returns from a week-long vacation complaining of cough, watery diarrhea, nausea, vomiting, and headache. She was informed that a few people in the hotel she stayed at experienced similar symptoms. On examination, fine crackles heard. Labs are significant for
- serum sodium 130 mEq/L (135-145)
- Aspartate aminotransferase 50 IU/L (8-38)
- Alanine aminotransferase 60 IU/L (4-44)

Radiographs are obtained (see photo)

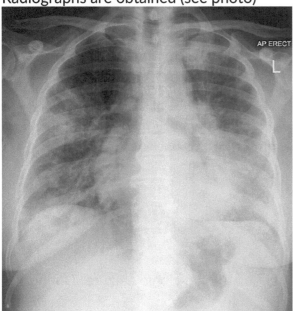

Which of the following is the initial management of choice?
a. Ceftriaxone
b. Piperacillin/tazobactam
c. Azithromycin
d. Amoxicillin
e. Vancomycin

Photo credit:
Case courtesy of Henry Knipe, Radiopaedia.org, rID: 31816

55. A 21-year-old female is referred to the gastroenterologist for a 5-month history of episodes of crampy abdominal pain that is frequently associated with loose stools. She experiences lower abdominal pain that is often relieved with defecation, sometimes accompanied by intermittent nonbloody watery diarrhea. A colonoscopy reveals areas of transmural inflammation and stricture. Which of the following is the most likely etiology of her symptoms?
a. Celiac disease
b. Irritable bowel syndrome
c. Ulcerative colitis
d. Crohn disease
e. Somatic symptom disorder

56. A 58-year-old male presents with acute onset of painless vision loss in his left eye as if "a curtain came down on my eye". The vision loss lasted for 10 minutes and spontaneously resolved on its own. He denies weakness, slurred speech, blurred vision, ocular pain, motor or sensory deficits. CT scan of the head is within normal limits. Which of the following diagnostic tests would be most helpful based on his symptoms at this time?
a. Echocardiogram
b. Tonometry
c. 24-hour Holter monitor
d. CT carotid angiography
e. Electrophysiology study

57. A 28-year-old woman is being evaluated after an inversion injury to the ankle stepping off of a curve. She is complaining of moderate pain with weightbearing. Physical examination is notable for swelling, tenderness, and ecchymosis to the lateral aspect of the ankle, without evidence of joint instability. Radiographs show soft tissue swelling with no evidence of fracture or dislocation. Which of the following is the best next step in management of this patient's injury?
a. Nonweightbearing short leg cast
b. Rest, observation, and follow up in 10 days
c. Referred to an orthopedic surgeon
d. Elastic wrap (eg, ACE bandage) or compression sleeve for a few days
e. Functional ankle brace, ice, elevation, and rest

58. A 55-year-old male is being evaluated for a generalized tonic-clonic seizure. During the workup, neuroimaging is performed (see photo).

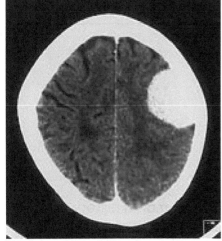

Which of the following is the most likely diagnosis?
a. Glioblastoma multiforme
b. Meningioma
c. Ependymoma
d. Oligodendroglioma
e. Hemangioma

Photo credit:
Glitzy queen00, Public domain, via Wikimedia Commons

59. A 26-year-old female with no significant past medical history presents to her primary care provider for her annual physical. She denies any symptoms. Her last Pap smear at 24 years of age was negative. Results of this Pap smear reveal Atypical squamous cells of undetermined significance (ASCUS). Which of the following is the preferred next step?
a. Repeat Pap and cervical cytology in 1 year
b. Reflex HPV testing
c. Colposcopy
d. Cotesting (Pap testing & HPV) in 3 years
e. Pap smear in 3 years

60. A 22-year-old man presents to his physician with back pain, fever, myalgia, and incessant nonproductive cough for 1 week. He denies acid reflux and has not been vaccinated for Influenza or SARS-CoV-2. He has a 5-pack year smoking history. On physical examination, there are scattered wheezes and rhonchi on auscultation without tachypnea, rales, tactile fremitus, nor dullness to percussion. Chest radiograph is obtained.

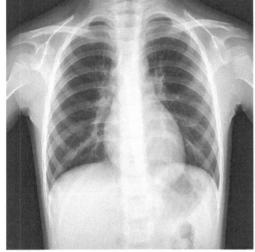

In addition to recommending smoking cessation or avoidance, which of the following is the initial management of choice?
a. Oral Prednisone
b. Azithromycin
c. Throat lozenges, hot tea; SARS-CoV-2 and Influenza testing
d. Levofloxacin
e. Ceftriaxone and Azithromycin

61. A 25-year-old woman presents to the clinic to establish care. She denies any symptoms and exercises regularly without experiencing dyspnea, chest pain, or palpitations. Physical examination is notable for mid-systolic click that occurs earlier with Valsalva maneuvering, narrow anteroposterior chest diameter, and a pectus excavatum deformity. Based on the most likely diagnosis, which of the following is the recommended management of this patient?
a. Prophylaxis for thromboembolism when undergoing surgical procedures
b. Prophylaxis for endocarditis if undergoing dental and respiratory procedures
c. Metoprolol
d. Reassure the patient of the benign nature of the disease

e. Mitral valve repair

62. A 67-year-old man is complaining of sudden-onset of chest tightness and dyspnea. He has experienced prior episodes of chest tightness with activity, but this episode occurred at rest. His medical history is significant for Hypertension and type II Diabetes mellitus. Vitals are stable. An electrocardiogram obtained reveals deep symmetric T wave inversions in V2 and V3 with ST depressions and T wave flattening in leads I, II, and V6. Which of the following is the most appropriate next step in the management of this patient?
a. IV Nitroglycerin
b. Oral Metoprolol
c. IV Alteplase
d. Oral Aspirin
e. IV Unfractionated Heparin

63. A 29-year-old male is complaining of subjective fever, malaise, fatigue, and cough for 3 weeks. He reports a few episodes of night sweats, decreased appetite, and weight loss. He currently lives with many roommates in a small apartment. A chest radiograph is obtained (see photo).

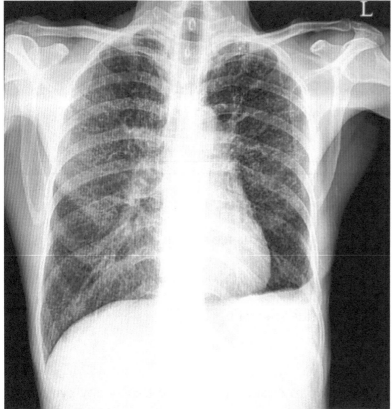

Which of the following is most appropriate next step to establish the most likely diagnosis?
a. Legionella urine antigen
b. Direct Coombs test and cold-agglutinin titers
c. Routine gram stain of sputum samples and sputum cultures
d. Acid-fast bacilli stain on sputum smears and culture
e. Bronchoscopy and bronchoalveolar lavage

Photo credit:

Shutterstock (used with permission)

64. A 20-year-old male suddenly collapsed while playing basketball. There are no palpable femoral or carotid pulses. High quality CPR is performed, and the following is noted (see photo).

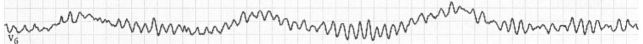

Which of the following is the most appropriate next step?
a. Synchronized cardioversion
b. IV Amiodarone
c. IV Magnesium sulfate
d. Unsynchronized cardioversion
e. IV Epinephrine

65. A 17-year-old ballerina is being evaluated for muscle weakness. Her last menstrual period was 4 months ago. Physical examination is notable for lanugo. Her BMI is 16 kg/m^2. Her abdomen is distended. Which of the following would most likely be seen on physical examination of this patient?
a. Hyperactive bowel sounds
b. Hyperthermia
c. Bradycardia
d. Hypertension
e. Smooth moist skin

66. A 3-year-old boy is brought in by his parents due to restricted vocabulary. He does not maintain eye contact, spends hours playing with the wheels of one of his trucks despite having many, is easily agitated by bright lights and loud sounds, and is preoccupied with ceiling fans. He does not interact with his older sister even with numerous attempts to engage play with him. He inspects things visually out of the corner of his eyes. Which of the following would most likely be seen on examination of this patient?
a. Short palpebral fissures, thin vermillion border, and smooth philtrum
b. Normal imaginative play
c. Exaggerated startle response
d. Always eating particular foods in a specific order
e. Enlarged testes

67. A 5-year-old boy presents to the clinic with his parents because he has been scratching his buttocks and anus for 6 days, often making it difficult for him to sleep at night. Physical examination reveals perianal excoriations. Cellophane tape testing is positive. Which of the following is the recommended initial management?
a. Diphenhydramine cream
b. Albendazole oral
c. Ivermectin oral
d. Lindane lotion
e. Hydrocortisone cream

68. A 54-year-old male with no significant past medical history presents with partial right side facial weakness and a painful rash in his right ear. On examination, there is a vesicular eruption along the auricle of the right ear. This condition is associated with a reactivation of the varicella-zoster virus in which of the following ganglia?
a. Trigeminal
b. Pterygopalatine (maxillary nerve)
c. Otic
d. Geniculate
e. Sphenopalatine

69. A 59-year-old male presents with left knee pain and swelling. He is not unable to bear weight on the affected knee due to severe pain. He has a history of type I Diabetes mellitus. Vitals are temperature 102°F (38.89°C), pulse 100/min, and blood pressure 140/92 mmHg. There is decreased range of motion of the knee with joint effusion. Arthrocentesis demonstrates a white cell count of 59,000 cells/µL. Which of the following organisms is most likely to grow out of culture?
a. *Pseudomonas aeruginosa*
b. *Staphylococcus aureus*
c. *Streptococcus pneumoniae*
d. Salmonella spp.
e. *Streptococcus pyogenes*

70. A 35-year-old female presents to the clinic with fatigue, headache, galactorrhea, and oligomenorrhea. She denies sore throat. Physical examination is notable for a diffuse goiter. Labs reveal
  • TSH: 4.5 µIU/ml (0.27–4.2)
  • Free T4: 4.98 ng/ml (0.72–1.56)
Thyroid scintigraphy reveals the following:

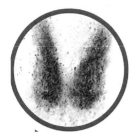

Normal   **Patient**

Which of the following would most likely be a finding on examination of this patient?
a. Bitemporal hemianopia on visual field testing
b. Tenderness with palpation of the thyroid gland
c. Bulging of the eyes with visualization of the upper sclera
d. Loss of the outer third of the eyebrows
e. Delayed sluggish deep tendon reflexes

Photo credit:
Petros Perros, CC BY-SA 3.0 <https://creativecommons.org/licenses/by-sa/3.0>, via Wikimedia Commons

71. A 32-year-old female presents with constant right upper quadrant pain for 5 hours after eating fried food. Vitals reveal a temperature of 101.6°F (38.67°C) and pulse 108/min. Her sclerae are white. Labs reveal:
WBC count: 16,000/mm^3 (5,000-10,000) neutrophil predominance
Total bilirubin: 0.9 mg/dL (up to 1.2)
ALT: 171 U/L (7-55)
Alkaline phosphatase: 50 U/L (44-147)
GGT: 20 IU/L (0-30).
Which of the following is the most likely diagnosis?
a. Acute Hepatitis
b. Choledocholithiasis
c. Acute Cholecystitis
d. Acute Cholangitis
e. Cholelithiasis

72. A 14-year-old boy is being evaluated after being elbowed in the face while playing football. He developed left periorbital swelling that worsens when he blows his nose. He is experiencing numbness below the left eye. Which of the following physical exam findings would most likely be seen in this patient?
a. Diplopia especially with upward gaze
b. Bilateral visual changes in the outer visual fields
c. Visual changes consistent with a "curtain" over the eye
d. Constriction of the visual field resulting in loss of peripheral vision
e. Central scotoma

73. A 20-year-old male presents to the ED after being bitten by a raccoon when he went jogging this morning. He cleansed the wound immediately when he got home. He has no past medical history. On examination, there is a superficial bite wound to the lower leg with no warmth, tenderness, or discharge. Tetanus vaccination is up to date. Which of the following is the most appropriate management?
a. Reassurance that no further management is needed
b. HDCV and Rabies immunoglobulin today followed by HDCV on days 3, 7, and 14
c. HDCV and Rabies immunoglobulin today followed by HDCV on days 3,7, 14, and 28
d. Rabies Immune Globulin half in the wound and half IM in the deltoid
e. HDCV only on days 0 & 3

74. Which of the following is the most common type of tic seen in individuals with Tourette syndrome?
a. Blinking
b. Sniffling
c. Grunting
d. Repetitive phrases
e. Biting of the lips

75. A 66-year-old man presents to his primary care physician with fatigue, generalized weakness, and lower back pain. Physical examination is notable for conjunctival pallor and midline point tenderness upon palpation of the lower spine. Laboratory studies are notable for:
- Hemoglobin: 9.9 g/dL (13.5-17.5)
- MCV: 84 fL (80-100)
- Serum calcium 14 mg/dL (8.5-10)
- Creatinine: 1.6 mg/dL (0.6-1.2)
- Blood urea nitrogen: 26 mg/dL (7-20)

The following is seen on peripheral smear (see photo).

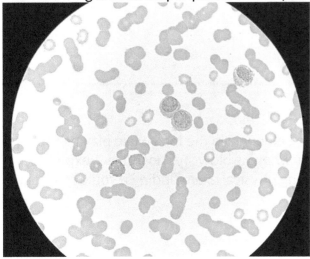

Which of the following is the most appropriate next step?
a. Bone marrow aspiration
b. Genetic testing for JAK2 mutation
c. Nuclear bone scan
d. Serum protein electrophoresis
e. Cross-sectional imaging with a CT scan

76. A 43-year-old male presents to the clinic with muscle cramps and generalized muscle weakness that began in his legs, progressing to the trunk and upper extremities. His medical history included newly diagnosed hypertension, and his medications include Hydrochlorothiazide. ECG showed normal sinus rhythm and the following (see photo).

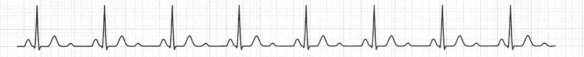

Which of the following is the most likely etiology of his presentation?
a. Hypokalemia
b. Hyperkalemia
c. Hypercalcemia
d. Hypocalcemia
e. Hypomagnesemia

Photo credit:
Shutterstock (used with permission)

77. A 19-year-old boy presents after an intentional overdose. He was found next to an empty bottle of Paroxetine. Vital signs are temperature 99.6° F (37.5° C), heart rate 120 bpm, and blood pressure 136/82. On physical examination, he is agitated, and inducible generalized clonus is noted. Which of the following is the treatment of choice for the agitation?
a. Haloperidol
b. Lorazepam
c. Diphenhydramine
d. Quetiapine
e. Dantrolene

78. A 23-year-old male is being evaluated for fatigue, difficulty falling asleep, back and muscle tension, recurrent headaches, and always feeling "on edge". He is constantly worried about his overall physical and mental health, he is very concerned about his relationship with his family, he dwells on thoughts if he will be able to perform sexually sufficient for his girlfriend, and he distresses over ideas of whether or not he will succeed in his academic studies at college. This uncontrollable worry has led to increased restlessness, irritability with others, and difficulty concentrating at school. Which of the following is the most likely diagnosis?
a. Somatic symptom disorder
b. Panic disorder
c. Major depressive disorder
d. Generalized anxiety disorder
e. Obsessive-Compulsive disorder

79. A 22-year-old male presents with intermittent periorbital edema, "foamy" urine, night sweats, and weight loss. Physical examination is notable for enlarged cervical lymph nodes with a rubbery consistency. Urinalysis reveals 3+ proteinuria and lymph node biopsy reveals the following

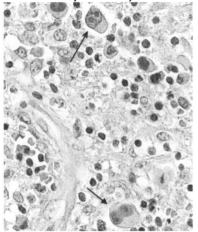

If a renal biopsy is performed, which of the following would most likely be seen?
a. Thickened glomerular basement membrane
b. Sclerosis of focal segments of the glomeruli
c. Fusion and effacement of podocytes
d. Apple green birefringence under polarized light on Congo red stain
e. Hypercellular glomeruli with many neutrophils

Photo credit:
Shutterstock (used with permission)

80. A 22-year-old male presents to the clinic for assistance. He was nominated the valedictorian of his class, which means he has to give a speech. He has to do his oral dissertation next week. He has a 3-year history of experiencing flushing, palpitations, shaking of his hands, and sweating when presenting class projects or when he play instruments in public. Physical examination is unremarkable. Which of the following is the most appropriate pharmacotherapy for this patient?
a. Lorazepam
b. Propranolol
c. Fluoxetine
d. Bupropion
e. Cannabinoids

81. A 42-year-old female presents with worsening heel pain exacerbated by standing on her feet all day as a cashier. The pain is worse in the morning with the first few steps of walking after getting out of bed and worsens at the end of the day. The pain improves after the first hour and with rest. On examination, there is local point tenderness near the medial tuberosity with maximal tenderness elicited on palpation over the inferior heel. There is pain with passive dorsiflexion of the toes. Which of the following is next step in the diagnosis?
a. MRI of the feet and ankle
b. No additional laboratory testing or imaging needed
c. Ultrasonography of the foot
d. Plain radiographs of the feet
e. CT scan of the feet and ankle

82. A 9-month-old previously healthy infant is being evaluated for fatigue, fever, and severe pain in the hands and feet. Physical examination is notable for edema and tenderness to the fingers and toes, tachycardia, and pallor. Labs reveal:
Hemoglobin 7.8 g/dL (9.5-14)
MCV: 87.5 (80-100)
Peripheral smear:

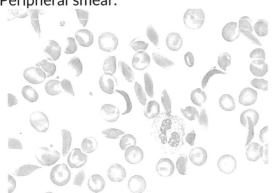

In addition to fluids, oxygen therapy, and pain relief, which of the following interventions is first line to reduce the risk of future pain episodes in this patient?
a. Penicillin
b. Red cell transfusions
c. Hydroxyurea
d. Rituximab
e. Periodic phlebotomy

83. A 66-year-old female presents to a clinic with back pain. The pain is dull and occurred after lifting a box. Sitting, spine extension, Valsalva maneuver, and movement aggravate the pain. She denies fever, chills, radiation of pain into the legs, urinary or fecal incontinence. Vitals are stable. On physical examination, midline and low back tenderness without paravertebral tenderness or lower extremity weakness are noted. Which of the following is the most likely diagnosis?
a. Spinal epidural abscess
b. Cauda equina syndrome
c. Vertebral compression fracture
d. Lumbar strain
e. Herniated disc

84. A 47-year-old woman presents to the office with concerns about urine leakage. She leaks a small amount of urine when she lifts heavy objects, coughs, sneezes, or laughs, which is embarrassing for her. Which of the following is the most significant predisposing factor for her underlying condition?
a. History of multiple vaginal births
b. Lower urinary tract infection
c. Increased or altered bladder microbiome
d. Bladder outlet obstruction
e. Damage to the spinal detrusor efferent nerves

85. A 55-year-old man presents to his primary care physician for evaluation of difficulty achieving and maintaining erections. He denies having any psychological stressors. He reports having no morning or night-time erections. Laboratory workup is negative, and first line therapy is to be described. What is the primary mechanism of action of first line therapy?
a. Synthetic testosterone analog
b. 5-alpha reductase inhibition
c. Phosphodiesterase-5 inhibition
d. Selective Alpha-adrenergic antagonist
e. Prostaglandin E1 analog

86. A 22-year-old male presents complaining of excruciating eye pain and an inability to open the right eye due to photophobia and foreign body sensation. The pain and photophobia make him too uncomfortable to drive or read. The symptoms occurred after being outside on a windy day. Visual acuity is 20/20 bilaterally and fundus examination is unremarkable. Which of the following is the most appropriate next step in the management of this patient?
a. Amsler grid visual assessment
b. Tonometry
c. Slit lamp examination with fluorescein
d. CT scan of the orbits
e. Emergent ophthalmologic consultation

87. A 32-year-old male returns to the clinic for follow-up. He has been experiencing ejaculation soon after initial vaginal penetration, which has caused emotional distress for him and his partner. He has tried to the start-stop method and squeezing the area between the shaft of the penis and glans without much success. He denies difficulty achieving or maintaining an erection. He is requesting pharmacological therapy. Which of the following is the most appropriate initial therapy for this patient?
a. Bupropion
b. Clomipramine
c. Tramadol
d. Paroxetine
e. Sildenafil

88. A 21-year-old man is being evaluated for excessive daytime sleepiness. He sometimes uncontrollably falls asleep during inappropriate times, such as during conversations or at work and feels refreshed after a brief nap. At times, emotions such as laughter and anger can trigger transient muscle weakness and loss of muscle tone of his face and neck. As he falls asleep, he experiences sensations of suffocation or falling or feeling as if someone is in the room with him. The sensations are vivid although he knows they are not real. Physical examination is unremarkable. Based on the most likely diagnosis, which of the following is the first-line management of his condition?
a. Zolpidem
b. Carbamazepine
c. Clonazepam
d. Venlafaxine
e. Modafinil

89. A 25-year-old previously healthy male is complaining of fever, dyspnea, chest pain, easy fatigability, and swelling of the ankles. He has no past medical history or cardiovascular history and is physically active at baseline On examination, he is tachycardic. Bilateral bibasilar pulmonary rales and elevated jugular venous pressure are noted. ECG reveals tachycardia and ventricular ectopic beats without ST changes. Troponin I is 1.2 (0-0.4) and SARS-CoV-2 antigen via nasopharyngeal swab is positive. Which of the following is the criterion standard in establishing the most likely diagnosis?
a. Analysis of pericardial fluid
b. Endomyocardial biopsy
c. Echocardiography
d. Cardiac magnetic resonance imaging
e. Cardiac catheterization

90. Which of the following has been shown to have the greatest impact on reducing the incidence of Hepatitis A?
a. Antivirals
b. Vaccination
c. Use of protected sexual intercourse
d. Needle exchange programs
e. Sanitation

91. A 30-year-old male undergoes a chest radiograph to rule out a rib fracture after a traumatic fall. The chest radiograph reveals no fracture, but a small pulmonary nodule is seen. He is a nonsmoker and has no significant medical history. He denies chest pain, hemoptysis, dyspnea, cough, weight loss, or wheezing. Physical examination is unremarkable. A chest radiograph shows a well-demarcated, fully calcified nodule in the right upper lobe.

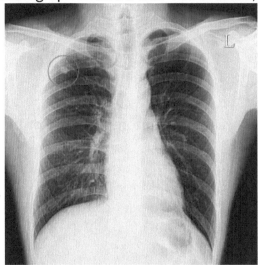

Which of the following is the most appropriate next step?
a. Provide reassurance with no further follow-up
b. Obtain a Tuberculin skin test
c. Perform a transthoracic biopsy
d. Obtain a computed tomography of the chest
e. Repeat chest radiograph in 3 months

Photo credit:
Shutterstock (used with permission)

92. A 37-year-old male presents to the clinic after noticing a small lump under the skin of his scalp, which is slowly increasing in size. He denies pain. On physical examination, there is a discrete 3-cm soft swollen nodule on the temple, with an overlying central punctum. It is freely mobile, ballotable, and nontender. Which of the following is the most likely diagnosis?
a. Epidermoid (epidermal inclusion) cyst
b. Lipoma
c. Abscess
d. Dermoid cyst
e. Keloid

93. A 51-year-old male presents to the clinic to establish care. He has no first-degree relatives or other risk factors for Colon cancer. Which of the following is the recommended screening for this patient according to the USPSTF?
a. First colonoscopy now and if normal schedule colonoscopy in 1 year
b. First colonoscopy now and if normal, schedule colonoscopy in 5 years
c. First colonoscopy now and if normal, schedule colonoscopy in 10 years
d. First colonoscopy now and if normal, schedule colonoscopy in 20 years
e. No colonoscopy needed until he is 60 years old or fecal occult blood positive

94. A 68-year-old male presents to the clinic for a persistent oral lesion despite brushing. He has a 40 pack-year smoking history and drinks 1 beer daily. Physical examination is notable for a uniformly white plaque on the anterior surface of the body of the tongue with a regular texture and well-defined margin. It cannot be scraped off with a tongue depressor or wiped off with gauze. Which of the following is the most likely diagnosis?
a. Hairy leukoplakia
b. Lichen planus
c. Oral Squamous cell carcinoma
d. Candidiasis
e. Leukoplakia

95. A 33-year-old male is placed on Amitriptyline for Major depressive disorder. Which of the following are the most common adverse effects of therapy?
a. Polyuria and polydipsia
b. Dry mouth and constipation
c. Weight loss and decreased appetite
d. Insomnia and agitation
e. Diaphoresis and hypertension

96. A 43-year-old female returns to the clinic for evaluation of nausea, vomiting of undigested material, abdominal pain, early satiety, and bloating. She has a longstanding history of type 1 Diabetes mellitus and was found to have delayed gastric emptying on scintigraphy. She has optimized her glycemic control and tried dietary modifications, including eating multiple smaller meals more frequently and blenderizing food. Which of the following is the most appropriate initial medical therapy for this patient?
a. Omeprazole
b. Metoclopramide
c. Erythromycin
d. Diphenhydramine
e. Ondansetron

97. A 34-year-old man presents to the clinic with decreased urinary stream, feeling of incomplete voiding, dribbling, hesitancy, and urinary spraying. He was recently evaluated for a pelvic fracture sustained in a motor vehicle collision, which was treated with conservatively with pelvic rest and Ibuprofen. Genitourinary examination is unremarkable. Which of the following is the most appropriate initial investigation to diagnose this patient's most likely condition?
a. CT scan of the pelvis
b. Uroflowmetry
c. Renal ultrasound
d. Retrograde urethrography
e. Voiding cystourethrogram

98. A 25-year-old male presents to the clinic for follow-up of Major depressive disorder. He is being treated with low-dose Fluoxetine. He was recently doing research about the adverse effect of pharmacotherapy and is really concerned about weight gain and sexual dysfunction from therapy. Which of the following is recommended next step?
a. Continue Fluoxetine; augment with Bupropion
b. Discontinue Fluoxetine; switch to Mirtazapine
c. Continue Fluoxetine; augment with Venlafaxine
d. Continue Fluoxetine dose
e. Discontinue Sertraline; switch to Paroxetine

99. A 66-year-old man presents to the clinic with a 3-month history of worsening dull, crampy epigastric pain, usually within the first hour after eating and subsiding within 2 hours of onset. He has adapted his eating pattern to eating less frequently in an effort to avoid the pain, which has resulted in a 10-lb. weight loss over the last 5 weeks. He denies bloody stool, early satiety, fatty food intolerance, nausea, or vomiting. He has a 30-pack year smoking history and Dyslipidemia. Physical examination is unremarkable. His last Colonoscopy was 5 years ago. Which of the following is the best next step in the evaluation of this patient?
a. Abdominal and pelvic CT angiography
b. Abdominal arteriography
c. Colonoscopy
d. Duplex ultrasonography of the abdomen and pelvis
e. Upper endoscopy

100. A 25-year-old male presents to the clinic with complaints of headache and weakness in his legs. He has been distressed because despite seeing a headache specialist, a neurologist, and a neurosurgeon, they have not been able to help him. Over the last 10 months, he has undergone numerous neuroimaging, electromyography, lumbar puncture, and laboratory evaluation, all of which were negative. On examination, he appears healthy and physical examination is unremarkable. Which of the following is the most likely diagnosis?
a. Factitious disorder
b. Body dysmorphic disorder
c. Somatic symptom disorder
d. Illness anxiety disorder
e. Functional neurological symptom disorder

END OF EXAM 4

1. INFECTIOUS DISEASE – RHEUMATIC FEVER [HISTORY AND PHYSICAL EXAMINATION]
The minor Jones criteria include:
- **fever (≥38.5°F) [choice E]**
- arthralgia (joint pain without inflammation)
- sedimentation rate ≥60 mm and/or C-reactive protein (CRP) ≥3.0 mg/dl,
- and prolonged PR interval (unless carditis is a major criterion)

The 5 major Jones criteria include "JONES"
- **J**oint pain with swelling (arthritis) most common
- "**O**h, my heart" Carditis
- **N**odules (subcutaneous)
- **E**rythema marginatum
- **S**ydenham chorea

2. DERMATOLOGY – SCABIES [PHARMACOLOGY]
First line agents for Scabies include:
- **Topical Permethrin [choice C]**
- **Oral Ivermectin** is an alternative that is cheaper and easier to use.

Topical Permethrin cream has a high cure rate >90%. It interferes with the function of voltage-gated sodium channels in insects and *S. scabiei*, interfering with neurotransmission.
It is safe in infants >2 months of age, children, adults, and pregnant or lactating women.
It is applied from the neck down and rinsed off 8-14 hours afterwards. A second application 7-14 days to ensure eradication is often recommended.
Scabies is classically associated with intensely pruritic erythematous papules, nodules, and linear burrows that may include the webspace.

Choice A [Topical Lindane] use has fallen out of favor due to increased risk of neurotoxicity.
Choice B [Clotrimazole cream] is used for Tinea fungal skin infections.
Choice D [Topical Hydrocortisone] may be used for pruritus but only after eradication with a scabicide.
Choice E [Oral Prednisone] is not used in the management of Scabies.

3. CARDIOLOGY – CHRONIC VENOUS INSUFFICIENCY [HISTORY AND PHYSICAL]
Classic physical examination findings of Chronic venous insufficiency include:
- **dependent pitting edema [choice A]**
- leg discomfort, fatigue, and itching
- reticular veins, varicose veins
- symptoms that improve with rest and leg elevation and not associated with exercise
- skin changes (blanched skin lesion, dermal atrophy, hyperpigmentation due to venous stasis dermatitis)
- ulcer formation, most commonly overlying the medial malleolus.

All of the other choices listed are classic for Peripheral arterial disease.
Peripheral arterial disease associated with:

- pallor on leg elevation, dependent rubor
- lateral malleolar ulcers
- atrophic skin changes
- decreased peripheral pulses.

4. GASTROINTESTINAL AND NUTRITION/CARDIOLOGY – PEANUT ALLERGY/ANAPHYLACTIC SHOCK [pharmacology]

The first and most important treatment in Anaphylaxis is aggressive and early management with intramuscular (IM) Epinephrine [choice B] without delay once the diagnosis of Anaphylaxis is suspected.

Intramuscular (IM) injection of Epinephrine is administered in the mid-outer aspect of the thigh.

- Pediatric dosing: 0.01 mg/kg 1:1,000 (1 mg/mL) solution IM q 5–15 minutes (or more frequently), maximum 0,5 mg per dose.
- Adult dosing: 0.3 to 0.5 mL 1:1,000 (1 mg/mL) solution IM q5–15 minutes

If signs of poor perfusion are present or symptoms are not responsive to Epinephrine injections (patients should respond to at most, 3 injections), IV Epinephrine infusion may be required.

Anaphylactic shock

- **Reduced blood pressure/hypotension** or associated symptoms and signs of end-organ malperfusion (eg, hypotonia, syncope, incontinence)
- **Respiratory compromise** (eg, stridor, dyspnea, wheezing (bronchospasm), hypoxemia, cyanosis.

Adjunctive therapy to Epinephrine may include:

- Albuterol [Choice A] for bronchospasm resistant to Epinephrine.
- Methylprednisolone [Choice C] 1 mg/kg (maximum 125 mg) IV
- Cetirizine [Choice D]
- Diphenhydramine [Choice E]
- H2 antihistamine (eg, IV Famotidine)
- IV fluids.

5. PULMONARY – LUNG CANCER SCREENING [HEALTH MAINTENANCE]

The US Preventative Services Task Force recommends annual low-dose CT screening [choice C] for those 50–80 years old who are at high risk of lung cancer:

- **at least a 20 pack-year smoking history and are**
- **either current smokers or former smokers having quit within the past 15 years.**

Screening should be discontinued once a person has not smoked for >15 years or develops a health condition substantially limiting life expectancy, or ability or willingness to undergo curative surgery.

Choice A [Colonoscopy] is performed every 10 years in those with average risk. His last colonoscopy 5 years ago was normal.
Choice B [Chest radiography] is not recommended as a screening tool for Bronchogenic carcinoma because it lacks sensitivity.

Choice D [Abdominal ultrasonography] is performed in men who ever smoked between the ages of 65-75 years.

Choice E [Pulmonary function testing] can be performed if an obstructive or restrictive lung disease is suspected.

6. GASTROINTESTINAL AND NUTRITION – CIRRHOSIS/HEPATIC ENCEPHALOPATHY [HISTORY AND PHYSICAL]

Patients with Hepatic encephalopathy may have other stigmata of Cirrhosis, including:
- **Ascites: shifting dullness [choice A], positive fluid wave test**
- **Spider angiomata**
- **Palmar erythema**
- **Jaundice.**

Hepatic encephalopathy is characterized by various neuropsychiatric and neuromuscular abnormalities resulting from the accumulation of toxic substances in the bloodstream (eg, ammonia), affecting brain function as a result of liver dysfunction.

Hepatic encephalopathy is characterized by:
- Asterixis: flapping tremor of the wrists
- CNS symptoms: altered mental status, change in mood, unsteadiness, decreased responsiveness.

Choice B (Ecchymosis to the flank) is Grey Turner sign, seen with Acute pancreatitis.

Choice C [Papilledema] is associated with Hypertensive encephalopathy.

Choice D [Palpable nontender gallbladder] describes Courvoisier sign, associated with Pancreatic cancer.

Choice E [Tenderness in the right upper quadrant with deep palpation] is hallmark of Murphy sign, associated with Acute cholecystitis.

7. PULMONARY – BRONCHIECTASIS [MOST LIKELY]

Characteristic CT features of Bronchiectasis [choice D] include:
- lack of airway tapering (parallel or "tram" track appearance) [arrowheads]
- signet ring sign: appearance of a cross-section of a dilated, air-filled bronchus with the smaller opacity of a pulmonary artery (white arrows)
- airway dilatation (airway lumen-artery diameter ratio ≥1.5)
- airway visibility at the lung periphery
- bronchial wall thickening.

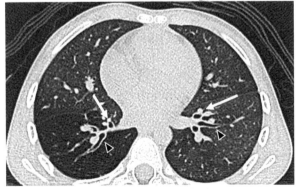

The classic clinical manifestations of Bronchiectasis include

- cough on most days of the week
- daily production of mucopurulent and tenacious sputum, and
- history of exacerbations.

Patients may also complain of dyspnea, hemoptysis, wheezing, and pleuritic chest pain.

8. ENDOCRINOLOGY – PHEOCHROMOCYTOMA [CLINICAL INTERVENTION]

An alpha-adrenergic blocker [eg, nonselective alpha blockers such as Phenoxybenzamine (choice B), or selective alpha blockers, such as Doxazosin] is given for at least 7 days preoperatively to normalize blood pressure in Pheochromocytoma.

Although Adrenalectomy is the definitive management of Pheochromocytoma, preoperative alpha-adrenergic and beta-adrenergic blockade must be done in specific order to prevent malignant hypertension from cutting into the tumor or from unopposed alpha blockade from initiating beta blockers before alpha blockers.

The order of therapy is:

- [1] Alpha-adrenergic blockade at least 7 days preoperatively,
- [2] Beta-adrenergic blockade [choice C] AFTER adequate alpha-adrenergic blockade has been achieved, beta-adrenergic blockade is begun. The beta-adrenergic blocker should **never** be started first.
- [3] Adrenalectomy [choice A] for definitive surgical management.

9. ENDOCRINOLOGY – CUSHING DISEASE [LABS AND DIAGNOSTIC STUDIES]

In patients with ACTH-independent Cushing syndrome (low baseline ACTH <5 pg/mL) not on glucocorticoid therapy, thin-section CT imaging of the adrenal glands [choice B] is the next step in the evaluation, looking for an adrenal mass.

This is because the increased cortisol in both Glucocorticoid therapy and Adrenal disease would result in negative feedback on the pituitary gland, resulting in a low ACTH.

Choice A [CT chest] is used to evaluate for an Ectopic ACTH-producing tumor (eg, Small cell carcinoma of the lung) in patients with [1] elevated baseline ACTH and [2] no suppression of cortisol (≤50% suppression of cortisol) after performing a High-dose Dexamethasone suppression test.

Choice C [Low dose dexamethasone suppression test] is used as an initial screening test for Cushing syndrome. The patient already underwent screening for Cushing syndrome with a 24-hour cortisol and nighttime cortisol level.

Choice D [High dose dexamethasone suppression test] is used in patients with an elevated baseline ACTH to distinguish between the 2 ACTH-dependent causes of Cushing syndrome (eg, Cushing disease due to a pituitary adenoma or an ectopic ACTH-producing tumor).

Choice E [MRI pituitary] is used to diagnose Cushing disease in a patient with [1] an elevated baseline ACTH and [2] suppression of cortisol (≤50% suppression of cortisol) after performing a High-dose Dexamethasone suppression test.

10. ENDOCRINOLOGY – HYPEROSMOLAR HYPERGLYCEMIC SYNDROME (HHS) [CLINICAL INTERVENTION]

Fluid replacement with isotonic solution (Lactated ringer or 0.9% sodium chloride) [choice E] is essential for Hyperosmolar hyperglycemic syndrome (HHS) and Diabetic ketoacidosis (DKA) for aggressive volume replacement to correct hypovolemia and hyperosmolality.
Patients with HHS are estimated to have a fluid deficit of 5–10 L.
In addition to fluid resuscitation, electrolyte repletion is essential.
Hyperosmolar hyperglycemic syndrome (HHS) most commonly occurs in type 2 Diabetes and presents with CNS changes (eg, altered mental status, lethargy, coma) severe hyperglycemia, dehydration, and no acidosis.

Choice A [Metoprolol] may be used for rate control of Atrial flutter, but fluid repletion is the most important next step.
Choice B [Insulin bolus followed by continuous infusion] is also important for treatment of HHS and DKA but should be instituted after some fluid repletion.
Choice D [IV Potassium chloride] should be held in patients with serum potassium ≥5.5. Once levels drop to <5.5, potassium should be given as patients have a total body potassium deficit and insulin administration will lower serum potassium levels.
Choice D [IV Calcium gluconate] is used in the management of severe Hyperkalemia (>6.5 mEq/L) or ECG changes (eg, peaked T waves or sine waves).

11. HEMATOLOGY – HEMOCHROMATOSIS [MOST LIKELY]
Hereditary hemochromatosis [choice C] should be suspected in patients >40 years of age with symptoms and findings of iron overload in organs and tissues:
- **Liver: hepatosplenomegaly, mild transaminitis,** Cirrhosis
- **Heart: Restrictive cardiomyopathy (as seen in this patient);** Dilated cardiomyopathy
- **Skin: bronze color of the skin and hyperpigmentation**
- **Pancreas: glucose intolerance and type 2 Diabetes mellitus**
- Joints: arthropathy.

In HH, *HFE* gene C282Y homozygosity results in decreased Hepcidin (which normally prevents excess iron absorption), increasing intestinal absorption of iron. This leads to iron overload and subsequent accumulation of iron into organs, resulting in organ damage.

Choice A [Sarcoidosis] is another cause of Restrictive cardiomyopathy but does not cause hyperglycemia and bronze-colored skin.
Choice B [Wilson disease] is due to copper overload in tissue, which can present with similar hepatic abnormalities in addition to the Kayser-Fleischer rings (brown rings encircling the cornea along the periphery of the iris).
Choice D [Nonalcoholic fatty liver disease] may cause a transaminitis but it not associated with bronze coloring of the skin.
Choice E [Primary Adrenal insufficiency] may result in skin hyperpigmentation but would more likely be associated with hypoglycemia, hyponatremia, and hyperkalemia due to cortisol and aldosterone deficiency. This patient's hyperglycemia and normal electrolytes makes Primary AI less likely.

12. MUSCULOSKELETAL – FIBROMYALGIA [PHARMACOLOGY]

Low-dose Tricyclic antidepressants (eg, Amitriptyline) [choice C] is a first-line pharmacological agent in patients with Fibromyalgia not responsive to conservative measures, especially for diffuse widespread muscle pain.

Cyclobenzaprine is an alternative to Amitriptyline.

SNRI (eg, Duloxetine) or Milnacipran can be used in patients with prominent fatigue &/or depression.

Pregabalin is especially helpful for sleep disturbances (Gabapentin alternative).

Cognitive behavioral therapy is also recommended.

Fibromyalgia is associated with:
- widespread muscle pain and tenderness
- fatigue
- cognitive and sleep disturbances.
- normal laboratory findings.

Choice A [Low-dose Prednisone] can be used in the management of Polymyalgia rheumatica, which is associated with achiness and stiffness of the hip and shoulder girdle and elevated ESR &/or CRP.

Choice B [High-dose Prednisone] is used for Polymyositis, which is associated with muscle weakness objectively on examination.

Choice D [Indomethacin], other Nonsteroidal anti-inflammatory drugs (NSAIDs), and glucocorticoids [choices A and B] have little benefit in Fibromyalgia unless there is evidence of peripheral pain, because Fibromyalgia is not an inflammatory conditions.

Choice E [Tramadol] has little benefit in the management of Fibromyalgia.

13. NEUROLOGY – CLUSTER HEADACHE [HISTORY AND PHYSICAL]

Cluster headache is a condition characterized by attacks of severe unilateral pain, accompanied by ipsilateral cranial autonomic symptoms (eg, ptosis, miosis, rhinorrhea, conjunctivitis) [choice A] and/or restlessness or agitation.

Triggers include alcohol intake, sexual activity, and glare.

Choice B [Vision loss] may be associated with Giant cell (Temporal) arteritis.

Choice C [Photophobia and nausea] are associated with Migraine.

Choice D [Papilledema and right cranial nerve IV palsy] may occur with the headache associated with Idiopathic intracranial hypertension.

Choice E [Reproduction of the pain with stroking the face on trigger zones] is associated with Trigeminal neuralgia.

14. MUSCULOSKELETAL – SCOLIOSIS [HISTORY AND PHYSICAL]

Observation is recommended for adolescents with Scoliosis with Cobb angles of 11 to 19° [choice C].

Patients are monitored every 6-9 months until skeletal maturity.

Bracing [choice E] may be indicated if the Cobb angle increases by ≥5° or progresses to ≥20° during observation. Bracing is usually contraindicated in patients with a Cobb angles of <20°.

Observation may also be recommended for Cobb angles of 20 to 24°, with clinical follow-up every 4-6 months until skeletal maturity.

Magnetic resonance imaging (MRI) of the spine [choice A] may be indicated in patients with Scoliosis and clinical or radiographic findings consistent with intraspinal pathology (eg, infection, tumor).

Bracing [choice E] may be indicated for patients with Cobb angles of 25 to 39°. Bracing may also be used in patients with Cobb angles between 40 and 49° and Risser grade 0 to 2 or Sanders stage 1 to 3 at the time of presentation, although surgery may be an option for some if >45°.

Surgery [choice B] may be indicated if Cobb angles progress to ≥50° during bracing.

15. MUSCULOSKELETAL – COLLES FRACTURE [HISTORY AND PHYSICAL]

Most Colles fractures are secondary to a Fall on an outstretched hand (FOOSH) with a pronated forearm in wrist extension (the position one assumes when trying to break a forward fall) [choice C].

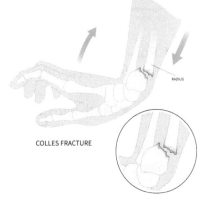

The force is then transmitted dorsally, resulting dorsal angulation of the distal fragment.

Photo credit:
Shutterstock (used with permission)

In healthy young patients, distal radius fractures often occur after violent injuries directly to the bone or by a compression load driving the scaphoid or lunate into the distal radius [choice E], more commonly resulting in a comminuted intraarticular fracture (Barton fracture).

Choice A Fall forward landing on the back of their wrist with their hand flexed or bent in toward their body, results in a Smith fracture (reverse Colles).

Choice B [Direct blow to the anterior or posterior aspect of the wrist and hand] is most likely to result in carpal bone fracture.

Choice D [Punching a stationary object with a clenched fist] results in a Boxer fracture to the fifth metacarpal neck.

16. NEUROLOGY – FOCAL IMPAIRED AWARENESS SEIZURES [MOST LIKELY]

Focal impaired awareness seizures [choice C] are characterized by:
- **Inability to respond with altered consciousness**; patients may have a blank stare and are unarousable
- **Automatisms** including oroalimentary automatisms (eg, lip-smacking, chewing, or swallowing).

Choice A [Myoclonic seizure] is associated with quick, uncontrollable muscle movement without changes in the level of awareness of consciousness.

Choice B [Absence seizure] is associated with staring episodes without loss of postural tone, often lasting 10-15 seconds.

Choice D [Tonic–clonic seizure] is associated with rigidity initially, followed by rhythmic jerking.

Choice E [Atonic seizure] is associated with sudden onset of loss of postural tone.

17. REPRODUCTIVE – ECTOPIC PREGNANCY [PROFESSIONAL PRACTICE]

Because the patient presents with symptoms that may be consistent with an Ectopic pregnancy (lower abdominal pain, dizziness, tachycardia) in a female with a missed pregnancy, a urine pregnancy test should be performed next [choice D].

Although the mother insists the child is not sexually active, pregnancy should be ruled out.

18. RENAL – ACUTE TUBULAR NECROSIS (ATN) – MOST LIKELY

The classic urinalysis in Acute tubular necrosis (ATN) reveals muddy brown granular, epithelial cell casts [choice D], and free renal tubular epithelial cells.

Ischemic or toxic injury to the tubular epithelial cells can lead to cell sloughing into the tubular lumen due either to cell death or to defective cell-to-cell or cell-to-basement membrane adhesion.

ATN occurs due to prolonged prerenal ischemia or toxic damage to the renal tubules due to nephrotoxins (eg, Vancomycin and Gentamicin).

Other findings of ATN reflect the renal tubules inability to conserve water and electrolytes:

- Fractional excretion of sodium (FENa) >2%
- Increased urine sodium >40 mEq/L
- BUN: creatinine ratio <15:1
- Low specific gravity 1.007-1.015 (isosthenuria)
- Low urine osmolality: 300-500 mOsm/Kg

Choice A [Broad waxy casts] are hallmark of End stage renal disease.

Choice B [Red cell casts] are hallmark of Acute glomerulonephritis.

Choice C [White cell casts] are hallmark of Acute interstitial nephritis.

Choice E [Fatty casts] are hallmark of Nephrotic syndrome.

19. PULMONARY/CARDIOLOGY – PULMONARY EMBOLISM/OBSTRUCTIVE SHOCK [CLINICAL INTERVENTION]

Systemic thrombolytic therapy (eg, Alteplase) [choice A] is first line treatment for patients with PE who present with, or whose course is complicated by, hemodynamic instability, especially with a presumptive diagnosis of PE on bedside lower extremity ultrasonography or transthoracic echocardiography.

Most cases of obstructive shock are due to right ventricular failure from hemodynamically significant pulmonary embolism (PE) or severe pulmonary hypertension (PH).

Embolectomy is appropriate for those in whom thrombolysis is either contraindicated or unsuccessful (surgical or catheter-based).

This patient has increased risk factors for PE (malignancy and recent surgery) with evidence of Obstructive shock (distended neck veins, hypotension, and RV strain on echocardiogram).

In Hemodynamically unstable patients despite resuscitation, definitive testing [choice C] is often considered unsafe.

Choice B [CT head] can be performed but should not delay treatment of this patient in Obstructive shock, especially with risk factors for PE and imaging suggestive of PE.
Choice D [D-dimer] is useful for its negative predictive value in patients with low risk for PE. Malignancy and surgery are both associated with elevated D-dimer levels.
Choice E [IV Heparin] is used in the management of hemodynamically stable PE. This patient has severe hypotension consistent with obstructive shock.

20. REPRODUCTIVE SYSTEM – CERVICITIS [PHARMACOLOGY]
A single intramuscular dose of Ceftriaxone [choice C] is the first line treatment for Cervicitis due to Gonorrhea.
- Weight <150 kg – Ceftriaxone 500 mg intramuscularly once
- Weight ≥150 kg (300 lbs.) – Ceftriaxone 1 g intramuscularly once.

Gram stain may reveal gram-negative intracellular diplococci if *N. gonorroheae* is the cause.

If Chlamydia testing is positive or if Chlamydia-specific test results are not available, patient should also be treated with Doxycycline 100 mg orally twice a day for 7 days.
If a Chlamydia-specific test has been performed and is negative, then Doxycycline treatment is not needed.

For treatment of Gonorrhea, Fluoroquinolones and Doxycycline are not appropriate alternatives due to increasing resistance to these antibiotics.
Monotherapy with Azithromycin alone is also not indicated.

Choice D [Metronidazole] is used in the management of Trichomoniasis and Bacterial vaginosis.
Choice E [Penicillin G] is used in the management of Syphilis.

21. PULMONARY – MESOTHELIOMA/ASBESTOSIS [HISTORY AND PHYSICAL]
Asbestos is the only known risk factor for malignant Mesothelioma [choice B].
The two main complications of Asbestosis are [1] respiratory failure and [2] malignancy (eg, Bronchogenic carcinoma, malignant Mesothelioma).
Occupational exposure to Asbestosis include renovation or demolition of asbestos-containing buildings, as seen in this patient.
Asbestosis exposure most commonly presents with a restricted pattern on PFT [normal or increased FEV1/FVC and decreased lung volumes (eg, RV, TLC, and RV/TLC)].
Classic radiograph findings include pleural plaques, as seen in this patient.

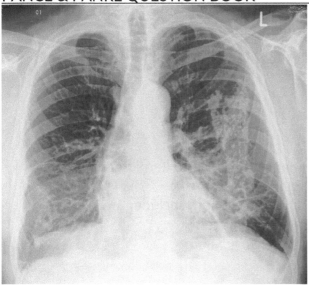

Choice A [Caplan syndrome] is the presence of Rheumatoid arthritis in patients with Silicosis.

Choice C [Lofgren syndrome] is characterized by the triad of arthritis, hilar lymphadenopathy, and erythema nodosum in patients with Sarcoidosis.

Choice D [Emphysema] is an obstructive disease most commonly associated with smoking. It is associated with an obstructive pattern on PFTs (this patient has a restrictive pattern).

Choice E [Bronchiectasis] is an obstructive disease most commonly associated with recurrent infections or Cystic fibrosis. It is associated with an obstructive pattern on PFTs (this patient has a restrictive pattern).

22. CARDIOLOGY – SUPRAVENTRICULAR TACHYCARDIA [CLINICAL INTERVENTION]

For the acute termination of symptomatic narrow complex Supraventricular tachycardia (SVT) in a hemodynamically stable patient, carotid sinus massage [choice D] or another vagal maneuver is the initial therapy.

In patients not responsive to Vagal maneuvers, Adenosine [choice A] is the first line medical therapy for stable SVT.

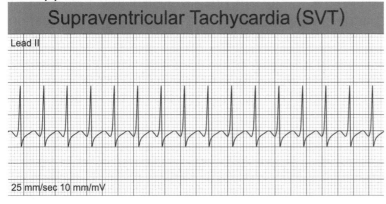

Choice B [Synchronized (direct current) cardioversion] is used in patients with hemodynamically unstable tachycardia with a pulse (eg, hypotension, altered mental status).

Choice C [IV Amiodarone] is usually reserved for wide complex tachycardia (Ventricular tachycardia).

Choice E [IV Esmolol] may be used for SVT after Adenosine has been tried 3 times.

23. REPRODUCTIVE SYSTEM – CYSTITIS DURING PREGNANCY [PHARMACOLOGY]

Medications safe for the treatment of Cystitis during pregnancy include:
- <u>Cephalosporin</u>: eg, Cephalexin [choice C]
- **Amoxicillin**
- **Amoxicillin-clavulanate**
- **Cefpodoxime**
- **Nitrofurantoin**
- **Fosfomycin**
- Sulfisoxazole is safe except in last days of pregnancy (can lead to kernicterus).

Medications for Cystitis that are usually avoided during pregnancy include:
- Trimethoprim-sulfamethoxazole in the first trimester & at term
- Aminoglycosides
- Fluoroquinolones
- Doxycycline.

24. HEMATOLOGY – ESSENTIAL THROMBOCYTHEMIA/THROMBOCYTOSIS [ET] [FOUNDATIONAL CONCEPTS]

~50% of patients with Essential thrombocythemia/thrombocytosis [ET] have a mutation of the JAK2 gene [choice E] in their blood-forming cells, which is the most common mutation associated with ET.

This mutation leads to hyperactive JAK (Janus kinase) signaling of bone marrow hematopoietic stem cells, causing the body to make increased number of myeloid cells. Homozygous JAK2 mutations present with more severe complications, such as a greater incidence of thrombotic events.

The 3 main diver mutations for ET include:
- JAK 2: ~50%
- CALR : 23.5% of cases [choice A]
- MPL: up 5% of cases [choice C]

ET is an uncommon indolent myeloproliferative neoplasm due to an isolated elevation of platelets and proliferation of enlarged, mature megakaryocytes with hyperloculated nuclei on bone marrow biopsy.

Choice B [BCR-ABL] fusion gene occurs due to a translocation between chromosomes 9 and 22, resulting in the Philadelphia chromosome, most commonly associated with Chronic myelogenous leukemia.
Choice D [t(15;17)] is associated with Acute myelogenous leukemia.

25. NEUROLOGY – CONCUSSION/MILD TRAUMATIC BRAIN INJURY [HEALTH MAINTENANCE]

For children and adolescents with Concussions, a brief period of physical and relative neurocognitive rest lasting 24 to 48 hours [choice B] is recommended, followed by a gradual and progressive return to non-contact, supervised, aerobic activity individualized to prevent symptom exacerbation until full recovery.
Cognitive and physical relative rest are the primary initial interventions for concussion.

Prior to returning to full participation in sports, athletes recovered from a Concussion should complete a course of non-contact exercise challenges of gradually increasing intensity and should not return until full resolution of symptoms off medication.

This approach is preferred rather than strict physical rest [choice A]

26. HEMATOLOGY – ALPHA THALASSEMIA TRAIT [MOST LIKELY]
Alpha thalassemia trait [choice D] should be suspected in patients with:
- **Mild or no anemia**
- **CBC: Microcytic hypochromic anemia (MCV 60-75) despite the mild anemia; occasional target cells**
- **Normal or increased red cell count; normal reticulocyte count**
- **Hemoglobin electrophoresis: normal ratios of Hb A, Hb A2, and HbF.**

Therefore, Alpha-thalassemia trait is usually diagnosed by exclusion or if genetic testing is performed.

Choice A [Hemochromatosis] usually presents in older adults >40 years of age and is associated with iron overload (increased serum ferritin).
Choice B [Beta thalassemia minor] presents similar to Alpha thalassemia minor and has similar CBC findings but is associated with increased Hb A2 and Hb F on electrophoresis.
Choice C [Alpha thalassemia intermedia/Hemoglobin H disease] is usually associated with symptoms from birth and by adulthood would have the stigmata of major Thalassemia (frontal bossing, chipmunk facies, hepatosplenomegaly). Hb H disease is associated with Hb H on peripheral smear disease.
Choice E [Iron deficiency anemia] is associated with decreased ferritin.

27. NEUROLOGY – ENCEPHALITIS [APPLYING FOUNDATIONAL CONCEPTS]
Herpes simplex virus (HSV) type 1 [choice D] is the most common viral cause of Encephalitis.
Temporal lobe involvement is strongly suggestive of Herpes simplex virus [HSV]-1.
Because of the brain parenchymal involvement, Encephalitis may present with focal neurological deficits (eg, cranial nerve palsies, hemiparesis), altered mental status, personality changes, and meningismus.
Early treatment for HSV encephalitis with IV Acyclovir is critical when it is suspected.

Choice A [*Neisseria meningitidis*] is associated with Viral meningitis. Although both are associated with the same CSF findings, the presence of focal deficits and temporal lobe enhancement makes Encephalitis the more likely diagnosis.
Choice B [*Streptococcus pneumoniae*] is associated with bacterial meningitis.
Choice C [Enterovirus] is associated with Viral meningitis. Although both are associated with the same CSF findings, the presence of focal deficits and temporal lobe enhancement makes Encephalitis the more likely diagnosis.
Choice E [*Cryptococcus neoformans*] is associated with

28. REPRODUCTIVE – MOLAR PREGNANCY [CLINICAL INTERVENTION]

Treatment of Hydatidiform molar (HM) pregnancy is surgical removal of the HM, which can be achieved by either Uterine evacuation [choice A] or in some cases by hysterectomy.

Uterine evacuation is comprised of mechanical dilation of the cervix, followed by suction aspiration (regardless of uterine size), and then sharp curettage to assure complete removal of molar tissue.

After surgical removal, serial human chorionic gonadotropin (hCG) levels are performed to confirm resolution of disease or to identify development of Gestational trophoblastic neoplasia (eg, invasive mole, choriocarcinoma).

The classic finding of a Complete mole on transvaginal Ultrasound is a central heterogeneous mass with numerous discrete anechoic spaces ("cluster of grapes", "snowstorm", or "honeycombed uterus").

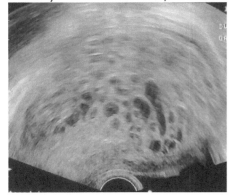

Choice B [Repeat ultrasound in 1 week] is inappropriate as surgical evacuation is essential.
Choice C [Administer Methotrexate] is not used in the initial management as treatment for Molar pregnancy is surgical not medical.
Choice D [Observation and serial B-hCG levels] is inappropriate as surgical evacuation is the most appropriate next step.
Choice E [Diagnostic laparoscopy] is not needed as surgical evacuation is the most appropriate next step.

29. CARDIOLOGY – TETRALOGY OF FALLOT [MOST LIKELY]

The classic finding of Tetralogy of Fallot (TOF) [choice C] is a "boot shaped" heart (upturned apex and a concave main pulmonary artery segment).

The echocardiogram is the diagnostic test of choice. Many patients are diagnosed prenatally (this patient did not seek prenatal care).

TOF is characterized by:
- [1] Large unrestricted ventricular septal defect (VSD)
- [2] RV outflow obstruction
- [3] RV hypertrophy
- [4] Overriding aorta.

Cyanosis is the most common presentation of TOF.

Choice A [Transposition of the great vessels] is associated with the "egg on a string" (cardiomegaly with a narrowed mediastinum) on chest radiographs.
Choice B [Atrial septal defect] is associated with pulmonary Hypertension on chest radiograph (prominent vascular markings, prominent hilum, with right atrial and ventricular enlargement).

Choice D [Coarctation of the aorta] is associated with the reverse 3 sign and rib notching on chest radiographs.

Choice E [Hypoplastic left heart syndrome] is associated with cardiomegaly and increased pulmonary vasculature on chest radiographs.

30. CARDIOLOGY – JUNCTIONAL ESCAPE RHYTHM/BRADYCARDIA [HEALTH MAINTENANCE]

Otherwise, healthy individuals who have junctional rhythms and are asymptomatic need no medical management [choice B] as the rhythm is usually a result of their increased vagal tone suppressing the SA node intrinsic automaticity.

A junctional escape rhythm occurs when the electrical activity of the SA node is blocked or is less than the automaticity of the AV node/His bundle (junction) and the junction assumes pacemaking responsibility.

Junctional escape rhythms are characterized by:
- Bradycardia, typically with a rate of 40 to 60 bpm.
- The QRS complex is narrow, <120 ms.
- P waves are absent before the QRS complex (occur simultaneously with the QRS complex), retrograde (inverted), very slow, or unrelated to the QRS complex.

Junctional Rhythm (Escape Rhythm)

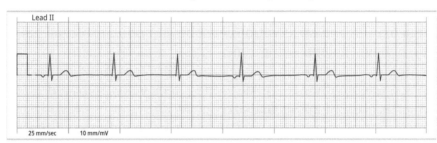

Classification of Junctional rhythm is determined by the heart rate:
- Junctional bradycardia: rate <40 beats per minute
- Junction escape rhythm: rate 40 to 60 beats per minute
- Accelerated junctional rhythm: rate of 60 to 100 beats per minute
- Junctional tachycardia: rate >100 beats per minute

Choice A [Atropine] is the first line management of symptomatic or unstable bradycardia.

Choice C [Transcutaneous pacing] and Choice D [Epinephrine] are options for symptomatic or unstable bradycardia unresponsive to Atropine.

Choice E [Permanent pacemaker placement] is definitive management of symptomatic or unstable bradycardia in which an inciting cause is not found or cannot be corrected.

31. PULMONARY – TUBERCULOSIS [PHARMACOLOGY]

Optic neuropathy (including optic neuritis and retrobulbar neuritis) is a rare but classic adverse effect of Ethambutol [choice A] and is often bilateral.

The toxic optic neuropathy is believed to result from the drug's metal-chelating effects, resulting in mitochondrial toxicity.

The development of Ethambutol optic neuropathy may be delayed, and vision loss is often reversible, improving over months after cessation of therapy.

Choice B [Rifampin] is associated with flu-like symptoms, thrombocytopenia, and orange-colored secretions.
Choice C [Streptomycin] and other Aminoglycosides are associated with nephrotoxicity and ototoxicity.
Choice D [Isoniazid] is associated with drug-induced Lupus, neuropathy (often prevented with coadministration of Pyridoxine/Vitamin B6), and hepatitis.
Choice E [Pyrazinamide] is associated with hepatitis, hyperuricemia, photosensitive skin rashes, GI symptoms, and arthritis.

32. PULMONARY – PNEUMOTHORAX [CLINICAL INTERVENTION]
Prompt drainage with a chest tube or catheter (eg, pigtail catheter) thoracostomy [choice D] is the first line management of a large Secondary spontaneous Pneumothorax (SSP) [≥2 cm from the pleural line to the chest wall at the apex).
Patients are often hospitalized to due to the increased risk for respiratory deterioration.
Secondary spontaneous Pneumothorax occurs in patients with underlying lung disease (the patient has a history of Asthma).

Chest tube or catheter (eg, pigtail catheter) thoracostomy is generally preferred over simple aspiration for drainage of air [choice C] in patients with SSP because thoracostomy is more likely to be successful.

Choice A [Supplemental oxygen and observation] may be an option for small SSP or patients who are asymptomatic or have minimal symptoms.
Choice B [Needle decompression followed by chest tube thoracostomy] is used in the management of a Tension pneumothorax (eg, distended neck veins, hypotension, tracheal deviation), none of which is present in this patient.
Choice E [Video-assisted thoracoscopic surgery (VATS)] may be indicated if there is persistent leak after chest tube placement or no regression with chest tube, as well as persistent or recurrent pneumothoracies.

33. ENDOCRINOLOGY – GRAVES' DISEASE [APPLYING FOUNDATIONAL CONCEPTS]
Graves' disease, the most common cause of Hyperthyroidism in the US, is caused by autoantibodies to the thyrotropin receptor (TRAb) [choice E] that stimulate the receptor, thereby promoting thyroid hormone synthesis and secretion and thyroid growth (causing a diffuse goiter).
Therefore, these antibodies are also known as Thyroid stimulating immunoglobulins [TSIs].
The presence of TRAb in the serum and thyroid eye disease (due to TRAb effect on the orbital muscle tissue) distinguishes Graves' disease from other causes of hyperthyroidism.

Thyroid peroxidase antibodies (TPOAb) [choice B] are suggestive of Hashimoto's disease, the most common cause of Hypothyroidism in the US.
Thyroglobulin antibodies (TgAb) [choice C] are suggestive of Hashimoto's disease, the most common cause of Hypothyroidism in the US.
TSH receptor blocking [choice D] antibodies would lead to Hypothyroidism.

34. ENDOCRINOLOGY – ADRENAL (ADDISONIAN) CRISIS [CLINICAL INTERVENTION]

IV isotonic fluid infusion (eg, 0.9% normal saline or 5% dextrose in 0.9% normal saline) and parenteral glucocorticoid therapy (eg, IV Hydrocortisone) [choice C] is the first line management of Adrenal crisis.

Hydrocortisone is often the preferred parenteral glucocorticoid due its dual glucocorticoid and mineralocorticoid activity.

Adrenal crisis is a severe form of Acute adrenal insufficiency and should be considered in any patient with shock.

35. EENT – KERATITIS [CLINICAL INTERVENTION]

Treatment of Infectious keratitis requires urgent ophthalmological referral [choice D] and prompt initiation of topical bactericidal antibiotics (optimally after obtaining cultures).

Antibiotic preparations for Bacterial keratitis used for Bacterial keratitis are often fortified.

Choice A [Initiate ophthalmic Prednisolone] should be left to the ophthalmologist to decide to administer, as the role of topical glucocorticoid use is controversial in Bacteria keratitis.

Choice B [Apply an eye patch to the right eye for comfort] should not be performed with suspected Pseudomonal keratitis in a contact lens wearer as it may cause the condition to progress rapidly.

Choice C [Irrigate the eye with Lactated ringers or normal saline] is used in the management of Chemical injuries to the eye.

Choice E [Initiate Moxifloxacin, discharge the patient, and inform the patient to use glasses until the symptoms resolve] is incorrect as it does not include immediate referral to the ophthalmologist.

36. EENT – ACUTE OTITIS MEDIA [PHARMACOLOGY]

High-dose Amoxicillin (80-90 mg/kg/day) [choice A] is the first line agent for uncomplicated Acute otitis media. Infants <6 months are at increased risk of severe infection, complications, or recurrence.

Amoxicillin has activity against the most common bacterial otopathogens: *Streptococcus pneumoniae*, nontypeable *Haemophilus influenzae*, and *Moraxella catarrhalis*.

Choice B [Observation with a scheduled follow up appointment in 48-72 hours] may be used in children with milder AOM.

Choice C [High-dose amoxicillin with clavulanate] can be used in patients not responsive to Amoxicillin or in AOM at increased risk for beta-lactamase-producing nontypeable *Haemophilus influenzae.*

Choice D [Tympanocentesis with culture] may be used to establish the etiologic diagnosis in children who appears toxic, is immunocompromised, or has failed previous courses of antibiotic therapy.

Choice E [Cefdinir] is an alternative to Acute otitis media in patients with mild non-IgE-mediated reaction to Penicillin.

37. EENT – ALLERGIC RHINITIS [APPLYING FOUNDATIONAL CONCEPTS]

Common indoor allergens [choice B] associated with Allergic rhinitis include house dust mites, cockroaches, allergens from household pets with fur, rodents, and fungi if recurring.

Common outdoor allergens associated with seasonal Allergic rhinitis include tree, grass, and weed pollens, as well as outdoor molds.

The nasal mucosa in patients with allergic rhinitis classically appears edematous and pale or bluish. Cobblestone when present is also hallmark of Allergic rhinitis.

The nasal mucosa in patients with nonallergic rhinitis is usually normal in color.
The nasal mucosa in Acute viral rhinosinusitis [choice A] or rhinitis medicamentosa is usually beefy red.

38. PSYCHIATRY/BEHAVIORAL SCIENCE – COCAINE USE DISORDER [HISTORY AND PHYSICAL]
Hallmarks of Cocaine use disorder [choice B] include:
- **Psychomotor: agitation, paranoia, unexplained weight loss, mood changes, seizures**
- **Examination findings (CNS activation): Hypertension, tachycardia, tremors, and dilated pupils that are reactive.**

Cocaine is a stimulate that activates alpha-1, alpha-2, beta-1, and beta-2 adrenergic receptors through increased levels of norepinephrine.

Choice A [Alcohol withdrawal syndrome] is an acute event that may result in similar symptoms. The patient's chronicity of symptoms suggests Cocaine use disorder.
Choice C [Bipolar disorder with manic episode] can present with paranoia but is not classically associated with the abnormal vital signs (hypertension, tachycardia), dilated pupils, and tremors.
Choice D [Phencyclidine intoxication] is also associated with altered mental status, psychomotor agitation, hypertension, and tachycardia, but is often associated with multidirectional nystagmus (horizontal, vertical, or rotatory nystagmus), which is not present in this patient.
Choice E [Heroin withdrawal] can also present with mydriasis, but is also associated with GI symptoms, excessive tearing, and piloerections without the psychotic features.

39. REPRODUCTIVE SYSTEM – CERVICAL INSUFFICIENCY [CLINICAL INTERVENTION]
A history-indicated cerclage [choice B] at 12 to 14 weeks of gestation is recommended in patients with recurrent (>1) second-trimester pregnancy losses or extremely preterm births (<28 weeks) preceded by painless cervical dilatation.
Cerclage provides structural support for weakness of the cervix.
At 16 weeks of gestation, daily vaginal Progesterone supplementation [choice D] may also be indicated for all patients with a history-indicated cerclage continued until 36+6 weeks of gestation.

40. MUSCULOSKELETAL – ANKYLOSING SPONDYLITIS [HISTORY AND PHYSICAL]
Anterior uveitis [choice A] is the most common extraarticular manifestation of Ankylosing spondylitis (AS), occurring in 20-30% of patients with AS.
Uveitis classically presents as acute unilateral pain, photophobia, and blurring of vision, and may be the first presenting manifestation.

Extraarticular manifestations of AS include:
- Anterior uveitis: 25-35%
- Aortic regurgitation (insufficiency) [choice B] 6-10%
- Inflammatory bowel disease [choice D] 5-10%
- Psoriasis [choice E] 10-25%

- Renal abnormalities 10-30%
- Osteoporosis [choice C] 11-18%.

41. RENAL – RHABDOMYOLYSIS [CLINICAL INTERVENTION]
Early and aggressive fluid resuscitation with isotonic crystalloid fluids, such as 0.9% saline [choice C], is the mainstay of treatment of Rhabdomyolysis.
IV crystalloid maintains or enhances kidney perfusion, thereby minimizing ischemic injury, increases the urine flow rate, and promotes urinary dilation, which will limit intratubular cast formation and increase excretion of the nephrotoxic myoglobin and heme pigments.

Choice A [Emergent hemodialysis] is not routinely used to remove myoglobin, hemoglobin, or uric acid.
Choice B [Infusion of Sodium bicarbonate] for urinary alkalinization can be an adjunct to crystalloid fluids in select patients after an appropriate diuresis occurs with Isotonic saline administration.
Choice D [Intravenous Furosemide] does not prevent AKI in patients with Rhabdomyolysis and can worsen hypocalcemia, increasing cast formation.
Choice E [Infusion of 0.45% saline with 5% dextrose] and other hypotonic fluids are not usually used in the management of Rhabdomyolysis.

42. REPRODUCTIVE SYSTEM – FIBROADENOMA [MOST LIKELY]
Fibroadenomas [choice D] are the most common benign tumor in the breast, accounting for >50% all breast biopsies.
A classic Fibroadenoma is a round or ovoid, rubbery, discrete, relatively movable, nontender mass 1–5 cm.

Choice A [Fibrocystic changes] is often bilateral, associated with waxing and waning in size in response to menstruation.
Choice B [Intraductal papilloma] are not as common as fibroadenomas. Nipple discharge, especially bloody nipple discharge, is a frequent clinical presentation.
Choice C [Infiltrative ductal carcinoma] classically presents with a breast mass and axillary lymphadenopathy.
Choice E [Galactocele] presents as soft cystic masses on physical examination.

43. INFECTIOUS DISEASE – ASCARIASIS [APPLYING FOUNDATIONAL CONCEPTS]
During the larval migratory phase of Ascariasis (active migration to the lungs), an acute transient Eosinophilic pneumonitis [choice C], known as Loeffler's syndrome, may develop, characterized by fever, cough, wheeze (hypersensitivity) and marked eosinophilia.
In the adult stage, under the stress of anesthesia, erratic migration of the worms, especially into upper airway and life-threatening complications like airway obstruction during or after extubation, or migration into endotracheal tube may occur as anesthesia causes the worm to become hypermobile.
Therefore, in patients with Ascariasis, deworming patients presenting for surgery with high eosinophil counts is important.

44. CARDIOLOGY – ENDOCARDITIS/MRSA [PHARMACOLOGY]
Empiric regimen for suspected Native valve endocarditis includes:

- **Vancomycin [choice C] for coverage of Methicillin resistant *Staphylococcus aureus* (especially in IV drug users), streptococci, and enterococci**
- **Ceftriaxone** for gram-negative and gram-positive coverage.

Vancomycin is preferred over Daptomycin-based regimen for MRSA coverage in Endocarditis.

Choice A [Penicillin G plus Gentamicin] is incorrect because Penicillin G does not have MRSA coverage.

Choice B [Amphotericin B] may be indicated as adjunctive therapy to empiric antibiotics if a fungal cause is suspected.

Choice D [Nafcillin] has excellent coverage of Methicillin-sensitive *S. aureus* (MSSA) but does not cover MRSA.

Choice E [Clindamycin] has excellent MRSA coverage for soft tissue infections, but Vancomycin has more effective MRSA coverage in Endocarditis.

45. RENAL – POSTINFECTIOUS GLOMERULONEPHRITIS – HISTORY AND PHYSICAL EXAMINATION

Postinfectious glomerulonephritis is associated with an antecedent history of a GAS skin or throat infection, such as Impetigo [choice D] or Streptococcal pharyngitis.

The latent period between GAS infection and PSGN is between one- and three-weeks following GAS pharyngitis and between three- and six-weeks following GAS skin infection.

Key features of Glomerulonephritis include red to brown urine (hematuria), proteinuria (which can reach the nephrotic range), edema, hypertension, and an elevation in serum creatinine.

Choice A [Diarrheal illness] may precede Hemolytic uremic syndrome in children.

Choice B [Protracted vomiting] may result in Prerenal azotemia.

Choice C [Recent Antibiotic use] may result in Acute tubular necrosis or Acute interstitial nephritis, depending on the antibiotic used.

Choice E [Recent allergies] may precede Minimal change disease, the most common cause of Nephrotic syndrome in children.

46. DERMATOLOGY – TOXIC EPIDERMAL NECROLYSIS (TENS) [MOST LIKELY]

Toxic epidermal necrolysis (TENS) [choice E] involves >30% of the total body surface area [entire trunk (18) + and both arms in their entirety (18) – 36%] **and is characterized by:**

- <u>**prodrome of fever and influenza-like symptoms**</u> 1-3 days before the development of mucocutaneous and skin lesions.
- <u>cutaneous lesions</u>: ill-defined, coalescing, erythematous macules with **atypical target lesions (flat).**
- <u>positive Nikolsky sign</u>: **vesicles and bullae form, and within days the skin begins to slough.**
- <u>mucosal involvement</u> seen in >90% following the skin lesions.

Medications are the most common trigger for Stevens Johnson syndrome (SJS) and TEN, such as Allopurinol (which this patient takes), anticonvulsants, & antibacterial sulfonamides.

If the involved skin is <10% of the total body surface area, it is referred to as Stevens Johnson syndrome.

Choice A [Bullous pemphigoid] is characterized by deep-seated bullae that do not rupture easy and a negative Nikolsky sign.

Choice B [Erythema multiforme major] is associated with raised target lesions (circular papules and plaques with three distinct rings) and negative Nikolsky sign.

Choice D [Staphylococcal scalded skin syndrome] is characterized by painful erythema, extensive peeling, and erosions without mucous membrane involvement.

47. RENAL – OBSTRUCTIVE UROPATHY – [CLINICAL INTERVENTION]

Foley catheter placement [choice B] can be used to relieve the obstruction of Obstructive uropathy (acute urinary obstruction) due to Benign prostatic hypertrophy, a common cause of urinary obstruction.

Patients with acute obstructive uropathy will most likely regain normal renal function after removing the obstruction. If the obstruction is prolonged, permanent bladder and/or renal damage may occur. Obstructive uropathy care characterized by an elevated postvoid residual and hydronephrosis [hypoechoic fluid accumulation (urine) that displaces the echogenic renal sinus fat in a branching pattern].

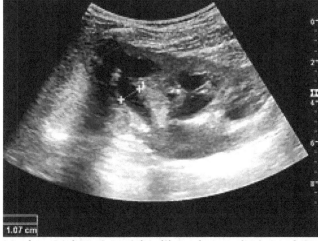

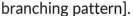

Hydronephrosis with dilated anechoic pelvis and calyces, along with cortical atrophy. The width of a calyx is measured on the US image in the longitudinal scan plane and illustrated by '+' and a dashed line.

Choice A [Suprapubic catheterization] may be used if there is a contraindication for performing Foley catheter.

Choice C [IV Normal saline] is used in the management of Prerenal azotemia and Acute tubular necrosis.

Choice D [Initiate Finasteride] is used in the long-term management of BPH to reduce the size of the prostate but takes 6-12 months to take full effect.

Choice E [Emergent hemodialysis] is not the management of Obstructive uropathy.

48. REPRODUCTIVE SYSTEM – MULTIPLE GESTATION [APPLYING FOUNDATIONAL CONCEPTS]

Although Ultrasound is needed to establish the diagnosis of multiple gestation, it may be suggested based on elevated levels of beta-hCG & maternal serum alpha-fetoprotein higher than normal [choice B].

Routine ultrasound examination in the first or early second trimester is the best method to ensure early diagnosis of a twin pregnancy, establish an accurate gestational age, and determine amnionicity and chorionicity.

49. PROFESSIONAL PRACTICE/PSYCHIATRY/BEHAVIORAL SCIENCE – ELDER ABUSE [CLINICAL INTERVENTION]

If a health care worker has reason to believe that an older adult is in a state of elder abuse or self-neglect, appropriate medical interventions should be offered, and reporting should be promptly initiated [choice B].

Adult Protective Services (APS) and Long-Term Care Ombudsman programs (LTCOP) exist in all United States jurisdictions. If there is doubt about where and how to report, one of these agencies or law enforcement can provide the needed information regarding how to report suspected elder abuse or self-neglect.

Reporting of elder abuse or self-neglect is said to be an effective and important intervention in the management of elder abuse.

Elder abuse including may include physical abuse, sexual abuse, neglect, emotional or psychological abuse, abandonment, and financial or material exploitation.

Unlike child abuse, interventions cannot be made against the abused person's wishes. Adults have the right to refuse intervention even if that means returning to a dangerous situation. neglect but adult protective services should still be informed.

The son cannot be called to discuss the patient's situation without the patient's expressed permission to do so.

50. CARDIOLOGY – AMYLOIDOSIS [MOST LIKELY]

Amyloidosis [choice E] is the most common cause of Restrictive cardiomyopathy (RCM).

The 3 leading causes of RCM, [1] cardiac Amyloidosis, [2] Sarcoidosis, & [3] Hemochromatosis, lead to a build-up of a substance (amyloid fibril deposition, granulomas, & iron respectively) in the myocardium, making the ventricles stiff (decreased compliance & diastolic dysfunction).

The classic findings of RCM on echocardiogram include diastolic dysfunction and biatrial enlargement.

The myocardium may have a granular (speckled) appearance) with Cardiac amyloid.

Choice A [Previous treatment with Doxorubicin] is a cause of Dilated cardiomyopathy, which is associated with systolic dysfunction on echocardiogram.

Choice B [Autosomal dominant mutation of genes that encode for cardiac cell sarcomere proteins] is the cause of Hypertrophic cardiomyopathy, which is associated with diastolic dysfunction and asymmetric septal hypertrophy on echocardiogram.

Choice C [Coxsackie virus infection] is a cause of Dilated cardiomyopathy, which is associated with systolic dysfunction on echocardiogram.

Choice D [Chronic inflammation of the pericardium] is associated with Constrictive pericarditis, which is associated with pericardial thickening &/or calcification on echocardiogram.

51. DERMATOLOGY – PSORIASIS [HISTORY AND PHYSICAL]

Nail changes associated with Psoriasis include:
- **pitting of the nails [choice B],** leukonychia, and crumbling of the nail plate.
- **circular tan-brown discoloration ("oil drop sign").**

Choice A [Concave shaped nails] describes spooning of the nails (koilonychia) seen with Iron deficiency anemia.

Choice C [Banded longitudinal brown to black pigmentation of the nail] may be a normal finding in patients with darker skin complexions.

Choice D (convex curving of the nails) describes clubbing, which can be associated with chronic pulmonary diseases.

Choice E [Transverse grooves of the nail plate], also known as Beau's lines, may be seen with Kawasaki disease.

52. CARDIOLOGY – STATINS [PHARMACOLOGY]
Myopathy (eg, myalgia) [choice B] is the most common significant adverse effect of Statins (up 10% patients experience myopathy).

Myositis (increased creatine kinase) and Rhabdomyolysis (rare) may also occur, especially with concomitant use Fibrates or Niacin.

Rosuvastatin & Pravastatin are safest in patients with history of Myopathy once symptoms resolve.

In patients who develop muscle adverse effects on Pravastatin or Fluvastatin, decrease the dose.

53. GASTROINTESTINAL AND NUTRITION – GASTROESOPHAGEAL REFLUX DISEASE [CLINICAL INTERVENTION]
Proton pump inhibitors such as Pantoprazole [choice E] are the first-line medical treatment for patients with classic symptoms of Gastroesophageal reflux disease (heartburn &/or reflux) that is persistent (≥2 times weekly) without alarm symptoms.

In addition, lifestyle and dietary modification is the backbone of therapy for both classic intermittent and persistent GERD (eg, weight loss, elevation of the head of the bed, reduction of triggers, etc.).

Choice A [Upper GI series (Barium esophagram)] is used to evaluate for esophageal motility disorders, which classically presents with chest pain and dysphagia to solids &/or liquids.

Choice B [Ambulatory 24-hour pH monitoring] is the criterion standard test for the diagnosis of GERD in patients with persistent symptoms (typical or atypical), especially if a trial of twice-daily PPI therapy has failed. It can also be used to determine the effectiveness of treatment for patients with persistent symptoms.

Choice C [Upper endoscopy] is used to assess for complications of GERD (eg, esophagitis, Barret's, Esophageal adenocarcinoma, stricture) in patients with alarm symptoms — dysphagia, odynophagia, recurrent vomiting, weight loss, hematemesis, anemia, melena, or increased age).

Choice D [Famotidine] or other Histamine 2 receptor antagonist can be used for Intermittent classic GERD (<2 times weekly).

54. PULMONARY – LEGIONELLA PNEUMONIA [PHARMACOLOGY]
Azithromycin [choice C] and Levofloxacin are the preferred initial empiric agents for the management of Legionella pneumonia.

They are effective at infiltrating lung tissue, achieve excellent intracellular concentrations, and are bactericidal.

Legionella infection should be suspected in patients with:

- <u>gastrointestinal symptoms</u> eg, nausea, vomiting, and diarrhea
- CNS symptoms
- Hyponatremia
- elevated hepatic transaminases

Because Legionella is spread via contaminated water sources, outbreaks may occur in large facilities (eg, cruise ships, hospitals, hotels [as in this patient], or apartment buildings.

Choice A [Ceftriaxone], Choice B [Piperacillin/tazobactam], Choice D [Amoxicillin], and other beta lactams are not used in the management of Legionella infections.
Choice E [Vancomycin] can be added if MRSA is the suspected organism.

55. GASTROINTESTINAL AND NUTRITION – CROHN DISEASE [MOST LIKELY]
The classic findings of Crohn disease [choice D] include:
<u>Histology:</u>
- **transmural inflammation, resulting in strictures**
- **granulomas**
<u>Colonoscopy:</u>
- **<u>cobblestone appearance</u>**: focal ulcerations and adjacent to areas of normal appearing mucosa along with nodular mucosal change
- **<u>skip areas</u>** of involvement with segments of normal-appearing bowel interrupted by large areas of disease.
- normal appearing rectal mucosa (eg, rectal sparing) is common.

Choice A [Celiac disease] is associated with increased intraepithelial lymphocytes, atrophic mucosa with loss of villi, enhanced epithelial apoptosis, and crypt hyperplasia on endoscopy.
Choice B [Irritable bowel syndrome] is a diagnosis of exclusion in patients with normal labs and normal bowel imaging.
Choice C [Ulcerative colitis] is associated with engorgement of the mucosa, giving it an erythematous friable appearance on colonoscopy. Histology findings include crypt abscesses and increased lamina propria cellularity.
Choice E [Somatic symptom disorder] is not associated with findings on workup.

56. NEUROLOGY – TRANSIENT ISCHEMIC ATTACK [LABS AND DIAGNOSTIC STUDIES]
Noninvasive imaging of the carotid arteries (or vertebral arteries for patients with posterior circulation symptoms) with angiography [eg, CTA (choice D) or MRA can be used to establish an arterial source of the embolism or low flow in patients with suspected TIA.
2/3 of all ischemic strokes and TIAs are due to carotid artery disease.
Selected patients found to have symptomatic cervical internal carotid artery stenosis of 50-99% with a life expectancy of at least 5 years are generally treated with revascularization via carotid endarterectomy or carotid artery stenting.

Choice B [Tonometry] is useful for assessing for Glaucoma by measuring the intraocular pressure.
Choice A [Echocardiogram], Choice C [24-hour Holter monitor], and choice E [Electrophysiology study] can be used to assess for a possible cardiac source in patients with TIA or ischemic stroke caused by embolism.

57. MUSCULOSKELETAL – ANKLE SPRAINS [CLINICAL INTERVENTION]

The management of Grade II Ankle sprains include RICE, NSAIDs, and ankle support (eg, elastic wrap + air cast, ankle brace, or similar splint [choice E] for up to a few weeks.

Ankle support in patients with mild or moderate sprains should not interfere with early rehabilitation.

The patient's history and physical examination is consistent with grade 2 Ankle sprain (incomplete tear), characterized by moderate pain, swelling, tenderness, and ecchymosis with mild to moderate joint instability as well some loss of range and function. Weightbearing is often painful for these patients.

Choice A [Nonweightbearing short leg cast] may be used in some patients with a Grade III Ankle sprain.

Choice B [Rest, observation, and follow up in 10 days] is usually insufficient for Grade II Ankle sprains since it is associated with an incomplete tear.

Choice C [Referral to an orthopedic surgeon] may be indicated for severe medial ankle sprain involving a full rupture of both the superficial and deep deltoid ligament, which is rare.

Choice D [Elastic wrap (eg, ACE bandage) or compression sleeve for a few days] may be used in mild (grade I) lateral or medial Ankle sprains.

58. NEUROLOGY – MENINGIOMA [MOST LIKELY]

On non-contrast head CT, Meningiomas [choice B] appear as hyperdense or isodense lesions attached to the dura as they form along the dura mater. The dura mater is one of the three layers that form the meninges.

Brain MRI with contrast is the best neuroimaging to detect a Meningioma.

Meningioma is a benign central nervous system tumor commonly arising from the meninges of the brain and spinal cord.

Most meningiomas are sporadic, benign, and slowly growing.

Choice A [Glioblastoma multiforme] is characterized by heterogeneous masses centered in the white matter with irregular peripheral enhancement, central necrosis, and surrounding vasogenic edema.

Choice C [Ependymoma] involves the fourth ventricle and most commonly occurs in children.

Choice D [Oligodendroglioma] is characterized by masses with calcifications on CT scan, which are neither sensitive nor specific.

Choice E [Hemangioma] is characterized by large inhomogeneous masses.

59. REPRODUCTIVE SYSTEM – CERVICAL CANCER SCREENING [HEALTH MAINTENANCE]

In women ≥25 years of age with Atypical squamous cells of undetermined significance (ASCUS) management includes:
- **(1) Reflex HPV testing (preferred) [choice B]**
- (2) Pap test in 1 year (acceptable alternative) [choice A]

Atypical squamous cells of undetermined significance (ASCUS) is the most common abnormal Pap test result.

It is characterized by atypical cells that demonstrate reactive changes but do not meet cytologic criteria for premalignant disease.

Choice C [Colposcopy] is performed in women ≥25 years of age with ASCUS who are HPV positive after reflex HPV testing.

Choice D [Perform Pap smear with HPV cotesting in 3 years] is used in the evaluation of ASCUS in women ≥25 years of age with ASCUS who are HPV negative after reflex HPV testing.

60. PULMONARY – ACUTE BRONCHITIS [HEALTH MAINTENANCE]

The mainstay of treatment of Acute bronchitis is patient education and symptoms control (eg, throat lozenges, hot tea, and smoking cessation or avoidance of secondhand smoke) [choice C].

Over the counter cough medications, such as Dextromethorphan or Guaifenesin can be added if additional cough relief is needed.

For most patients, Acute bronchitis is usually due to a viral respiratory infection, is self-limited, and often resolves in one to three weeks without therapy.

Testing for COVID-19 and Influenza are often performed in all patients presenting with respiratory tract infection symptoms when appropriate.

Treating with empiric antibiotic therapy [choices B, D, and E] are not recommended for Acute bronchitis in most cases as it is one of the main causes of inappropriate antibiotic overuse. This patient has a negative chest radiograph, so bacterial Pneumonia is unlikely.

61. CARDIOLOGY – MITRAL VALVE PROLAPSE [HEALTH MAINTENANCE]

In asymptomatic patients with Mitral valve prolapse (MVP), no intervention is needed besides reassuring the patient of the benign nature of the disease with a low risk of complications [choice D].

Depending on the severity of MVP, regular follow-up visits to assess for complications in conjunction with echocardiograms can be used to monitor patients with MVP.

The classic finding of MVP is a systolic ejection click that may be heard earlier with maneuvers that decrease LV volume (eg, Valsalva, standing).

Noncardiac findings may include skeletal changes (eg, pectus excavatum, narrow AP diameter, scoliosis).

Choice A [Prophylaxis for thromboembolism when undergoing surgical procedures] is not required in patients with MVP without a prior thromboembolic event.

Choice B [Prophylaxis for endocarditis if undergoing dental and respiratory procedures] is no longer recommended for patients with MVP.

Choice C [Metoprolol] and other Beta blockers may be used in select patients with autonomic dysfunction (eg, MVP syndrome with atypical chest pain, dyspnea, palpitations, tachyarrhythmias). This patient is asymptomatic.

Choice E [Mitral valve repair] can be used for severe MVP associated with Mitral regurgitation or severe symptomatic MVP.

62. CARDIOLOGY – UNSTABLE ANGINA [PHARMACOLOGY]

Early antiplatelet therapy with a loading dose of 325 mg of nonenteric coated Aspirin [choice D], chewed or crushed for faster absorption, should be administered in most patients presenting with Acute coronary syndrome.

Aspirin is a first line antiplatelet agent in ACS which significantly lowers the risk of serious cardiovascular events and also reduces mortality in Acute ST elevation MI.

Unstable angina should be suspected in patients with chest pain >30 minutes, new in onset, or worsening + ECG evidence of ischemia without infarction (eg, ST depressions, T wave inversions, &/or flattened T waves without ST elevation).

Sublingual nitroglycerin is administered in patients with ischemic chest pain, followed by IV Nitroglycerin [choice A] in patients with persistent pain after three sublingual Nitroglycerin tablets, Hypertension, or Heart failure.
Choice B [Oral Metoprolol], Atenolol, or other Beta blockers can be given in patients without contraindications within 24 hours.
Choice D [IV Alteplase] and other fibrinolytic therapy are not used in Unstable angina and Non-ST elevation MI due to no evidence of benefit (and possible harm) of fibrinolytic therapy. Fibrinolytic therapy is an alternative to catheterization for reperfusion therapy in ST elevation MI (STEMI).
Choice E [IV Unfractionated Heparin] should also be initiated as soon as possible after the diagnosis but placing an IV to administer Heparin should not delay administering Aspirin orally.

63. INFECTIOUS DISEASES/PULMONARY – TUBERCULOSIS/MILIARY TB [LABS AND DIAGNOSTIC STUDIES]

In patients with imaging and clinical presentation suspicious of Tuberculosis (TB), 3 sputum specimens should be submitted for acid fast bacilli (AFB) smear [choice D], mycobacterial culture, and NAA testing (obtained via cough or induction) at least 8 hours apart and including at least one early-morning specimen.
The detection of Acid-fast bacilli (AFB) on microscopic examination of stained sputum smears is the most rapid and inexpensive tool to establish the diagnosis of TB.

Tuberculosis should be suspected in patients with
- cough >2 to 3 weeks' duration, lymphadenopathy, fevers, night sweats, weight loss) and associated epidemiologic factors (this patient lives in a crowded environment).
- Chest radiographs revealing lobar consolidation, pleural effusions (1/3 of patients), or small fibronodular lesions (Miliary TB). This patient has left-sided effusion with a Miliary pattern.

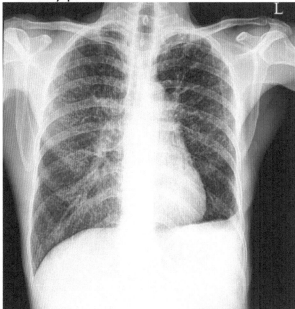

-

Choice A (Legionella urine antigen) classically presents with pulmonary symptoms, gastrointestinal symptoms (nausea, vomiting, diarrhea), CNS symptoms, Hyponatremia, and increased LFTs. It is transmitted via contaminated water sources, not from person to person.

Choice B [Direct Coombs test and Cold-agglutinin titers] is supportive of the diagnosis of *Mycoplasma pneumoniae.*

Choice C [Routine gram stain of sputum samples and sputum cultures] should be part of the routine workup but would not be able to detect *Mycobacterium.* Acid fast staining is required to identify TB.

Choice E (Bronchoscopy and bronchoalveolar lavage) is invasive and is usually reserved to establish the diagnosis of Tuberculosis in patients who unable to produce adequate amounts of sputum via either expectoration or induction of sputum.

64. CARDIOLOGY – VENTRICULAR FIBRILLATION [CLINICAL INTERVENTION]

Excellent cardiopulmonary resuscitation (CPR) and Rapid defibrillation (Unsynchronized cardioversion) [choice D] is the management of choice for Pulseless Ventricular tachycardia (VT) and Ventricular fibrillation (VF).

Pulseless VT and VF are the only 2 "shockable" non-perfusing rhythms. They both originate from the ventricles.

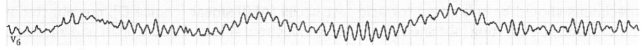

Photo credit:
Jer5150, CC BY-SA 3.0 <https://creativecommons.org/licenses/by-sa/3.0>, via Wikimedia Commons

Choice A [Synchronized cardioversion] is used to stabilize most unstable tachyarrythmias with a pulse.

Choice B [IV Amiodarone] can be used for most stable wide-complex tachycardias.

Choice C [IV Magnesium sulfate] is used in the management of Torsades de pointes.

Choice E [IV Epinephrine] is administered, along with CPR, in patients with Pulseless electrical activity and Asystole.

65. PSYCHIATRY/BEHAVIORAL SCIENCE – ANOREXIA NERVOSA [HISTORY AND PHYSICAL]

Classic findings associated with Anorexia nervosa include:
- **Bradycardia (pulse <60 beats per minute) [choice C]**
- Hypothermia (core temperature <35°C or 95°F)
- Hypotension (systolic blood pressure <90 mmHg and/or a diastolic blood pressure <50 mmHg)
- Hypoactive bowel sounds and bowel distention
- Xerosis (dry, scaly skin)
- Brittle hair and hair loss
- Lanugo hair growth
- Abdominal distention
- Proximal muscle weakness.

66. PSYCHIATRY/BEHAVIORAL SCIENCE – AUTISM SPECTRUM DISORDER [HISTORY AND PHYSICAL]

Features of Autism spectrum disorder include:
- **Insistence on sameness and routines; inflexible behavior, such as always eating particular foods in a specific order [choice D]**
- restricted, repetitive patterns of behavior, interests, or activities.
- patterns of special interest and leisure activities (eg, very specific and often mechanical interests such as ceiling fans)
- visual inspection of objects out of the corner of the eyes.

Autism spectrum disorder (ASD) is a group of neurodevelopmental disorder characterized by persistent deficits in social communication and social interaction, and repetitive, restricted patterns of behavior, interests, or activities.

Choice A [Short palpebral fissures, thin vermillion border, and smooth philtrum] are features of Fetal alcohol syndrome.

Choice B [Normal imaginative play] is often absent or impaired in children with ASD. They often engage in "scripted" play activities (eg, mimicking verbatim what has been seen on television or in other types of media).

Choice C [Exaggerated startle response] is a classic feature of Tay-Sachs disease.

Choice E [Macroorchidism] may occur in adolescents with Fragile X syndrome, which can also present with ASD, but is a feature seen in adolescents (after puberty), not young children.

67. INFECTIOUS DISEASE – ENTEROBIASIS/PINWORM [CLINICAL INTERVENTION]

Albendazole [choice B], Mebendazole, or Pyrantel pamoate are first line agents against Enterobiasis (Pinworm infection). A repeated dose is often given after 2 weeks.

Due to high rate of household transmission, concurrent treatment of the entire household is recommended.

Although most Pinworm infections are asymptomatic, perianal itching especially at night is the classic presentation.

Egg examination of cellophane tape or plastic paddle (coated with an adhesive surface) placed on the perianal skin helps to confirm the diagnosis.

Ivermectin [choice C] is not generally used to treat Pinworm infections although Ivermectin has efficacy against *E. vermicularis.*

68. INFECTIOUS DISEASE – RAMSAY-HUNT SYNDROME (HERPES ZOSTER OTICUS) [APPLYING FOUNDATIONAL CONCEPTS]

Ramsay-Hunt syndrome (Herpes zoster oticus) is reactivation of Varicella zoster virus in the geniculate ganglion [choice D] of the sensory branch of cranial nerve 7 (facial nerve) with or without subsequent spread to cranial nerve (CN) 8.

Ramsay-Hunt syndrome (Herpes zoster oticus) classically presents with the triad of:
- [1] ipsilateral facial paralysis (often more severe than Bell's palsy),
- [2] ear pain, and
- [3] vesicles in the auditory canal or on the auricle.

Other findings may include taste perception disturbances, tongue lesions, and hearing changes (decreased hearing, tinnitus, hyperacusis).

Choice A [Trigeminal] ganglion is associated with Herpes Zoster ophthalmicus.
Choice B [Pterygopalatine] ganglion is associated with facial nerve and innervates the lacrimal glands, mucous membrane glands of the nose, sinuses, and mouth.
Choice C [Otic] ganglion innervates the parotid gland for salivation and is associated with the parotid gland.
Choice E [Sphenopalatine] is a group of nerves linked to the trigeminal nerve.

69. MUSCULOSKELETAL – SEPTIC ARTHRITIS [APPLYING FOUNDATIONAL CONCEPTS]

Staphylococcus aureus **[choice B] is the most common cause of bacterial arthritis detected by culture in all age groups.**
S. aureus (including Methicillin-resistant S. aureus) is the most common cause of Septic arthritis in adults.
Other gram-positive organisms such as streptococci are also important potential causes of Septic arthritis.

Streptococcus pneumoniae [choice C] s responsible for a small percentage of cases of septic arthritis in adults.
Salmonella species [choice D] may cause bacterial arthritis in children with Sickle cell disease and related hemoglobinopathies.
Septic arthritis due to gram-negative bacilli [choices D and E] generally occurs in older adults, in patients with underlying immunosuppression, intravenous drug users or as a sequelae of trauma.

70. ENDOCRINOLOGY – PITUITARY ADENOMA/TSH SECRETING ADENOMA [HISTORY AND PHYSICAL EXAMINATION]

Pituitary tumors, such as TSH-secreting adenoma can lead to visual defects in 25-35%, including bitemporal hemianopia (hemianopsia) [choice A] when the pituitary lesions compress the optic chiasm.
A TSH-secreting pituitary adenoma should be suspected in
- hyperthyroid patients with diffuse goiter and no extrathyroidal manifestations of Graves' disease [choice C], who have
- **high serum free T4 and T3 concentrations and inappropriately unsuppressed (normal or high) serum TSH concentrations (both in the same direction),** especially in the presence of headache or clinical features of concomitant hypersecretion of other pituitary hormones: eg, symptoms of prolactinoma (this patient has galactorrhea) and acromegaly.

The thyroid appearance on ultrasound and radioiodine imaging is similar to that in Graves' disease (diffuse homogeneous enlargement, normal or high radioiodine uptake, increased color Doppler flow).

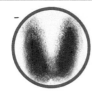

Normal   **Patient**

Choice B [Tenderness with palpation of the thyroid gland] occurs with infection of the thyroid gland (eg, Subacute/DeQuervain thyroiditis due to viral infection or Suppurative thyroiditis due to bacterial infection), radiation, or trauma to the thyroid gland.
Choice C [Bulging of the eyes with visualization of the upper sclera] is hallmark of Graves' disease, which can also present with diffuse increased uptake of RAIU scan but is associated with a primary hyperthyroid profile (eg, normal or decreased TSH, elevated serum free T4).
Choice D [Loss of the outer third of the eyebrows] and choice E [Delayed sluggish deep tendon reflexes] are hallmark of Hypothyroidism.

71. GASTROINTESTINAL AND NUTRITION – ACUTE CHOLECYSTITIS [MOST LIKELY]
Acute cholecystitis [choice C] should be suspected in patients with the classic triad:
- **[1] Fever** due to infection and inflammation
- **[2] Elevated white count** due to infection and inflammation
- **[3] RUQ pain that is continuous >4-6 hours.**

Acute calculous cholecystitis refers to inflammation of the gallbladder due to a stone blocking the cystic duct.

Choice A [Acute Hepatitis] can present similar with fever and RUQ pain but is associated with a lymphocytosis.
Choice B [Choledocholithiasis] is associated with jaundice and a cholestatic pattern (elevated alkaline phosphatase and GGT) with a normal white count and without fever.
Choice D Acute Cholangitis] is associated with Charcot triad: (1) fever/chills, (2) RUQ pain, and (3) jaundice. It is associated with a cholestatic pattern (elevated alkaline phosphatase and GGT) with a normal white count and without fever.
Choice E [Cholelithiasis] is associated with RUQ pain <4-6 hours, normal examination, and normal labs.

72. EENT – ORBITAL FLOOR FRACTURE [HISTORY AND PHYSICAL]
Diplopia, particularly with upward gaze [choice A] (due to entrapment of the inferior rectus muscles), and numbness below the eye (due to involvement of the infraorbital nerve) may occur with fractures of the orbital floor.
Orbital subcutaneous emphysema from air from the maxillary sinus — eyelid swelling that worsens especially after blowing the nose or with sneezing and periorbital ecchymosis are other common findings.

Choice B [Bilateral visual changes in the outer visual fields] characterizes bitemporal hemianopia, associated with lesions compressing the optic chiasm (eg, pituitary tumors).
Choice C [Visual changes consistent with a "curtain" over the eye] describes visual loss associated with Retinal detachment.
Choice D [Constriction of the visual field resulting in loss of peripheral vision] describes tunnel vision associated with Glaucoma.

Choice E [Central scotoma] is associated with Optic neuritis.

73. INFECTIOUS DISEASE – RABIES [HEALTH MAINTENANCE]
Postexposure prophylaxis for Rabies in unvaccinated individuals include both passive and active immunization with
- **Immunocompetent: Rabies immune globulin administered on day 0; HDCV or PCECV total of 4 doses: one dose (1 mL) IM on days 0, 3, 7, and 14 [choice B].**
- Immunocompromised: Rabies immune globulin administered on day 0; HDCV or PCECV total of 5 doses: one dose (1 mL) IM on days 0, 3, 7, 14, and 28 [choice C].

Previously vaccinated:
- HDCV or PCECV total of 5 doses: one dose (1 mL) on days 0 and 3 [choice E].

74. NEUROLOGY – TOURETTE SYNDROME [HISTORY AND PHYSICAL EXAMINATION]
Motor tics are the most common initial symptoms of Tourette syndrome, with blinking being the most common motor tic [choice A].
Tics may include:
- **Motor tics** usually involves the face, head or neck (eg, **blinking most common initial symptom**, facial grimacing, shrugging, head thrusting, sniffling)
- **Verbal or phonetic tics** eg, grunts, throat-clearing, sniffing, barking, moaning, coughing, obscene words (coprolalia), repetitive phrases, repeating the phrases of others (echolalia)
- **Self-mutilating tics** eg, Hair pulling, nail biting, biting of the lips etc.

75. HEMATOLOGY – MULTIPLE MYELOMA [LABS AND DIAGNOSTIC STUDIES]
Serum protein electrophoresis (SPEP) with immunofixation [choice D] is one of the initial tests for suspected Multiple myeloma to assess for a monoclonal (M) spike, most commonly IgG (60%).
Multiple myeloma should be suspected in older patients who present with "CRAB" symptoms due to end organ damage: **C**alcium elevations, **R**enal insufficiency, **A**nemia, and **B**one pain.
Not specific to Multiple myeloma, but the classic findings on CBC with peripheral smear is a normocytic normochromic anemia of chronic disease and Rouleaux formation (RBCs stacked like coins) due to hyperparaprotenemia.

The initial screen for suspected Multiple myeloma includes:
- Complete blood count
- Serum calcium and creatinine
- Serum protein electrophoresis (SPEP) with immunofixation
- Serum free light chain (FLC) assay to assess for Bence Jones proteins
- Quantitative immunoglobulins.

Cross-sectional imaging (CT, PET/CT, or MR) is also performed.

Choice A [Bone marrow aspiration] is indicated for definitive diagnosis if SPEP shows an M spike &/or Urine protein electrophoresis is positive for Bence Jones proteins.
Choice B [Genetic testing for JAK2 mutation] is useful if Polycythemia vera, Essential thrombocythemia, or Primary myelofibrosis are suspected.

Choice C [Nuclear bone scan] is not helpful for Multiple myeloma because the bone loss results in lytic lesions, which are not detected on a Nuclear bone scan. Radiographs may show punched out lytic lesions.

Choice E [Cross-sectional imaging with a CT scan] may be ordered based on abnormal results on SPEP &/or UPEP so it is not the best next step at this time.

76. RENAL – HYPOKALEMIA [MOST LIKELY]
The classic ECG findings of Hypokalemia [choice A] include depression of the ST segment, decrease in the amplitude of the T wave, and an increase in the amplitude of U waves which occur at the end of the T wave.

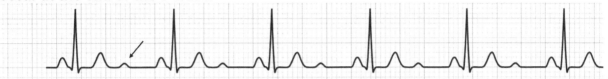

Hydrochlorothiazide can cause hypokalemia by indirectly stimulating renal K+ excretion via (1) increased distal Na and fluid delivery in the distal convoluted tubule resulting in physiological excretion of potassium, and (2) enhanced aldosterone secretion due to volume contraction, promoting potassium excretion.

Choice A [Hyperkalemia] is associated with peaked T waves and a sine wave pattern on ECG.
Choice C [Hypercalcemia] is associated with a shortened QT interval, which is not seen here. Thiazide diuretics can also cause Hypercalcemia.
Choice D [Hypocalcemia] is associated with a prolonged QT interval, which is not seen here.
Choice E [Hypomagnesemia] may result in prolonged QT interval, prolonged PR, QRS widening, atrial or ventricular fibrillation, ventricular tachycardia, and Torsades de pointes.

77. NEUROLOGY – SEROTONIN SYNDROME [PHARMACOLOGY]
**After discontinuing the offending agent, IV Benzodiazepines [choice B] are used for agitation to promote sedation as well as for correcting mild increases in heart rate and blood pressure.
Key features of Serotonin syndrome include:**
- <u>Autonomic instability</u>: eg, tachycardia and hypertension, hyperthermia, diaphoresis
- Agitation, dilated pupils
- <u>Neuromuscular hyperreactivity</u>: tremor, akathisia, deep tendon hyperreflexia, inducible or spontaneous clonus, muscle rigidity, , and. Neuromuscular findings are typically more pronounced in the lower extremities.

Choice A [Haloperidol] and choice C [Diphenhydramine] have anticholinergic properties, which may inhibit sweating, worsening the temperature.
Choice D [Quetiapine] is not the first line agent for the management of Serotonin syndrome.
Choice E [Dantrolene] can be used as adjunctive therapy for Neuroleptic malignant syndrome.

78. PSYCHIATRY/BEHAVIORAL SCIENCE – GENERALIZED ANXIETY DISORDER [MOST LIKELY]
In patients with Generalized anxiety disorder [choice D], excessive worry usually concerns day to day worries about multiple different aspects of life (physical symptoms, work, interpersonal, academics) for at least 6 months; they find it difficult to control the worry.
The anxiety is often associated with at least 3 of the following for at least 6 months:

- Difficulty controlling the worrying
- Restlessness, feeling keyed up or on edge; Being easily fatigued
- Difficulty in concentrating or mind going blank, irritability
- Muscle tension, Sleep disturbance, Irritability.

The anxiety results in significant distress or impairment in social and occupational areas and is not attributable to any physical cause or substance use.

Choice A [Somatic symptom disorder] are primarily worried about one or a few specific physical symptoms.

Choice B [Panic disorder] is associated with unexpected panic attacks that cause physical symptoms of sympathetic system activation during discrete episodes in addition to worry about future panic attacks.

Choice C [Major depressive disorder] share similar features but patients with GAD often worry about future events; patients with MDD often worry about past events.

Choice E [Obsessive-Compulsive disorder] is associated with intrusive thoughts that lead to compulsive behaviors to temporarily ease the thoughts that are time consuming.

79. RENAL – NEPHROTIC SYNDROME [LABS AND DIAGNOSTIC STUDIES]

Minimal change disease, characterized by fusion and effacement of podocytes [choice C] predominates as the cause of Nephrotic syndrome in individuals with hematologic malignancies, particularly Hodgkin lymphoma but also Non-Hodgkin lymphoma and Leukemia.

MCD in the setting of Hodgkin lymphoma may present with abrupt onset of massive proteinuria.

The patient has the classic Reed-Sternberg cell (multilobed or bilobed nuclei) on biopsy.

Choice A (Thickened glomerular basement membrane) is hallmark of Membranous nephropathy is more common with solid tumor malignancies than with Lymphoma.

Choice B [Sclerosis of focal segments of the glomeruli] is hallmark of Focal segmental sclerosis, common in patients with Hypertension, Black race, IV Heroin use, and HIV.

Choice D [Apple green birefringence under polarized light on Congo red stain] can be seen with Amyloidosis, which is most commonly associated with Multiple myeloma.

Choice E [Hypercellular glomeruli with many neutrophils] is hallmark of Postinfectious glomerulonephritis.

80. PSYCHIATRY/BEHAVIORAL SCIENCE – SOCIAL ANXIETY DISORDER [HEALTH MAINTENANCE]

Beta blockers [choice B] are the preferred pharmacologic agent in patients who experience significant physiological symptoms (eg, tremor, tachycardia) 30-60 minutes prior to the performance, especially for single or rarely recurring situations.

Cognitive-behavioral therapy (CBT) is preferred for patients who will experience recurring encounters of performance.

Benzodiazepines [choice A] are an alternative to Beta blockers but may not be suitable in which sedation or impaired cognition may be an issue during the performance (eg, giving an oral dissertation).

Choice C [Fluoxetine] and choice D [Bupropion] are more appropriate for patients with Generalized anxiety disorder as they are taken on a daily basis and this patient does not have to perform frequently.

Choice E [Cannabinoids] are not recommended for the management of SAD.

81. MUSCULOSKELETAL – PLANTAR FASCIITIS [HISTORY AND PHYSICAL]

The diagnosis of plantar fasciitis can usually be made on the basis of history and physical examination alone and imaging is generally not indicated for the evaluation of Plantar fasciitis, so no additional labs or imaging is needed [choice B].

Plantar fasciitis is a clinical diagnosis based on the presence of both:

- [1] plantar heel pain worse when initiating walking or after a period of inactivity
- [2] Local point tenderness near the origin of the plantar fascia at the medial tuberosity of the calcaneum.

Imaging studies may be indicated when the diagnosis is not clear, but the primary role of imaging is to evaluate for other causes of heel pain than to make the diagnosis of PF.

MRI [choice A] is a sensitive method for detecting Plantar fasciitis, but it is usually not required for establishing the diagnosis.

Ultrasonography [choice C] in Plantar fasciitis can demonstrate thickening of the fascia and diffuse hypoechogenicity, indicating edema at the attachment of the plantar fascia to the calcaneus.

Plain radiographs [choice D] may show heel spurs, which are of little diagnostic significance.

82. HEMATOLOGY – SICKLE CELL DISEASE [HEALTH MAINTENANCE]

Daily Hydroxyurea therapy [choice C] is the mainstay of treatment of patients with Sickle cell disease to reduce the incidence of acute vaso-occlusive pain episodes and other vaso-occlusive events including acute chest syndrome and in some cases stroke.

Hydroxyurea reduces hospitalization rates and prolongs survival.

Hydroxyurea increases production of Hb F (which does not sickle and has a higher affinity for oxygen), increases RBC water, reduces RBC sickling, alters RBC adhesion to the endothelium, and inhibits ribonucleotide reductase.

The peripheral smear shows many sickled cells.

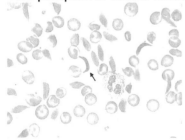

Choice [Penicillin] is administered in young children <5 years of age in addition to immunization is used to prevent infectious complications of SCD.

Choice B [Red cell transfusions] given monthly is second line to Hydroxyurea to treat and prevent the complications of SCD (eg if patients fail to respond to Hydroxyurea).

Choice D [Rituximab] is not routinely used in the management of Sickle cell disease.

Choice E [Periodic phlebotomy] is used in the management of Polycythemia vera and Hereditary hemochromatosis.

83. MUSCULOSKELETAL – VERTEBRAL FRACTURE [MOST LIKELY]

Acute vertebral body compression fracture [choice C] may occur with minimal or no trauma, such as lifting, coughing, bending, or a fall, are associated with pain.
It is often associated with pain and tenderness well localized to the midline spine at &/or near the fracture site.

Choice A [Spinal epidural abscess] often presents with subacute back pain, fever, and chills.
Choice B [Cauda equina syndrome] often presents with radiculopathy, urinary or bowel incontinence, or saddle anesthesia.
Choice D [Lumbar strain] presents with paravertebral tenderness along the muscles without midline tenderness.
Choice E [Herniated disc] presents with radiculopathy.

84. GENITOURINARY – STRESS INCONTINENCE [APPLYING FOUNDATIONAL CONCEPTS]

Risk factors for Stress incontinence include:
- **pregnancy and childbirth (particularly vaginal birth) [choice A]**
- **nerve injuries to the pelvis or lower back, and**
- **pelvic surgery, such as a hysterectomy.**

Causes of Stress incontinence include loss of support from pelvic floor musculature and connective tissue, such as pelvic floor trauma after vaginal delivery.
Pelvic floor muscle (Kegel) exercises are a key component in the initial management of women with urinary incontinence, especially Stress incontinence.
Pelvic muscle (Kegel) exercises strengthen the pelvic floor musculature and inhibit detrusor contractions.
Stress urinary incontinence have involuntary leakage of urine that occurs with increases in intra-abdominal pressure (eg, with exertion, sneezing, coughing, laughing) in the absence of a bladder contraction.

Choice B [Lower urinary tract infection] may result in Urge incontinence more likely.
Choice C [Increased or altered bladder microbiome] may result in Urge incontinence more likely.
Choice D [Bladder outlet obstruction] may result in Overflow incontinence more likely.
Choice E [Damage to the spinal detrusor efferent nerves] may result in Overflow incontinence more likely.

85. GENITOURINARY – ERECTILE DYSFUNCTION [PHARMACOLOGY]

Phosphodiesterase-5 (PDE5) inhibitors [choice C], such as Sildenafil, Tadalafil, or Vardenafil are the initial pharmacologic therapy for Erectile dysfunction because of their efficacy, ease of use, and favorable adverse effect profile.
Lifestyle modification (weight loss, physical activity) and medical management of cardiovascular risk factors may also improve sexual function in some men with ED.

In men with low testosterone, combination therapy with a PDE5 inhibitor and testosterone [choice A] may be considered.

Choice B [5-alpha reductase inhibition] medications are used to reduce the size of the prostate in Benign prostatic hyperplasia.

Choice D [Selective Alpha-adrenergic antagonist] medications are used for the symptoms of Benign prostatic hyperplasia and to facilitate the passage of kidney stones.

Choice E [Prostaglandin E1 analog] medications, such as intraurethral administration of Alprostadil, is an alternative medication in the management of Erectile dysfunction.

86. EENT – CORNEAL ABRASION [HISTORY AND PHYSICAL]

After completing visual acuity and fundus examination, Fluorescein examination [choice C] should be performed to assess for Corneal foreign body as Fluorescein staining is most helpful clinical tool to see a Corneal abrasion.

A Corneal abrasion is diagnosed by a staining defect, which can appear linear or geographic depending upon the epithelial defect as the dye collects in the abrasion and fluoresces under Cobalt blue light.

The lid should be everted to assess for foreign bodies; if present, foreign bodies should be removed.

Choice A [Amsler grid visual assessment] is used to assess Macular degeneration.

Choice B [Tonometry] is used to assess intraocular pressure of Glaucoma.

Choice D [CT scan of the orbits] is useful to diagnose Orbital cellulitis or in suspected Globe rupture.

Choice E [Emergent ophthalmologic consultation] is not necessary for corneal abrasion unless the foreign body is deeply embedded.

87. GENITOURINARY – PREMATURE EJACULATION [PHARMACOLOGY]

Selective serotonin reuptake inhibitors (SSRIs), such as Paroxetine [choice D] are the first line pharmacologic therapy for Premature ejaculation.

Paroxetine is probably the most effective SSRI for Premature ejaculation (9-minute ejection delay vs. baseline), but other SSRIs (eg, Sertraline, Fluoxetine, Citalopram, and Escitalopram) may also be used. Management depends upon the etiology, but the backbone of therapy include Selective serotonin reuptake inhibitors (SSRIs), topical anesthetics, and psychotherapy when psychogenic and/or relationship factors are present.

Choice A [Bupropion] is used for Depression in patients who experience sexual dysfunction on other typical antidepressants.

Choice B [Clomipramine] is a serotonergic tricyclic indicated for Premature ejaculation if SSRIs are ineffective or not tolerated.

Choice C [Tramadol] can be used as an alternative for Premature ejaculation if SSRIs and Clomipramine are ineffective or not tolerated. There is a risk of adverse effects and addiction risk.

Choice E [Sildenafil] and other Phosphodiesterase (PDE) 5 inhibitors may also be effective for the treatment of PE, but mainly in men with PE and coexisting ED

88. PSYCHIATRY/BEHAVIORAL SCIENCE – NARCOLEPSY [PHARMACOLOGY]

In addition to sleep hygiene, a trial of Modafinil [choice E], a wake-promoting medication, is a first line medication for patients with Narcolepsy with mild to moderate sleepiness.

Modafinil is a first-line pharmacologic agent in Narcolepsy because it is very effective in achieving good control of sleepiness, is generally well tolerated, and misuse is rare.

Classic features of Narcolepsy include:
- moderate to severe daytime sleepiness
- cataplexy: transient facial weakness or falls caused by episodes emotionally triggered muscle weakness)
- hypnagogic hallucinations: hallucinations when falling asleep or awakening
- sleep paralysis: inability to move for one or two minutes immediately after awakening.

Choice A [Zolpidem] is a nonbenzodiazepine hypnotic that may be useful in the management of Insomnia.

Choice B [Carbamazepine] is not used in the management of Narcolepsy.

Choice C [Clonazepam] are not routinely used in the management of Narcolepsy due to its ability to promote daytime sedation.

Choice D [Venlafaxine] can be used for residual cataplexy after use of wake promoting agents in selected individuals with Narcolepsy.

89. CARDIOLOGY – MYOCARDITIS [LABS AND DIAGNOSTIC STUDIES]

A Definitive diagnosis of Myocarditis is based upon identification of diagnostic findings on Endomyocardial biopsy [choice B], such as fibrosis and inflammation (eg, inflammatory infiltrate of the myocardium with necrosis or degeneration of myocytes) as described by the Dallas criteria.

Although rarely performed due to its invasive nature, Endomyocardial biopsy is reserved for patients with unexplained new-onset fulminant Heart failure with worsening cardiac function.

Myocarditis should be suspected in previously healthy young patients without a cardiac history that present with acute Heart failure.

Choice A [Analysis of pericardial fluid] is not necessary in patients without a Pericardial effusion.

Choice C [Echocardiography] is the most useful noninvasive test to assess ventricular function in Myocarditis, but it is not the criterion standard.

Choice D [Cardiac magnetic resonance imaging] has variable sensitivity and findings suggestive of Myocarditis are nonspecific.

Choice E [Cardiac catheterization] is not usually indicated unless there are findings that are indistinguishable from Acute coronary syndrome (eg, ST elevations).

90. GASTROINTESTINAL AND NUTRITION – HEPATITIS A VIRUS (HEALTH MAINTENANCE)

Globally, the rates of Hepatitis A virus (HAV) have decreased due to improvements in public healthcare policies, sanitation [choice E], and education.

Sanitation has had the greatest impact on reducing the incidence of HAV.

Because Hepatitis A is primarily transmitted through the fecal-oral route, the risk of Hepatitis A infection is associated with a lack of safe water and poor sanitation and poor personal hygiene (such as contaminated and dirty hands).

Improved sanitation, food safety and immunization are the most effective ways to combat hepatitis A.

The spread of Hepatitis A virus can be reduced by:
- adequate supplies of safe drinking water;
- proper disposal of sewage within communities; and

- personal hygiene practices (eg, regular handwashing before meals and after going to the restroom).

Choice B [Vaccination] has had a significant impact on HAV but not as great as sanitation. Prior to hepatitis A exposure, the primary personal protection is vaccination, especially those at high risk.

91. PULMONARY – SOLITARY PULMONARY NODULE [LABS AND DIAGNOSTIC STUDIES]

Computed tomography of the chest without contrast [choice D] using a lower than usual radiation dose technique is the preferred modality for initial evaluation for malignancy risk of an incidental pulmonary nodule.

CT is the most reliable modality for assessing nodule size, growth, and lobar location, and also allows visualization of nodule attenuation (density) and borders.

A solitary Pulmonary nodule is defined as a relatively well-defined round or oval pulmonary parenchymal lesion ≤30 mm in diameter.

Most nodules are benign, with the most common benign causes being infectious granulomas and benign tumors (eg, pulmonary hamartomas).

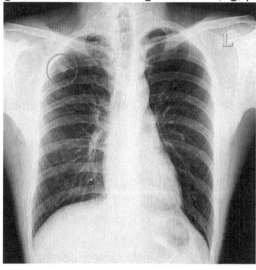

Choice A [Provide reassurance with no further follow-up] is inappropriate because the pulmonary nodule should be worked up via CT scan to assess malignancy risk and for further details of the nodule.

Choice B [Obtain a Tuberculin skin test] is not required in a patient without symptoms of Tuberculosis. The nodule was an incidental finding in this patient.

Choice C [Perform a transthoracic biopsy] is useful if the CT scan reveals a lesion suspicious for malignancy.

Choice E [Repeat chest radiograph in 3 months] can be performed if there is a low probability of lung cancer based on CT scan findings.

92. DERMATOLOGY – EPIDERMOID (EPIDERMAL INCLUSION) CYST [MOST LIKELY]

Epidermoid (epidermal inclusion) cyst [choice A] or improperly called "sebaceous cyst," most commonly presents as an asymptomatic skin colored nodule, often with a visible central punctum.

Epidermoid cysts may become secondarily infected by the normal skin flora.

Once infected, the cysts enlarge, become more erythematous, and painful.

Choice B [Lipoma] is soft, painless subcutaneous nodule without a central punctum.

Choice C [Abscess] is associated with erythema, tenderness, and fluctuance.

Choice D [Dermoid cyst] is a congenital subcutaneous nodule seen in infants and young children.

Choice E [Keloid] is an indurated, elevated, erythematous lesion with a glossy surface.

93. GASTROINTESTINAL AND NUTRITION – COLORECTAL CANCER [HEALTH MAINTENANCE]

The USPSTF recommends Colonoscopy as a screening test is usually performed every 10 years [choice C] for a patient at average risk of CRC, starting at age 50 years (Grade A).

- <u>Grade A recommendation</u>: screening for colorectal cancer in all adults aged 50-70 years.
- <u>Grade B recommendation</u>: screening for colorectal cancer in all adults aged 45-49 years.

<u>In patients with a first degree relative ≥60 years:</u>
- start at age 40 years [<u>OR</u> 10 years earlier than age which the family member developed CR cancer, whichever is EARLIER] & <u>every 10 years thereafter.</u>

<u>In patients with a first degree relative <60 years:</u>
- start at age 40 years [<u>OR</u> 10 years earlier than age which the family member developed CR cancer, whichever is EARLIER] & <u>every 5 years thereafter.</u>

94. EENT – LEUKOPLAKIA [HISTORY AND PHYSICAL]

Leukoplakia [choice E] classically presents as white patches or plaques that cannot be scraped off.

Alcohol and tobacco use are major risk factors. Leukoplakia represents hyperkeratoses in response to chronic irritation (eg, from dentures, tobacco).

Because 2–6% may represent either dysplasia or early invasive Squamous cell carcinoma, individuals with persistent lesions require biopsy for definitive diagnosis and histopathologic examination to assess for dysplasia and to exclude other oral disorders that present similar.

Choice A [Hairy leukoplakia] is seen with advanced HIV and presents with raised corrugated ('hairy") area most common on the lateral surface of the tongue.

Choice B [Lichen planus] is characterized by white lines, papules, or plaques in a reticulated or lacy pattern on the oral mucosa ("Wickham striae).

Choice C [Oral Squamous cell carcinoma] classically presents with an ulcer, nodule, or indurated plaque involving the oral cavity. The floor of the mouth and lateral or ventral tongue are the most common sites.

Choice D [Candidiasis] presents with white plaques on the buccal mucosa, palate, tongue, and/or the oropharynx that can be scraped off from the surface where it adheres, leaving behind an erythematous surface.

95. PSYCHIATRY/BEHAVIORAL SCIENCE – TRICYCLIC ANTIDEPRESSANTS [PHARMACOLOGY]

<u>Antimuscarinic (anticholinergic) effects</u> **are the most common adverse effects of Tricyclic antidepressants (TCAs) — eg, dry mouth, constipation [choice B], urinary retention, tachycardia, blurred vision, & orthostatic hypotension. The elderly may experience confusion or hallucinations.**

Other classic adverse effects of Tricyclic antidepressants include:
- <u>Antihistamine effects</u>: sedation, weight gain, confusion
- <u>Alpha-adrenergic blockade</u>: orthostatic hypotension, dizziness
- <u>CNS stimulation</u>: lowered seizure threshold
- SIADH
- Sexual dysfunction, Increased suicidality on initiation (especially <25 years of age).
- <u>Prolonged QT interval</u>: best indicator of overdose.

96. ENDOCRINE/GASTROINTESTINAL AND NUTRITION – GASTROPARESIS [PHARMACOLOGY]

Metoclopramide [choice B] is first line prokinetic therapy for Gastroparesis in patients with symptoms despite lifestyle modification.

Metoclopramide, a dopamine 2 receptor antagonist, a 5-HT4 agonist, and a weak 5-HT3 receptor antagonist, enhances gastric emptying by improving gastric antral contractions and decreasing postprandial fundus relaxation.

Patients who fail to respond to a trial of Metoclopramide may be treated with oral Erythromycin [choice C] liquid formulation, 40 to 250 mg three times daily.
Patients with persistent nausea and vomiting despite prokinetics may be treated with antihistamines, such as Diphenhydramine [choice D], and if persistent, Serotonin 5HT3 antagonists, such as Ondansetron [choice E].
If symptoms are persistent, Prochlorperazine may be used.
Proton pump inhibitors [choice A] do not reliably treat the symptoms of Gastroparesis.

97. GENITOURINARY – URETHRAL STRICTURE [LABS AND DIAGNOSTIC STUDIES]

Noninvasive studies, such as uroflowmetry [choice B] and ultrasound postvoid residual [PVR] measurement are initial tests for suspected Urethral stricture.

Stricture of the male urethra should be suspected if noninvasive studies elicit poor bladder emptying with low peak rate of urine flow.

Patients with abnormal noninvasive studies should undergo cystourethroscopy, retrograde urethrogram [choice D], voiding cystourethrogram [choice E], or ultrasound urethrography [choice C] to establish the diagnosis.

98. PSYCHIATRY/BEHAVIORAL – MAJOR DEPRESSIVE DISORDER [PHARMACOLOGY]

Bupropion [choice A] is the antidepressant of choice in patients with Major depressive disorder in patients who are
- **fearful of weight gain with other antidepressants**
- **fearful of sexual adverse effects with other antidepressants**
- **desire smoking cessation.**

Bupropion has less GI, weight gain, & sexual adverse effects compared to SSRIs, SNRIs [choice C], and TCAs.

Treatment options for sexual dysfunction on antidepressant therapy include:
- (1) lowering the antidepressant dose, if feasible
- (2) switching to another antidepressant (eg, Bupropion, Mirtazapine)
- (3) augmenting with either Bupropion or a Phosphodiesterase-5 inhibitor (eg, Sildenafil).

Although Mirtazapine [choice B] is associated with less sexual adverse effects, weight gain is a frequent adverse effect due to antihistaminic properties, which is also a concern for this patient.

The usage of SSRIs and SNRIs simultaneously [choice C] increases the risk of Serotonin syndrome as both a serotonergic agents.

Choice D (Continuing the Fluoxetine) without addressing the patients concern is not recommended.

Paroxetine [choice E] has more sexual dysfunction, antihistaminic activity, & more significant anticholinergic activity (can cause more dry mouth, dizziness, and weight gain).

99. GASTROINTESTINAL AND NUTRITION – CHRONIC MESENTERIC ISCHEMIA [LABS AND DIAGNOSTICS]

Computed tomographic (CT) angiography of the abdomen and pelvis [choice A] is the best initial imaging study for Chronic mesenteric ischemia, as recommended by both The Society for Vascular Surgery and the American College of Radiology.

CT angiography helps to confirm or exclude the presence of mesenteric atherosclerotic vascular disease and excludes other abdominal pathologies as the etiology.

Chronic mesenteric ischemia (intestinal angina) refers to episodic or constant intestinal hypoperfusion most commonly resulting from mesenteric atherosclerotic disease from stenosis or occlusion of at least two mesenteric vessels.

Classic symptoms are postprandial abdominal pain and food aversion in anticipation of the pain, resulting in weight loss.

Choice B [Abdominal arteriography] is invasive imaging that may be used if the results of noninvasive CT angiography are inconclusive or if CT angiography suggests vascular intervention is needed.

Choice C [Colonoscopy] is not needed as the last one <10 years ago was negative.

Choice D [Duplex ultrasonography of the abdomen and pelvis] may be used to exclude mesenteric ischemia of the celiac and super mesenteric arteries but CT is the preferred initial modality.

Choice E [Upper endoscopy] is used to establish the diagnosis of Gastric ulcers, which classically presents with epigastric pain that worsens with eating, postprandial belching and epigastric fullness, early satiety, fatty food intolerance, nausea, and occasional vomiting.

100. PSYCHIATRY/BEHAVIORAL – SOMATIC SYMPTOM DISORDER [MOST LIKELY]
The 2 core features of Somatic symptom disorder [choice C] are:
- **≥1 current somatic (physical) symptoms that are long-standing (≥6 months)** and cause distress or psychosocial impairment.
- excessive thoughts, worrying, or behaviors (time and energy) related to the somatic symptoms or to health concerns.

Unlike Illness anxiety disorder, patients are not focused on a particular illness.

Choice A [Factitious disorder] is associated with intentionally falsifying symptoms and/or signs for primary gain.

Choice B [Body dysmorphic disorder] is the preoccupation with a perceived or exaggeration of a physical defect (eg, large nose, being deformed).

Choice D [Illness anxiety disorder] is associated with excessive worry about having or acquiring a serious undiagnosed general medical condition despite having little to no symptoms of that illness. If symptoms are present, they are minimal and are often due to an exaggeration of normal body functions.

Choice E [Functional neurological symptom disorder], previously known as conversion disorder, is characterized by abnormalities or deficits of motor or sensory function that are not medically explained (eg, paresis, blindness, mute). Patients are often not overly concerned with their neurological deficits.

1. A 42-year-old male presents with exertional dyspnea, fatigue, and intermittent leg edema. On examination, hoarseness of the voice is noted. Cardiac auscultation reveals a low-pitched diastolic rumbling murmur following an opening snap. The murmur is best heard between the fifth and sixth ribs at the left mid-clavicular line. Which of the following is most likely in this patient's history?
a. Infective endocarditis
b. Rheumatic fever
c. Myocardial infarction
d. Hypertension
e. Congenital heart defect

2. A 50-year-old male develops SARS-CoV-2 and is admitted to the hospital. He is quickly intubated and later becomes unresponsive. He is noncommunicative and his organs are shutting down. He did not designate a power of attorney and there is no documented advance directive. He is married and his husband of 15 years says that during many discussions, the patient mentioned he did not want to be resuscitated if he is dying. His mother states she remembered him saying as a kid he wants to be resuscitated. His adult daughter and his older brother are unsure of what his wishes are. Which of the following is the most appropriate action if he develops Asystole?
a. Defer to the sibling what would be the most appropriate course of action
b. Consult the hospital ethics committee
c. Defer to the adult daughter what would be the most appropriate course of action
d. Begin full resuscitation as per his mother's wishes
e. Assure the patient's comfort and allow his family to be there at the beside during his final moments of life

3. A 2-year-old boy is being evaluated for fever and rash that began on his face. The fever started 72 hours ago, followed by a rash that developed 2 days ago. He has not received any childhood vaccinations. Examination reveals a well-appearing child with fine pinpoint discrete maculopapules and prominent tender posterior cervical, suboccipital, and postauricular lymphadenopathy. Which of the following is the most likely diagnosis?
a. Rubella
b. Erythema infectiosum
c. Rubeola
d. Scarlet fever
e. Kawasaki disease

4. A 22-year-old female presents to the office for emergency contraception. She had unprotected sexual intercourse with a stranger 48 hours ago. Her last menstrual period was 14 days ago. Physical examination is unremarkable and urine hCG is negative. Which of the following is most effective at preventing pregnancy in this patient?
a. Combination oral contraceptives
b. Oral Levonorgestrel only pill
c. Etonogestrel subdermal implant
d. Copper-containing intrauterine device
e. Ulipristal acetate

5. A 22-year-old male is arrested after assaulting an elderly male. When asked about the incident, he describes with excitement how he hit him with his own cane. He showed no remorse for his actions. Which of the following is most likely in his childhood history?
a. Conduct disorder
b. Attention-deficit Hyperactivity disorder
c. Oppositional defiant disorder
d. Disruptive mood regulation disorder
e. Intermittent explosive disorder

6. A 25-year-old female presents to the clinic complaining of intermittent episodes of wheezing, nonbloody diarrhea, coughing, and hemoptysis. Chest radiograph shows a centrally located pulmonary mass. Bronchoscopy shows a pink well-vascularized mass. The presence of which of the following is most consistent with the most likely diagnosis?
a. Hypoactive bowel sounds
b. Peripheral cyanosis
c. Clubbing of the finger
d. Cutaneous flushing
e. Hematochezia

7. A 22-year-old male presents with pain to the dorsum of the right hand. Radiographs are obtained (see photo).

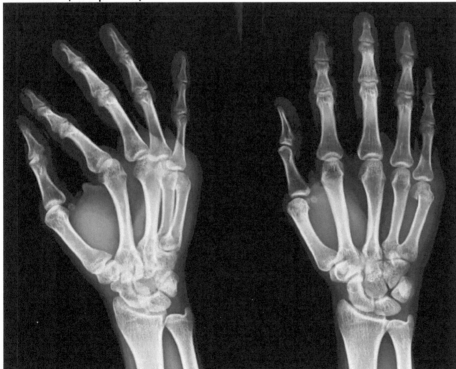

Which of the following describes the most likely mechanism of injury?
a. Fall on an outstretched hand with hyperextension
b. Direct blow to the volar aspect (palm) of the hand
c. Torsional injury to the base of the finger
d. Direct trauma to a clenched fist
e. Fall on an outstretched hand with hyperextension

8. A 23-year-old female presents to the clinic with a 12-month history of frequent menstruation associated with heavy bleeding. Menarche occurred at age 14, and she had light periods every 28-30 days, lasting 6-9 days with minimal cramping. During her cycle, she bleeds through a menstrual pad every 2-3 hours for the first 4-5 days. Her last menstrual period began 2 weeks ago. Initial workup including transvaginal ultrasound is negative and beta-hCG is negative. Which of the following medications would be most helpful in managing this patient's symptoms?
a. Letrozole
b. Danazol
c. Leuprolide
d. Ethinyl estradiol
e. Levonorgestrel IUD

9. A 79-year-old male presents to the clinic for back pain and unintentional 15 lb. weight loss. He eats a diet low in vegetables. He has a history of Benign prostatic hyperplasia. Social history is positive for a 20-pack year smoking history, and he does not exercise regularly. Physical examination reveals an obese male. Digital rectal examination reveals a rock hard asymmetric nodular prostate. Prostate specific antigen is 12.5 ng/mL (0-6.5 ng/ml aged 70-79). Transrectal biopsy is positive for adenocarcinoma. Which of the following risk factors is most strongly related to the development of cancer in this patient?
a. Cigarette smoking
b. Obesity
c. Diet low in vegetables
d. Benign prostatic hyperplasia
e. Advanced age

10. A 24-year-old male is brought to the emergency department after being ejected from his motorcycle and suffering a hyperflexion injury to the neck. On examination, he is incontinent of urine and has no movement of the lower extremities. There is also loss of temperature, light touch, and pain sensation in the lower extremities. Proprioception, vibration, fine touch, and pressure sensation are intact in all extremities. Which of the following is the most likely diagnosis?
a. Posterior cord syndrome
b. Anterior cord syndrome
c. Central cord syndrome
d. Brown Sequard syndrome
e. Middle cerebral artery stroke

11. Compared to Type 2 Diabetes mellitus, which of the following symptoms is most specific for Type 1 Diabetes mellitus?
a. Fatigue
b. Polyuria
c. Polydipsia
d. Weight loss
e. Vulvovaginal infection

12. A 10-year-old boy presents to the clinic for jaundice. He is recovering from a recent upper respiratory tract infection. Physical examination is notable for pallor, scleral icterus, and splenomegaly. Initial labs reveal:

Hemoglobin 9 g/dL (14-18)

Reticulocyte count 6.3% (0.5-1.5%)

MCHC 38 g/dl (31.5-35)

Indirect bilirubin 3.7 g/dL (0.2-0.8)

Direct antiglobulin test negative for IgG and C3

The following is seen on peripheral blood smear.

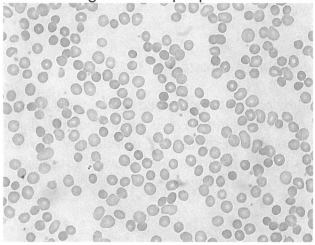

Which of the following is the most likely diagnosis?

a. Gilbert syndrome

b. Glucose-6-phosphate dehydrogenase deficiency

c. Warm autoimmune hemolytic anemia

d. Hereditary spherocytosis

e. Cold agglutinin disease

13. A 20-year-old male presents to the emergency department with abdominal pain. He is given appropriate management. 1 hour after initial management, his labs are as follows:

- Serum glucose 190 mg/dL (70-110)
- Serum sodium 140 mEq/L (135-145)
- Potassium 4.3 mEq/L (3.5-5)
- Bicarbonate 19 mEq/L (22-26)
- Chloride 100 mEq/L (96-106)
- Serum ketones: positive

Which of the following is the most appropriate next step in the management of this patient?

a. IV 0.9% sodium chloride, IV regular Insulin, IV Potassium chloride

b. Emergent hemodialysis

c. IV 5% Dextrose with 0.9% sodium chloride, IV regular Insulin, IV Potassium chloride

d. IV 0.9% sodium chloride and IV regular Insulin

e. IV 0.9% sodium chloride and IV Potassium chloride

14. A 27-year-old female presents to urgent care with a 3-day history of dysuria, urinary frequency and urgency, suprapubic pain, fever, chills, and hematuria. Vitals reveal a temperature of 101.2°F (38.4°C), BP: 120/70 mmHg, pulse 96/min, respirations 18/min, and pulse oximetry 98% on room air. There is suprapubic and left flank tenderness with mild palpation. She is able to eat and drink. Initial labs reveal a WBC count of 19,200/microL (5,000–10,000). Urinalysis shows 32 white blood cells per cubic millimeter, 25 RBCs/hpf, positive nitrites and leukocyte esterase, and white cell casts. A urine culture is sent, and results are pending. Beta hCG is negative. Which of the following is the first-line management?
a. Inpatient management with intravenous Ceftriaxone
b. Outpatient management with oral Nitrofurantoin
c. Outpatient management with oral Ciprofloxacin
d. Inpatient management with intravenous Daptomycin
e. Outpatient management with oral Trimethoprim/sulfamethoxazole

15. A 66-year-old female presents complaining of dysphagia to both solids and liquids as well as regurgitation of bland undigested food. Barium esophagram reveals dilation of the distal esophagus with a narrowed esophagogastric junction. Esophageal manometry reveals aperistalsis in the distal two-thirds of the esophagus and incomplete lower esophageal sphincter relaxation. Which of the following is the most likely diagnosis?
a. Distal esophageal spasm
b. Hypercontractile esophagus
c. Gastroesophageal reflux disease
d. Zenker diverticulum
e. Achalasia

16. Which of the following is a classic adverse effect of the second-generation neuroleptic Olanzapine?
a. Hypertension
b. Shortened QT interval
c. Serotonin syndrome
d. Weight gain
e. Hypoglycemia

17. An infant is delivered via vaginal delivery at 27+1 weeks of gestation. Physical examination of the infant reveals tachypnea, nasal flaring, expiratory grunting, intercostal and subxiphoid retractions, and cyanosis. There are decreased breath sounds and the infant is pale with decreased peripheral pulses. A chest radiograph reveals a diffuse reticulogranular ground-glass appearance. Which of the following is the most likely diagnosis?
a. Congenital cyanotic heart disease
b. Meconium aspiration
c. Respiratory distress syndrome in the newborn
d. Persistent pulmonary hypertension of the neonate
e. Transient tachypnea of the newborn

18. A 25-year-old male is brought to the ED via ambulance for confusion. He was recently diagnosed with Bipolar I disorder treated with Risperidone. Vital reveal temperature 38.3°C (100.94°F), blood pressure 160/92 mmHg, pulse 138 beats/min. Lead pipe rigidity, diaphoresis, hyporeflexia, and regular sized pupils are noted. Laboratory investigation reveal mild leukocytosis (leukocyte count 11.8 x 10^9/L) and creatine kinase (CK) level 1,280 U/L (55-170). Risperidone is discontinued and he is given IV Lorazepam with continued symptoms. Which of the following medications should be given next?
a. Haloperidol
b. Benztropine
c. Physostigmine
d. Cyproheptadine
e. Dantrolene

19. A mother brings her 9-month-old for recurrent "belly aches" for the past 10 days. The child experiences abrupt episodes of intermittent abdominal pain and vomiting, accompanied by crying and drawing up of his legs, which seems to relieve the pain. He has no complaints in between episodes. His mother became concerned when he developed several episodes of stool mixed with blood and mucus. An abdominal ultrasound is performed (see photo).

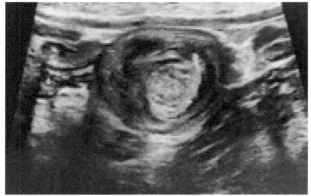

Which of the following is the recommended next step in the management of this patient?
a. Pneumatic enema
b. Rectal suction biopsy followed by transanal mucosal biopsy if negative
c. Barium swallow
d. 99m technetium pertechnetate (Meckel) scan
e. Rehydration and electrolyte replacement, followed by Pyloromyotomy

Photo credit:
Cerevisae, CC BY-SA 4.0 <https://creativecommons.org/licenses/by-sa/4.0>, via Wikimedia Commons

20. A 55-year-old male with a history of Myocardial infarction presents with increasing dyspnea on exertion. An echocardiogram is performed, revealing an ejection fraction of 39% (50-70%). Which of the following would most likely be seen on physical examination?
a. Diastolic knock
b. Pulsus bisferiens
c. Weak delayed carotid pulses
d. Third heart sound
e. Fourth heart sound

21. A 67-year-old female with a history of Chronic obstructive pulmonary disease presents to the emergency with right-sided pleuritic chest pain, fever, and cough. A chest radiograph is performed (see photo).

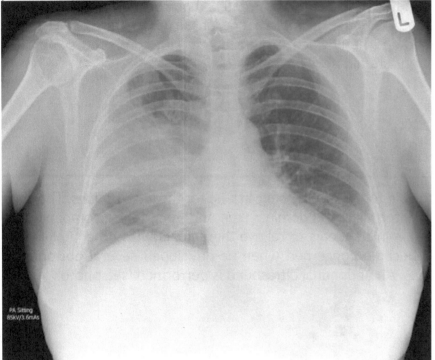

She is admitted to the hospital for Acute exacerbation of COPD. Which of the following is the recommended management of this patient?
a. Vancomycin
b. Piperacillin/tazobactam
c. Ceftriaxone plus Azithromycin
d. Doxycycline
e. Amoxicillin plus clavulanic acid

Photo credit:
Case courtesy of Jeremy Jones, Radiopaedia.org, rID: 13553

22. A 34-year-old woman presents to the clinic because she has not had her menses for the last 9 months. Prior to this, she had a regular menses every 28 days lasting 4-6 days. Physical exam is notable for thin, dry, fragile-appearing vaginal mucosa with vulvovaginal pallor. No hirsutism is noted. Labs reveal:
- serum estradiol (E2) of 10 pg/mL (30-400)
- follicle-stimulating hormone (FSH) of 63 mIU/L (4.7-21.5).

Transvaginal ultrasound reveals a thin endometrial stripe. Which of the following is the most likely etiology of this patient's amenorrhea?
a. Intrauterine adhesions
b. Functional hypothalamic amenorrhea
c. Primary ovarian insufficiency
d. Pituitary adenoma
e. Pituitary infarction (Sheehan syndrome)

23. A 50-year-old male is being evaluated for right foot pain and swelling. He denies any trauma. The following is seen on radiographs (see photo).

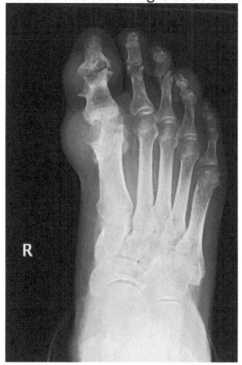

Which of the following is the most likely etiology of his presentation?
a. Calcium pyrophosphate crystal deposition
b. Bony destructive changes due to chronic bacterial infection of the bone
c. Localized inflammation of the joint from peripheral neuropathy due to Diabetes mellitus
d. The presence of a pannus resulting in joint destruction
e. Monosodium urate crystal deposition

Photo credit:
Case courtesy of Naim Qaqish, Radiopaedia.org, rID: 81562

24. A 22-year-old G2P1 female at 34 weeks gestation presents to labor and delivery triage with vaginal spotting. Over the last 45 minutes, she has experienced painless spotting without abdominal pain. There is no uterine tenderness on examination. An urgent transabdominal ultrasound is performed, showing a viable fetus and normal amniotic fluid. Fetal heart rate monitoring shows accelerations lasting 15-20 seconds but <2 minutes. Based on the history and findings, which of the following is the most likely diagnosis?
a. Uterine rupture
b. Vasa previa
c. Placenta previa
d. Abruptio placenta
e. Threatened abortion

25. A 70-year-old man presents with left-sided pleuritic chest pain and dyspnea. He is febrile and tachypneic. Physical examination reveals dullness to percussion, decreased fremitus, and decreased breath sounds in the left middle and lower lung fields. Chest radiograph is obtained (see photo).

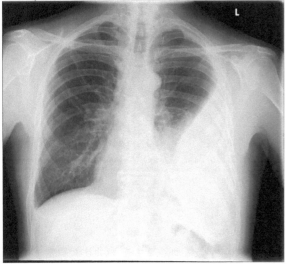

Thoracentesis is performed, with pleural fluid analysis revealing:
- pleural pH 6.88 (7.60-7.64)
- pleural fluid glucose 18 mg/dL (60)
- pleural fluid protein 5 g/dL (1-2 g/dL)
- gram stain: gram positive diplococci

In addition to systemic antibiotic therapy, which of the following is the best next step in management of this patient?
a. Thoracotomy
b. Prednisone
c. Chest tube thoracostomy
d. Video assisted thoracoscopy
e. Bronchoscopy

Photo credit:
Case courtesy of Ian Bickle, Radiopaedia.org, rID: 74921

26. A 40-year-old male presents with heel pain after suddenly pivoting on his foot while running. He felt as he had been struck in the back of the ankle and heard a "pop", followed by severe, acute pain. It has been over 10 years since his last run but recently, he has resumed exercising. Based on the most likely diagnosis, which of the following findings is most reliable?
a. Inability to evert the foot
b. Pain along the posterior aspect of the ankle
c. Absence of plantar flexion with squeezing of the calf
d. Tenderness along the base of the fifth metatarsal
e. Inability to ambulate

27. A 57-year-old male is complaining of 8/10 dull and constant colicky abdominal pain for 3 days. Associated symptoms include nausea, vomiting, and low-grade fever. He has a history of obesity and chronic constipation. Vital reveal a temperature 101°F (38.4°C), blood pressure 136/72 mmHg, pulse 104/min, and SaO_2 99% on room air. Abdominal examination demonstrates left lower quadrant abdominal tenderness without guarding or rigidity. Labs reveal a hemoglobin of 16 g/dL (13-17) and leukocyte count 13,200 cells/mm³ (5,000-10,000) with normal differential. Which of the following is the recommended next step in evaluation of this patient?
a. Amylase and lipase levels
b. Barium enema
c. Colonoscopy
d. Computed tomography scan of the abdomen and pelvis
e. Abdominal ultrasound

28. A 32-year-old male is complaining of chest fullness and shortness of breath for 3 days. Vital signs are temperature 98.8°F (37.11°C), blood pressure 118/70 mm Hg, and heart rate 92 beats/min. Examination reveals clear lungs and distant heart sounds. Chest radiograph reveals an enlarged cardiac silhouette with clear lung fields. Which of the following is most helpful to establish the most likely diagnosis?
a. Cardiac stress test
b. Electrocardiogram
c. Echocardiogram
d. Pericardiocentesis
e. Cardiac catheterization

29. A 44-year-old female is complaining of right upper quadrant pain that began about 8 hours ago and has been steadily increasing in intensity. It is associated with nausea and vomiting. Vitals are temperature 98.8°F (37.11°C), blood pressure 122/78 mmHg, and pulse 88/minute. Physical examination is notable for scleral icterus and right upper quadrant tenderness without rebound tenderness or guarding. Initial labs reveal:
  • white blood cell count 7,000/mm³ (5,000-10,000)
  • total bilirubin 7.2 mg/dL (≤1.2)
  • ALT 131 U/L (7-55)
  • alkaline phosphatase 640 U/L (44-147)
  • GGT 120 IU/L (0-30).
Which of the following is the most likely diagnosis?
a. Acute Hepatitis
b. Choledocholithiasis
c. Acute Cholecystitis
d. Acute Cholangitis
e. Cholelithiasis

30. A 70-year-old female presents to the clinic with a 3-month history of right-sided headache, pain with chewing food, low-grade fever, myalgias, and malaise. Vitals are stable. There is a palpable temporal artery with a normal neurological examination. An elevated erythrocyte sedimentation rate is noted. Prompt initiation of therapy in this patient is recommended to reduce which of the following complications?
a. Aortic dissection
b. Aortic aneurysm
c. Stroke
d. Anterior ischemic optic neuropathy
e. Cerebral ischemia

31. A 53-year-old man presents with chronic epigastric abdominal pain that often radiates to the back. It is often worse when recumbent and he experiences postprandial exacerbations. His stools have become bulky, oily, and difficult to flush. Review of systems is positive for a 15-lb. weight loss over the last 5 months. On examination, no jaundice or palpable masses are noted. Labs reveal mild elevation of lipase and amylase. A CT scan reveals pancreatic calcifications. Which of the following is most likely to be in this patient's medical history?
a. Cystic fibrosis
b. Cigarette smoking
c. Alcohol consumption
d. Family history of pancreatic cancer
e. Gallstones

32. A 23-year-old primigravid female is complaining of intermittent fever and left breast pain. She gave birth to a full-term healthy girl via spontaneous vaginal delivery. Physical examination is positive for a firm, erythematous, edematous, and warm area of the left breast with a 3-cm area of fluctuance. Left axillary lymphadenopathy is also noted. There is no nipple discharge. Which of the following is the best next step in management of this patient?
a. Warm compresses, use of supportive bra, and Cephalexin
b. Needle aspiration and Dicloxacillin
c. Warm compresses and use of a breast pump or manual pump
d. Mammogram
e. Core needle biopsy

33. A 49-year-old male with a history of Hypertension being treated with Captopril presents to the dermatology clinic with painful blisters that began on the lips 2 months ago. The pain is worsened with chewing and swallowing. Recently, he developed skin lesions on his trunk and arms. On examination, there are tender erosions on the buccal and palatine mucosa. There are numerous flaccid blisters on erythematous skin that rupture easily, producing painful denuded erosions that bleed easily. Extension of blistering is induced by applying mechanical pressure to on normal skin at the edge of the blister. There are no lesions on the palms and soles. Which of the following is the most likely diagnosis?
a. Toxic epidermal necrolysis
b. Bullous pemphigoid
c. Pemphigus vulgaris
d. Stevens-Johnson syndrome
e. Type IV hypersensitivity drug reaction

34. A 70-year-old male presents to the clinic for evaluation. On examination, there is a harsh holosystolic murmur that is best heard at the right upper sternal border that is associated with a weak, delayed pulse. An ECG is obtained.

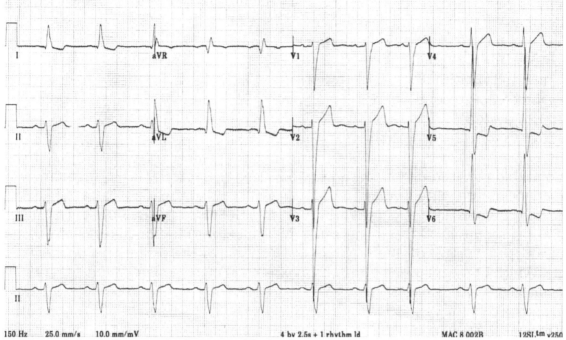

Which of the following is the most likely diagnosis?
a. Right bundle branch block
b. Right axis deviation
c. Left ventricular hypertrophy
d. Acute pericarditis
e. Brugada syndrome

35. A 10-year-old with a history of Intussusception and Asthma presents with an intensely itchy rash on the elbows. On examination, there are erythematous papules and vesicles on the antecubital fossae with exudation and crusting. There is a darkened transverse crease on the nasal bridge. Which of the following is the most likely diagnosis?
a. Nonbullous impetigo
b. Atopic dermatitis
c. Psoriasis
d. Scabies
e. Irritant contact dermatitis

36. A 44-year-old male presents with diarrhea and perioral paresthesias after a recent thyroidectomy for Follicular thyroid carcinoma. On physical examination, increased bowel sounds, and facial spasm is noted with tapping of the face. Which of the following laboratory values would most likely be increased?
a. serum calcium
b. serum phosphate
c. intact PTH
d. vitamin D
e. calcitonin

37. A 67-year-old male presents to the clinic with subacute worsening diarrhea, diffuse abdominal cramping, and fever. On examination, he is tachycardic and tachypneic. Initial labs are significant for a white blood cell count of 49,500 cells/microL (5,000-10,000). Sigmoidoscopy is performed, revealing elevated yellow-white plaques and nodules on the colonic mucosa, consist with pseudomembranes. Which of the following is the most likely predisposing factor for this patient's condition?
a. Use of Ibuprofen for back pain
b. Drinking untreated water
c. Consuming undercooked pork
d. Consuming raw oysters
e. Taking antibiotics for chronic prostatitis

38. An 18-month-old boy is brought to the emergency department for difficulty breathing. He has been experiencing intermittent cough, fever, hoarseness, rhinorrhea, and nasal congestion for the past 3 days. Vitals are temperature 37.7°C (99.9°F), respirations 30/min, and pulse oximetry 98% on room air. On examination, mild inspiratory stridor at rest, intercostal retractions, and harsh brassy cough are noted. Examination of the posterior oropharynx is unremarkable. Which of the following is the best next step in management of this patient?
a. Supplemental oxygen via face mask
b. Intubation and mechanical ventilation
c. Nebulized racemic Epinephrine
d. Nebulized Albuterol
e. Chest radiograph

39. A 56-year-old male presents to the emergency department with chest pressure for 90 minutes. He has a history of Dyslipidemia. An ECG is performed, revealing inverted T waves in leads III and ST segment depression in V1, V3, and V6. Troponin I is 0.154 ng/mL (0-0.04). Cardiac catheterization is performed, revealing 95% occlusion of the left anterior descending artery treated with angioplasty with a drug-eluting stent. He is placed on Lisinopril, Metoprolol, Aspirin, and Rosuvastatin. Which of the following should be added to this patient's regimen?
a. Rivaroxaban
b. Nifedipine
c. Alteplase
d. Clopidogrel
e. Verapamil

40. A 24-year-old male presents to his primary care provider for a six-week history of intrusive images and nightmares after he was held at gunpoint on his way to work. He has been having trouble concentrating in school and began taking the long way to school and work to avoid passing the area of the incident. He also reports waking up 3-4 times during the night from nightmares in a cold sweat with his heart racing. On mental status examination, he appears tired and avoids eye contact. Given the likely diagnosis, which of the following is the most appropriate treatment for this patient?
a. Emotionally focused therapy
b. Acceptance and commitment therapy
c. Psychodynamic therapy
d. Trauma-focused Dialectical behavioral therapy
e. Trauma-focused psychotherapy that includes exposure

41. A 20-year-old male presents with swelling to the forearm. He has a history of IV drug use and past infection with Methicillin resistant *Staphylococcus aureus*. Physical examination reveals an area of erythema, warmth, induration, and fluctuance. An incision and drainage is performed. Which of the following antibiotics should the patient be prescribed?
a. Azithromycin
b. Trimethoprim-sulfamethoxazole
c. Levofloxacin
d. Amoxicillin-clavulanate
e. Metronidazole

42. A previously healthy 5-year-old boy is being evaluated after experiencing a generalized tonic-clonic seizure at home. His parents state since last week, he had abdominal pain and diarrhea that was initially watery but after a few days, it became bloody with mucous. Vitals reveal fever and tachycardia. Initial labs reveal a white cell count of 23,000 cells/microL (5,000-10,000). Neurologic examination is normal. Which of the following is the most likely cause of this patient's symptoms?
a. Rotavirus
b. *Shigella sonnei*
c. *Vibrio cholerae*
d. Intussusception
e. Enterotoxigenic *Escherichia coli*

43. A 55-year-old male is being managed for Argatroban overdose. He is treated with Fresh frozen plasma (FFP). An uneventful transfusion of 2 FFP units took place. However, 3 hours after FFP transfusion, the patient experienced a sudden onset of fever, chills, and breathlessness. On examination, he is profusely diaphoretic, with BP: 100/50 mmHg, P: 120/min, T: 39°F (102.2°C), R: 34/min, and SaO$_2$: 77%. A chest radiograph is performed (see photo).

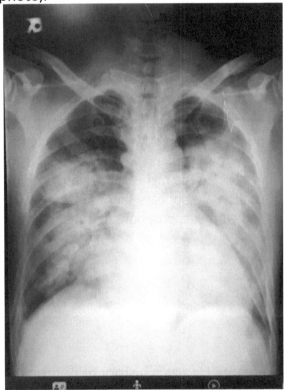

Which of the following is the most likely diagnosis?
a. Acute transfusion-related hemolytic reaction
b. Transfusion-related acute lung injury
c. Transfusion-associated circulatory overload
d. Acute febrile nonhemolytic transfusion reaction
e. Anaphylactic transfusion reaction

Photo credit:
Shutterstock (used with permission)

44. A 43-year-old man presents with a 5-week history of gradual decrease in hearing, deterioration of speech discrimination, and occasional ringing on the left side. Weber test reveals that the sound from the tuning fork placed on the patient's forehead localizes to the right side. Air conduction is better than bone conduction on both sides with Rinne testing. Which of the following is the most likely diagnosis in this patient?
a. Cerumen impaction
b. Vestibular schwannoma
c. Cholesteatoma
d. Benign paroxysmal positional vertigo
e. Otosclerosis

45. A 55-year-old male with no significant past medical history was seen in the emergency department for burning left-sided chest pain. He underwent a workup for Acute coronary syndrome, which was negative. 48 hours later, he developed erythematous papules that progressed to vesicles on an erythematous base located on a single dermatome. Which of the following is the first line management of this condition?
a. Topical Betamethasone
b. Oral Valacyclovir
c. Oral Fluconazole
d. Topical Butenafine
e. Topical Mupirocin

46. A 33-year-old male presents to the clinic for worsening fatigue, dyspnea on exertion, and generalized weakness. He has a history of AIDS for which he is on Trimethoprim-sulfamethoxazole for PCP and Toxoplasmosis prophylaxis and Seizure disorder on Phenytoin. Physical examination is notable for an enlarged erythematous tongue and conjunctival pallor without scleral icterus. Initial labs reveal a WBC count of 5,200/mm^3 (5,000-10,000), Hemoglobin 10 g/dL (11-15), and the following on peripheral blood smear (see photo).

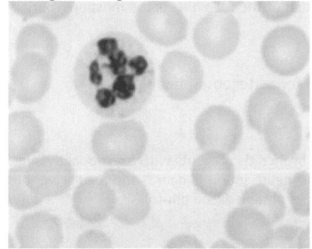

Which of the following labs would most likely be seen in this patient?
a. Megakaryocytes and decreased platelet count
b. Increased methylmalonic acid, increased homocysteine
c. Normal methylmalonic acid, increased homocysteine
d. Normal methylmalonic acid, decreased homocysteine
e. Elevated prothrombin time, decreased platelets

47. A 55-year-old male is complaining of cheek pain and burning sensation that was preceded 48 hours by low-grade fever, chills, and malaise. Physical examination reveals a raised area of bright erythema, warmth, shininess, and tenderness with clearly demarcated raised borders. Which of the following is the most likely causative organism of this patient's condition?
a. Group A Streptococcus
b. Staphylococcus aureus
c. Pseudomonas aeruginosa
d. Streptococcus pneumoniae
e. Clostridium perfringens

48. A full term neonate is being evaluated in the nursery shortly after vaginal birth. Examination of the genitalia reveals a urethra located at the ventral distal surface of the penis with incomplete foreskin closure around the glans, resulting in the appearance of a dorsal hooded prepuce. There is normal penile length without curvature. Both testicles are palpated in the scrotum. Normal development is otherwise noted, and cardiac and pulmonary examination are within normal limits. His mother requests that a circumcision be performed. Which of the following is the most appropriate next step in the management of this patient's condition?
a. Perform an echocardiogram
b. Ultrasound of the kidneys
c. Proceed with circumcision
d. Referral to for surgical correction at 6 months
e. Perform karyotype analysis

49. A 3-year-old boy presents to the emergency department for fever, worsening left ear pain, and lethargy. He was seen in urgent care 5 days ago and was diagnosed with Acute otitis media, for which he was placed on Cefdinir. Physical examination is notable for bulging of the tympanic membrane with postauricular erythema, postauricular tenderness, and protrusion of the pinna. There is auricular discharge noted. Which of the following is the most appropriate next step?
a. Tympanostomy tube placement
b. Otolaryngology consult
c. Ciprofloxacin otic and placement of an ear wick for better absorption
d. Switch oral Cefdinir to Amoxicillin-clavulanate
e. CT scan and IV Piperacillin-tazobactam

50. A 60-year-old male with a history of Chronic bronchitis presents with exertional dyspnea and fatigue. On examination, a fixed, split second heart sound is heard, and jugular venous pressure is measured at 12 cm H_2O (6-8). An ECG is obtained (see photo).

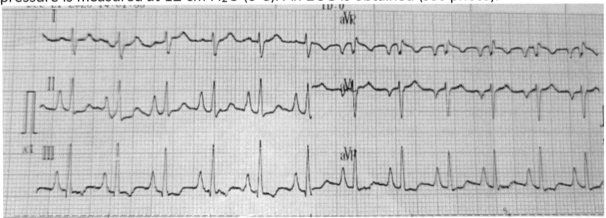

Which of the following is the most likely diagnosis?
a. Left atrial enlargement
b. Cor pulmonale
c. Wolff-Parkinson white
d. Multifocal atrial tachycardia
e. Wandering atrial pacemaker

51. A 35-year-old male presents with excessive thirst, urinary frequency, and nocturia. He denies fevers, chills, or headaches. Laboratory evaluation reveals:
- Serum glucose 90 mg/dL (70-110)
- Serum sodium 144 mEq/L (135-145)
- Serum osmolality 310 mOsm/kg (270-295)
- Urine specific gravity 1.001 (1.001-1.025)
- Urine osmolality 230 mOsm/kg
- Urine osmolality after water deprivation: 250 mOsm/kg

Which of the following is the most appropriate next step in the evaluation of this patient?
a. Dexamethasone suppression test
b. Glucose suppression test
c. Fasting plasma glucose test
d. Cosyntropin stimulation test
e. Desmopressin stimulation test

52. A 14-day-old neonate has persistent jaundice that was present since birth treated with phototherapy. On examination, severe pallor, irritability, frontal bossing, and hepatosplenomegaly are noted. Initial labs reveal:
- hemoglobin 9 g/dL (14-24)
- MCV 64 fL (80-100) with hypochromia
- increased RBC count
- elevated indirect hyperbilirubinemia
- elevated LDH levels
- reduced haptoglobin, and the following on peripheral smear (see photo)

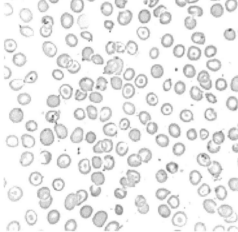

Which of the following is the most likely diagnosis?
a. Iron deficiency anemia
b. Alpha thalassemia minor
c. Hemoglobin Barts disease
d. Beta thalassemia major (Cooley anemia)
e. Alpha thalassemia intermedia (Hemoglobin H disease)

Photo credit:
Ed   Uthman   from   Houston,   TX,   USA,   CC   BY   2.0
<https://creativecommons.org/licenses/by/2.0>, via Wikimedia Commons

53. A 32-year-old female is complaining of recurrent paroxysms of severe right-sided facial pain described as a jolt of electricity and shooting in nature, lasting for a few seconds. The pain radiates to the right ear, temporal area, and jawline. The pain is provoked by talking, chewing, or cold wind gusts. She denies numbness or muscle weakness. Physical examination is unremarkable except for reproduction of the pain with light touching of the face. Which of the following tests should be part of the workup of this patient?
a. Noncontrast CT head
b. Temporal artery biopsy
c. MRI/MRA of the brain with and without contrast
d. Trigeminal reflex testing
e. Lumbar puncture

54. A 40-year-old male presents to the clinic with exertional dyspnea, malaise, weight loss, and chronic dry cough for the last 2 years. He denies smoking. He has been breeding carrier pigeons for the last 10 years. Physical examination reveals inspiratory squeaks and bibasilar crackles. Chest radiograph is obtained (see photo).

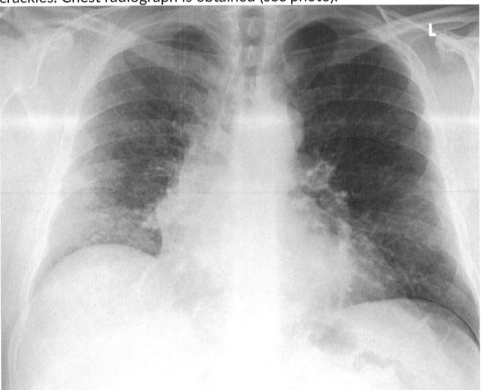

Pulmonary function testing reveals decreased FEV1, increased FEV1/FVC, as well as low diffusing lung capacity for carbon monoxide and partial pressure of oxygen. In addition to minimizing contact with potential inciting antigens, which of the following is recommended next step in the management of this patient?
a. Prednisone
b. Azithromycin
c. Albuterol
d. Lung transplantation
e. Montelukast

55. A 31-year-old male is referred to the endocrinology clinic for neck swelling. Vitals are stable. Physical examination is notable for a goiter. Initial labs reveal
- Serum TSH: 0.002 µIU/mL (0.4–4.8).
- Serum free T4: 2.82 ng/dL (0.8–1.71)

Thyroid scintigraphy is performed (see photo).

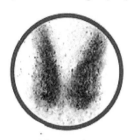 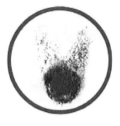

Normal   Patient

Which of the following is the most likely diagnosis?
a. Hashimoto thyroiditis
b. Toxic multinodular goiter
c. Graves' disease
d. Papillary thyroid carcinoma
e. Toxic adenoma

Photo credit:
Petros Perros, CC BY-SA 3.0 <https://creativecommons.org/licenses/by-sa/3.0>, via Wikimedia Commons

56. A 65-year-old male with a longstanding history of Chronic bronchitis is found to have a decrescendo diastolic high-pitched blowing murmur heard loudest at the left second intercostal space. The murmur increases in intensity with inspiration and decreases in intensity with Valsalva strain. Which of the following is the most likely diagnosis?
a. Aortic regurgitation
b. Aortic stenosis
c. Pulmonic stenosis
d. Mitral stenosis
e. Pulmonic regurgitation

57. A 3-month-old boy is brought to the clinic for multiple episodes of gagging and gasping for air after severe coughing over the last 48 hours. During the last event, he started coughing intensely during a feed, vomited, and then stopped breathing. He became cyanotic for about 10 seconds, then quickly returned to normal. He has history of clear rhinorrhea and increasing cough for 1 week. On examination, there is nasal congestion and clear rhinorrhea without crackles, wheezing, or stridor. Cardiopulmonary examination is normal. Which of the following is the most appropriate pharmacotherapy for this patient?
a. Oseltamivir
b. Azithromycin
c. Albuterol
d. Prednisone
e. Amoxicillin

58. A 64-year-old female presents to the ED complaining of epigastric discomfort that began during dinner 1 hour ago. The discomfort is associated with nausea and vomiting. The discomfort was not relieved with antacids. Vitals are stable. An ECG is performed (see photo).

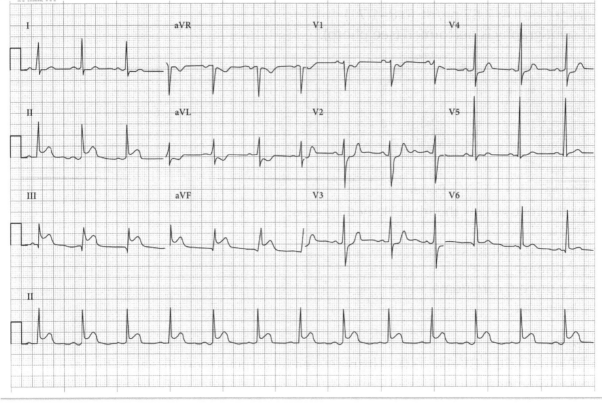

She is administered Aspirin, Clopidogrel, Heparin, and IV fluids. Which of the following is the most appropriate next step in the management of this patient?
a. Percutaneous coronary intervention
b. IV Alteplase
c. Add Verapamil
d. TIMI risk factor assessment
e. Add IV Morphine

59. A 25-year-old male presents to the clinic in December with a 3-day history of fever, myalgia, back pain, malaise, clear rhinorrhea, frontal headache, sore throat, and fatigue of abrupt onset. He has a past medical history of Asthma and has not received the Influenza vaccine this year. Vitals reveal a temperature 100°F (37.7°C), blood pressure 120/72 mmHg, pulse 104/min, and respiratory rate 20/min. Clear rhinorrhea, conjunctival erythema, erythematous pharynx, symmetrical chest expansion, and clear breath sounds are noted. Which of the following is the next best step in the management of this patient?
a. Influenza vaccination
b. Amantadine
c. Doxycycline
d. Ibuprofen
e. Oseltamivir and Acetaminophen

60. A 12-year-old male is being evaluated for frequent, bulky, foul-smelling stools that are oily and poor weight gain. He also has a history of frequent severe respiratory infections and chronic rhinosinusitis. Initial labs reveal serum 25-hydroxyvitamin D (25[OH]D) levels of 10 ng/mL (30-50). Initial stool studies show increased fecal fat and increased fecal elastase. Which of the following tests would be most helpful to establish the most likely diagnosis?
a. Transglutaminase antibodies
b. Anti-mitochondrial antibodies
c. Bronchial provocation testing
d. Parietal cell antibodies
e. Sweat chloride test

61. A 50-year-old male is admitted to the hospital for Myocardial infarction. He becomes unarousable. On examination, there are no palpable carotid, brachial, or femoral pulses. The following is seen on the monitor (see photo).

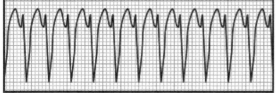

In addition to chest compressions, which of the following is the most appropriate next step?
a. Synchronized cardioversion
b. Unsynchronized cardioversion
c. Amiodarone
d. Magnesium sulfate
e. Verapamil

62. A 65-year-old male presents to the clinic for an annual physical examination. He has a history of Hypertension and a 20-pack year smoking history. He denies any symptoms. Physical examination is notable for an abdominal bruit. Abdominal ultrasonography reveals an abdominal aorta of 5.5 cm. Which of the following is the recommended next step as per the Society for Vascular Surgery guidelines?
a. No further management is needed
b. Repeat ultrasound in 3-6 months
c. Repeat ultrasound in 6-12 months
d. Surgical repair
e. Repeat ultrasound in 3 years

63. A 50-year-old female presents with fever and weight loss. She has a history of seropositive Rheumatoid arthritis. Physical examination is positive for mild splenomegaly. Felty syndrome is suspected. Which of the following diagnostic studies would be most helpful in establishing the most likely diagnosis?
a. Arthrocentesis
b. Absolute neutrophil count (ANC) <1500 mm^3
c. Chest radiograph revealing pulmonary nodules
d. Pulmonary function testing showing a restrictive pattern
e. Liver function testing showing AST:ALT ratio >2:1

64. A 30-year-old female at 12 weeks gestation presents with abrupt onset of dyspnea, pleuritic chest pain, and hemoptysis after a long plane ride. Physical examination reveals tachypnea and tachycardia. An ECG shows sinus tachycardia and SaO_2: 88% room air. Chest radiograph is normal. Initial labs reveal a BUN: 18 mg/dL (7-20), creatinine 1.9 (0.6-1.2), sodium 140 mEq/L (135-145), and K: 3.8 mEq/L (3.5-5). Pulmonary embolism is suspected. Which of the following is the most appropriate next step?
a. Lung scintigraphy (Ventilation perfusion scan)
b. D dimer
c. CT pulmonary angiography (High resolution CT scan)
d. Compressive Doppler ultrasonography of the lower extremities
e. Pulmonary function testing

65. A 57-year-old male presents to his primary care practitioner complaining of knee pain and stiffness. The pain worsens with activity throughout the day and with climbing stairs. He experiences morning stiffness lasting ~5-15 minutes after waking up. Physical examination is notable for crepitus and the knee joint is cool to touch. Radiographs are obtained (see photo).

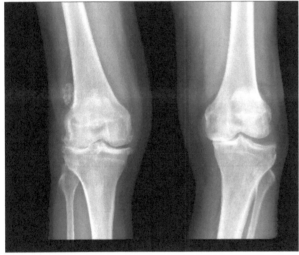

Which of the following is the recommended initial management in this patient?
a. Duloxetine
b. Intraarticular Triamcinolone
c. Topical Diclofenac
d. Topical Capsaicin
e. Naproxen

66. A 50-year-old male is to undergo a routine colonoscopy. He is informed that he will undergo anesthesia and is explained the potential risks of the colonoscopy. Which of the following types of consent is required?
a. Conditional
b. Verbal
c. Written
d. Passive
e. Implied

67. A 46-year-old male presents with trouble walking. Over the last 10 months, he has developed progressive weakness of his upper and lower extremities. Recently, he developed difficulties speaking and swallowing. He denies numbness, weakness, or paresthesia. On examination, flaccid weakness in the right arm, left forearm muscle atrophy, hyperreflexia on the right with right upgoing plantar responses, fasciculations of the muscles of his tongue, and right biceps atrophy are noted. His gait is spastic with spontaneous ankle clonus. Which of the following is the most likely diagnosis?
a. Amyotrophic lateral sclerosis
b. Guillain-Barre syndrome
c. Multiple sclerosis
d. Myasthenia gravis
e. Inflammatory myopathy

68. A 32-year-old woman is being evaluated for worsening heavy menstrual bleeding over the last 2 years. She is sexually active and uses condoms for contraception. She is planning on becoming pregnant in the next 12 months. Pelvic examination shows an asymmetrically enlarged and firm nontender uterus. Urine hCG is negative. Pelvic ultrasound reveals 2 submucosal fibroids. Which of the following is the recommended next step in the management of this patient's menorrhagia?
a. Endometrial ablation
b. Uterine artery embolization
c. Combination oral contraceptive pills
d. Copper-containing intrauterine device
e. Hysteroscopic myomectomy

69. A 20-year-old male presents to the emergency department with excruciating retrosternal and upper abdominal pain that radiates to the back. The pain is sharp and worsens with swallowing. He had been drinking alcohol heavily prior to forcefully retching and vomiting, which heralded the onset of pain. Vitals are notable for tachycardia and tachypnea. On physical examination, there is crepitus upon chest palpation and mediastinal crackling with each heartbeat. There is moderate epigastric tenderness without guarding, rigidity, or rebound tenderness. Which of the following is the most likely diagnosis?
a. Peptic ulcer perforation
b. Mallory-Weiss tear
c. Acute pancreatitis due to alcohol
d. Esophageal rupture
e. Aortic dissection

70. A 24-year-old female presents after a brief syncopal episode. She has had 3 prior episodes. She has no past medical history and does not take any medications. An ECG is performed, revealing a QTc interval of 520 msec. Which of the following is the first line management of choice?
a. Amiodarone
b. Sotalol
c. Propranolol
d. Quinidine
e. Procainamide

71. A 45-year-old male is diagnosed with severe Alcohol use disorder. He has begun alcohol counseling and has been participating in a mutual help group. He is requesting additional pharmacotherapy. Which of the following is a first line agent for this patient?
a. Naltrexone
b. Flumazenil
c. Naloxone
d. Methadone
e. Chlordiazepoxide

72. A 2-year-old male with a history of Hypospadias presents with mild abdominal pain and swelling. On examination, he is noted to have no irises, consistent with aniridia. There is a palpable, nontender mass on the right side of his abdomen. Urinalysis is positive for hematuria. Which of the following is the most likely diagnosis?
a. Nephroblastoma
b. Neuroblastoma
c. Pheochromocytoma
d. Ewing sarcoma
e. Renal cell carcinoma

73. An 18-year-old male presents with a painless "lump in his neck". Review of systems is positive for recurrent fever over the past month, fatigue, and decreased appetite. Examination reveals enlarged lymph nodes in the left cervical region only that are nontender, firm, rubbery, and mobile with swallowing with no overlying erythema or warmth. An excisional biopsy is performed (see photo).

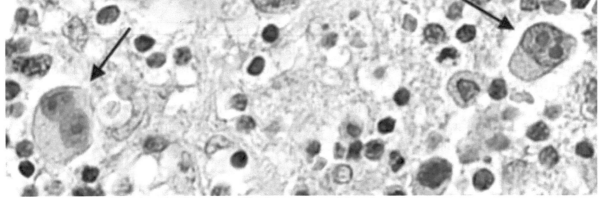

Which of the following is the most likely seen on histology?
a. Lymphocyte depleted
b. Nodular sclerosis
c. Diffuse large B cell
d. Lymphocyte rich
e. Follicular lymphoma

74. A 65-year-old man with a history of Hypertension presents to his primary care provider for blood pressure management. He is compliant with Hydrochlorothiazide and Amlodipine with minimal effect. Physical examination is notable for a bruit in the right flank. Initial labs reveal a normal serum creatinine. Doppler ultrasonography of both renal arteries reveals significant stenosis of 74% the right renal artery. Which of the following is the most appropriate management for this condition?
a. Initiate Lisinopril
b. Right renal artery stenting
c. Renal artery bypass graft
d. Right nephrectomy
e. Initiate Atenolol

75. A 70-year-old female presents to the clinic complaining of easy bruising, frequent respiratory infections, and fatigue. She has a history of Thyroid carcinoma treated with surgery followed by radiation 10 years ago. Labs reveal:
- hemoglobin 9.1 g/dL (12-16)
- white cell count 4,000/mm^3 (5,000-10,000)
- absolute neutrophil count 1,080/microL (2,500-7,000)
- platelet count: 88,000/mm^3 (150,000-450,000)
- reticulocyte count 0.1% (0.5-2.5%).

Peripheral smear reveals hypogranular neutrophils with reduced segmentation and bilobed nuclei (see photo).

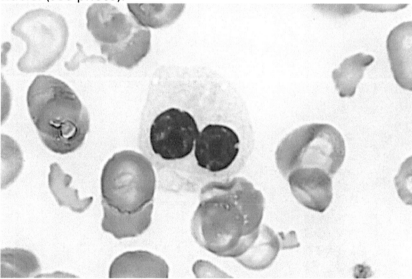

Which of the following is the most likely diagnosis?
a. Myelodysplastic syndrome
b. Primary myelofibrosis
c. Polycythemia vera
d. Chronic myelogenous leukemia
e. Hodgkin lymphoma

Photo credit:
The Armed Forces Institute of Pathology (AFIP), Public domain, via Wikimedia Commons

76. A 33-year-old female presents to the clinic complaining of episodes of substernal chest discomfort around midnight to early morning, often awakening her from sleep. The episodes are accompanied by nausea, sweating, and dizziness but not breathlessness. Each episode generally lasts 5 to 15 minutes and resolves spontaneously. ECG is normal but showed transient ST-segment elevations in leads V1, V2, and V3 during an episode. Cardiac arteriography reveals no significant coronary artery occlusion. Which of the following is the first line long-term management of choice?
a. Propranolol
b. Diltiazem
c. Aspirin plus Rosuvastatin
d. Cilostazol
e. Digoxin

77. A 25-year-old male presents with fever, sudden onset rigors, and right-sided pleuritic chest pain. Vitals are BP: 130/80 mmHg, P: 120/minute, and R: 20/min. Lung examination reveals decreased increased fremitus on the right, with bronchial breath sounds. A chest radiograph is obtained (see photo).

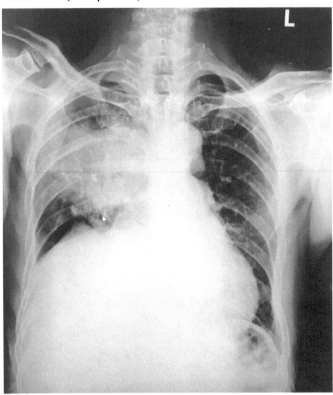

Which of the following is the most likely etiology of his presentation?
a. *Streptococcus pneumoniae*
b. *Mycoplasma pneumoniae*
c. *Klebsiella pneumoniae*
d. *Haemophilus influenzae*
e. *Chlamydophila pneumoniae*

Photo credit:
Shutterstock (used with permission)

78. A 35-year-old male presents with right knee pain and swelling while playing soccer. On examination, there is a joint effusion without ecchymosis. He has pain with walking but a normal gait. Valgus stress testing is positive. Which of the following is the most likely diagnosis?

a. Patellofemoral syndrome

b. Lateral collateral ligament injury

c. Anterior cruciate ligament injury

d. Medial collateral ligament injury

e. Posterior cruciate ligament injury

79. A 13-year-old male is incidentally noted to have a palpable 1 cm solitary midline neck mass. He denies pain, dysphagia, or dyspnea. There is no family history of thyroid nodules or cancer. He does not take any thyroid medications. Vitals are normal. The nodule is freely mobile with swallowing and nontender. No other neck masses or lymphadenopathy are noted. Labs reveal a serum TSH of 1.7 mIU/L (0.5-5.0). Which of the following is the next step in the workup of this patient?

a. Serum free T4 and Total T3

b. Iodine 131 nuclear medicine scan (scintigraphy)

c. Thyroid ultrasound

d. Fine needle aspiration

e. Serum calcitonin levels

80. A 64-year-old male is brought to the clinic for progressive cognitive deficits. He has a history of Alzheimer disease, for which he is on Donepezil. His Mini mental examination score is 16. Addition of which of the following is recommended in this patient?

a. Bromocriptine

b. Levodopa-Carbidopa

c. Memantine

d. Deutetrabenazine

e. Aducanumab

81. A 15-year-old male with no past medical history presents for a yearly physical examination. On examination, long, slender, and lanky fingers, joint laxity, pectus carinatum, and a midsystolic click are noted. Which of the following would most likely be seen on physical examination?

a. Upward and temporally displaced lenses

b. Skin hyperextensibility

c. Macroorchidism

d. Multiple soft tissue bruises

e. Hypertrophic scar formation

82. A 52-year-old male presents to his primary care provider complaining of pain in his legs after walking more than 10 blocks. He has a past medical history of Dyslipidemia, Hypertension, and a 30-pack year smoking history. On physical examination, the dorsalis pedis and posterior tibialis pulses are faint but palpable, Which of the following would most likely be seen on physical examination of this patient?
a. Skin that is warm to the touch
b. Eczematous patches or plaques with brownish discoloration
c. Medial malleolar ulcers
d. Peripheral edema
e. Erythema with leg dependency

83. A 50-year-old male returns to the clinic for localized eyelid swelling for 10 days. He denies pain, vision changes, ocular pruritus, or preceding injury. Physical examination is notable for a nontender rubbery nodule on the lateral aspect of the right upper eyelid without overlying erythema or warmth. He is told to apply frequent warm compresses to the area. He returns 2 months later, and the eyelid findings remain unchanged. Which of the following is the most appropriate next step in the management of this patient?
a. Prescribe topical Methylprednisolone acetate
b. Referral to an ophthalmologist
c. Prescribe Ciprofloxacin ophthalmic solution
d. Continue warm compresses and follow up in 8 weeks
e. Prescribe Amoxicillin-clavulanate

84. A 65-year-old male presents to the emergency department after a trip and fall. He is complaining of mild headache and dizziness. Physical examination reveals a superficial laceration to the scalp and a scalp hematoma. A Noncontrast CT of the head is performed.

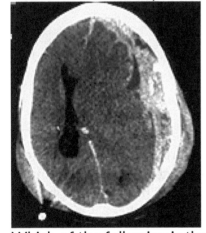

Which of the following is the most likely etiology of his presentation?
a. Rupture of a cortical bridging vein
b. Rupture of a Berry aneurysm
c. Rupture of the small cortical arteries
d. Arteriovenous malformations
e. Rupture of the middle meningeal artery

Photo credit:
Glitzy queen00 at English Wikipedia, Public domain, via Wikimedia Commons

85. A 56-year-old female presents with right wrist pain, swelling, and deformity to the wrist. He accidentally slipped and fell on the slippery floor after mopping and he landed with an outstretched hand on the ground. He is complaining of paresthesias to the hand. Radiographs are obtained (see photo).

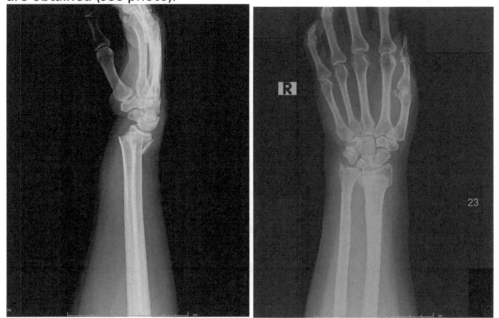

Which of the following is most likely present due to nerve injury associated with the radiograph findings?
a. Loss of two-point discrimination over the fifth finger
b. Loss of abduction and opposition of the thumb against resistance
c. Decreased extension of the wrist against resistance
d. Adduction of the index, fourth, and fifth digits
e. Inability to make the O.K. sign by touching the tips of the index finger and the thumb together

Photo credit:
Case courtesy of Rodolfo Antonio Perez Mackenzie, Radiopaedia.org, rID: 63525

86. A 40-year-old male with a history of uncontrolled Hypertension presents with bleeding from his left nostril. He also admits to nose picking. Topical Oxymetazoline is applied to the left nare and direct pressure to the nares is applied. He is instructed to sit with his head forward. 20 minutes later, he is now complaining of a sensation of blood trickling down his throat and blood emanating from both nares. Which of the following is the most common source of his bleeding?
a. Kiesselbach plexus
b. Anterior ethmoid artery
c. Sphenopalatine artery
d. Superior labial artery
e. Greater palatine artery

87. A 30-year-old male presents to the clinic for a follow-up appointment. He has a history of Schizophrenia, for which he was placed on Fluphenazine. Since his last visit he has gained 20 lbs. and has developed a fine hand tremor. He has been going to the gym 4 days a week, working out for 1 hour but has not been able to lose weight. His BMI is now 35. He desires to be switched to a new medication. Which of the following medications should the patient be switched to?
a. Olanzapine
b. Aripiprazole
c. Clozapine
d. Haloperidol
e. Chlorpromazine

88. A 30-year-old female with a history of a Gastrinoma treated with resection 3 years ago is complaining of nausea, malaise, and headache. Initial labs reveal
- serum calcium level of 11.5 mg/dL (8.5–10)
- serum intact parathyroid hormone (iPTH) measurement of 984 pg/mL (10–65)
- serum phosphate of 2.2 mg/dL (2.7-4.5).

Which of the following is most consistent with the lab findings?
a. increased deep tendon reflexes
b. prolonged QT interval
c. positive Chvostek's sign
d. circumoral paresthesias
e. absent bowel sounds

89. A 6-year-old boy presents with a 2-day history fever, urgency, and dysuria for 3 days. He denies any abdominal pain or hematuria. This is his third episode in 6 months. He was previously diagnosed with Acute cystitis and treated with appropriate antibiotics. Urinalysis shows pyuria and positive leukocyte esterase. BUN and creatinine are within normal limits. Ultrasound of the abdomen reveals fusion at the inferior pole of both kidneys. Which of the following is most commonly associated with this condition?
a. Aniridia
b. Ureteropelvic junction obstruction
c. Hypospadias
d. Renal malignancies
e. Absent ureters

90. A 27-year-old G1P2 at 32+2 weeks gestation presents to labor and delivery with contractions. She has been having 1 painful contraction every 15 minutes for the past 3 hours and reports mild spotting on her underwear. A transabdominal ultrasound is performed followed by a pelvic exam. Her cervix is effaced 82% and dilated 4 cm. Which of the following is the most recommended next step in the management of this patient?
a. Continue progression of labor
b. Nifedipine and Betamethasone
c. Indomethacin and Betamethasone
d. Observation and watchful waiting
e. Cesarean section

91. A 29-year-old auto mechanic presents to the emergency department (ED) with moderate right eye pain, blurred vision, and photophobia. He was working on a car engine when the battery ruptured, and battery fluid splashed into his right eye. He irrigated the eye for a few minutes at work and was brought to the ED by his supervisor. He has difficulty opening his eyelids and right conjunctival redness is noted. In addition to rapid determination of the ocular pH, which of the following is the most appropriate next step?
a. Topical Proparacaine 0.5% followed by copious irrigation with Lactated ringers
b. Perform a visual acuity test in both eyes
c. Pupil dilation and examination with slit lamp examination
d. Topical Erythromycin ointment 0.5% and ophthalmology consultation
e. Application of Fluorescein strip and slit lamp examination to assess for abrasion or ulcerations

92. A 55-year-old female presents to the clinic due to leakage of urine. She feels like she is "constantly wet". She experiences hesitancy and nocturia, frequently waking her up at night. She has a history of Diabetes mellitus and underwent menopause at age 50. On examination, dribbling of urine is noted and there is no leakage when she is asked to cough. There is reduced perineal sensation to pinprick testing. Urinalysis is negative for leukocyte esterase and nitrites. Which of the following is the most likely diagnosis?
a. Urge incontinence
b. Overflow incontinence
c. Genitourinary syndrome of menopause
d. Stress incontinence
e. Urethral hypomobility

93. A 33-year-old man presents with fever, chills, malaise, neck swelling, and swallowing difficulty. He has had pain in the lower left second molar since last week. He has a history of multiple dental caries. Extraoral examination shows bilateral submandibular tenderness, induration, and palpable crepitus without fluctuance involving the upper neck, chin, and floor of the mouth. Intraoral examination is limited due to trismus and tongue elevation, and he is drooling. Which of the following is the next best step in management of this patient?
a. Computed tomography (CT) of the neck with intravenous contrast
b. Magnetic resonance imaging (MRI) of the neck
c. Needle aspiration
d. Early surgical decompression
e. IV Methylprednisolone

94. A 50-year-old male presents with headache and bone pain. Initial labs reveal
- serum calcium 7.2 mg/dL (8.5-10)
- serum phosphate 5.3 mg/dL (3.5-4.5)
- serum intact parathyroid hormone (iPTH) 436 pg/mL (10-55)

Radiographs of the skull are obtained, revealing ground-glass densities (see photo).

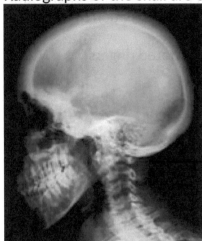

Which of the following is the most likely etiology of his presentation?
a. Parathyroid adenoma
b. Parathyroid hyperplasia
c. Chronic kidney disease
d. Multiple myeloma
e. Autoimmune destruction of the parathyroid gland

Photo credit:
Anish A. Patel, Rohit Ramanathan, Joshua Kuban, and Marc H. Willis, CC BY 3.0 <https://creativecommons.org/licenses/by/3.0>, via Wikimedia Commons

Choice E [Autoimmune destruction of the parathyroid gland] is associated with Primary hypoparathyroidism, associated with the triad of decreased iPTH, hypocalcemia, and increased serum phosphate.

95. A 50-year-old woman is complaining of gradual onset of muscle weakness for several months. She has difficulty getting up from a chair, climbing the stairs, and placing her groceries on the top shelves in her kitchen. She also reports fatigue. Physical examination is notable for 3/5 muscle strength in the deltoids and hip flexors without tenderness and 2+ biceps, triceps, patellar, and ankle tendon reflexes. Repeated use does not change the muscle weakness. Which of the following is the best to confirm the most likely diagnosis?

a. Electromyography

b. Aldolase levels

c. Acetylcholine receptor antibodies

d. Muscle biopsy

e. Erythrocyte sedimentation rate

96. A 25-year-old administrative assistant is complaining of pain, tingling described as a pins and needles sensation, and numbness on the left hand that sometimes wakes him up. The symptoms mildly improve with shaking of his hand. The symptoms primarily involve the left thumb, index, and middle fingers. On examination, pain and paresthesias are elicited when the clinician percusses the patient's wrist as well as when the patient is asked to flex both of his palms at the wrist. There is no hypothenar or thenar eminence atrophy. Which of the following is the most appropriate initial step in the management of this patient's condition?
a. Volar (cock-up) splint in neutral position at night
b. Place the patient in an ulnar gutter splint with orthopedic follow-up
c. Surgical decompression
d. Oral Prednisone
e. Naproxen

97. A 40-year-old male is complaining of dental pain for 3 days, worse with consumption of cold drinks. The pain is increasing in intensity and has become continuous. He has a history of dental caries but refused fillings. On physical exam, the patient has a localized area of swelling in the gum line adjacent to the right first premolar. The swelling is fluctuant and tender. Which of the following is the most appropriate next step?
a. Perform a root canal
b. Place a dental filling
c. Azithromycin
d. Trimethoprim-sulfamethoxazole
e. Penicillin V potassium

98. A 54-year-old male with a history of Hypertension presents to the clinic for an annual physical examination. He denies chest pain, shortness of breath, or dizziness. Vitals are blood pressure 132/72 mmHg, P: 50 bpm, O2 sat: 99% room air. The following is seen on heart monitoring (see photo).

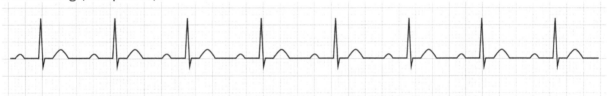

Which of the following is the most appropriate next step in this patient?
a. Atropine
b. No further management is needed
c. Transcutaneous pacing
d. Epinephrine
e. Permanent pacemaker placement

99. A 51-year-old female presents with pruritus to her left nipple, initially associated with a burning sensation. The lesion has worsened with darkening of the skin surrounding the nipple and has not resolved with Aloe vera gel application. She denies pain, bleeding, or nipple discharge. Physical examination is notable for a scaly vesicular lesion on the nipple extending to the areola. There are no palpable masses or axillary lymphadenopathy. Which of the following is the most likely diagnosis?
a. Intraductal papilloma
b. Paget disease of the breast
c. Contact dermatitis
d. Candida mastitis
e. Inflammatory breast cancer

100. A 28-year-old woman at 37+3 weeks gestation with an uncomplicated pregnancy presents to the emergency department after leakage of clear fluid from her vagina. She denies abdominal pain, uterine contraction, or bleeding. Nitrazine strip tests blue when a sample of the fluid is tested. Group B streptococcus testing is negative. Fetal nonstress testing is reassuring. The Obstetrician informs the patient that prompt induction of labor is recommended. The patent wants to wait to see if labor will "happen naturally". Which of the following is the most appropriate next step in the management of this patient?
a. Induction of labor
b. Explain to the patient the risks and benefits of induction vs. expectant management
c. Consult the hospital ethics committee
d. Consult with the husband to change her mind for what is best for the unborn child
e. Perform a Cesarean section

END OF EXAM 5

1. CARDIOLOGY – MITRAL STENOSIS [HISTORY AND PHYSICAL]
Rheumatic heart disease (RHD) [choice B] is by far the most common cause of Mitral stenosis (MS); other causes are much less frequent.
The onset of Rheumatic MS is usually between the third and fourth decades of life.
A mid-diastolic rumbling murmur with presystolic accentuation heard after the opening snap and a loud S1 are hallmark of MS.

Other much less frequent causes of Mitral stenosis include:
- Mitral annular calcification
- Radiation-associated valve disease
- Congenital heart disease is uncommon and usually present in childhood or infancy
- Infective endocarditis, mitral annular calcification,
- Systemic lupus erythematosus, Rheumatoid arthritis.

2. PROFESSIONAL PRACTICE – ADVANCED DIRECTIVES
In patient's without documented advanced directives, the patient's wishes as expressed by his spouse [choice E] is the most appropriate course of action.
In patients without documented advance directive, the order in which the actions should be followed are medical power of attorney > spouse or intimate partner > adult child > parent > adult sibling.

3. INFECTIOUS DISEASE – RUBELLA [HISTORY AND PHYSICAL]
Rubella [choice A] is a childhood exanthem characterized by typically characterized by
- **rash: maculopapular exanthem (discrete pinpoint lesions) that spares the palms and soles.**
- **fever**
- **lymphadenopathy: posterior cervical, suboccipital, and postauricular lymphadenopathy.**

Rubella should be suspected in a nonimmune individual who shows symptoms or signs consistent with rubella infection (eg, rash, fever, lymphadenopathy).

Choice A [Erythema infectiosum] presents with prodromal symptoms, followed facial erythema with circumoral pallor ("slapped cheek" appearance) followed by development of a lacy reticular rash on the extremities and trunk. It is not associated with the suboccipital lymphadenopathy.
Choice C [Rubeola] presents with the 3 C's (cough, coryza, conjunctivitis), followed by a brick red rash that starts on the face, spreads, and coalesces.
Choice D [Scarlet fever] presents with sore throat, erythematous rash with rough (sandpaper) texture, circumoral pallor, and a strawberry tongue. It is rare under the age of 3.
Choice E [Kawasaki disease] presents with "WARM + CREAM" — fever for ≥5 days with 4 of the following: conjunctivitis, rash, extremity edema, lymphadenopathy, and mucositis.

4. REPRODUCTIVE – EMERGENCY CONTRACEPTION [HEALTH MAINTENANCE]
The Copper-containing intrauterine device [choice D] is the most effective emergency contraception method.
In order of maximal to minimal efficacy: Copper TCu380A IUD (most effective) > Levonorgestrel IUD > Ulipristal acetate (UPA) > oral Levonorgestrel.

When used for emergency contraception, the copper TCu380A and Levonorgestrel 52 mg IUDs result in pregnancy rates of <1%.

The oral medication EC methods UPA [choice E] & oral Levonorgestrel [choice B] have pregnancy rates of ~1-3%.

5. PSYCHIATRY/BEHAVIORAL – ANTISOCIAL PERSONALITY DISORDER/ASPD [HISTORY AND PHYSICAL]

Although Antisocial personality is only diagnosed in adults (≥18 years of age), individuals with ASPD will have had symptoms in childhood consistent with Conduct disorder [choice A].
Although most children with Conduct disorder do not develop adult ASPD, 40% of boys and 25% of girls eventually develop ASPD.
Similar to ASPD, Conduct disorder is diagnosed in children and adolescents with a repetitive and persistent pattern of behavior violating basic rights of others or major societal norms or rules, including bullying, truancy, theft, etc.

6. PULMONOLOGY – BRONCHIAL CARCINOID TUMOR [HISTORY AND PHYSICAL]

Acute symptoms of Carcinoid syndrome include:
- <u>**Histamine release:**</u> **cutaneous flushing [choice D] and bronchospasm**
- <u>**Serotonin release:**</u> **diarrhea.**

Carcinoid syndrome may occur due to Bronchial carcinoid tumor, a neuroendocrine tumor caused by systemic release of vasoactive substances such as serotonin and other bioactive amines, such as histamine, serotonin, dopamine, and norepinephrine.
Patients may complain of cough or wheeze, hemoptysis, chest pain, or recurrent pneumonia.
The classic appearance of Bronchial carcinoid tumor on bronchoscopy is a typically pink to red vascular mass with intact overlying bronchial epithelium.

7. MUSCULOSKELETAL – BOXER FRACTURE [APPLYING FOUNDATIONAL CONCEPTS]

Direct trauma to the clenched fist [choice D] is the most common cause of fracture of the fifth metacarpal neck (Boxer fracture).
The energy is transferred through the fifth metacarpal axially and mostly results in apex dorsal angulation due to the pull of the interosseous muscles of the hand.

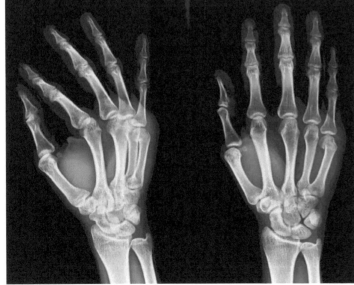

8. REPRODUCTIVE – ABNORMAL UTERINE BLEEDING [PHARMACOLOGY]

The Levonorgestrel intrauterine device (IUD) is the most effective hormonal therapy for Abnormal uterine bleeding.

The initial management of choice for Abnormal uterine bleeding include:
- Levonorgestrel IUD (most effective),
- Combined Oral contraceptives (OCPs), or
- Progestins.

9. GENITOURINARY – PROSTATE CANCER [HISTORY AND PHYSICAL]

Prostate cancer has one of the strongest relationship between age [choice E] than any other human malignancy.

Prostate cancer risk begins to rise sharply after age 55 years (99% of cases occur over the age of 50 years) and peaks at age 70–74, declining slightly after age 74.

The 3 most established risk factors for the development of Prostate cancer include [1] age, [2] race/ethnicity and [3] family history.

Other risk factors may include:
- Cigarette smoking and tobacco use -shows conflicting data on being an independent risk factor for Prostate cancer
- Obesity shows a small but statistically significant risk for Prostate cancer.
- Diet low in vegetables may be a for Prostate cancer as is a diet high in animal fat

Choice D [Benign prostatic hyperplasia] does not increase the risk for Prostate cancer.

10. NEUROLOGY – ANTERIOR CORD SYNDROME [MOST LIKELY]

Anterior cord syndrome [choice B] most commonly occurs after a hyperflexion injury and involves injury to the spinothalamic tract, and is characterized by:
- **<u>motor deficits</u> in the lower extremities**
- **bladder dysfunction**
- **<u>sensory deficits</u>: loss of temperature, pain, light touch sensation below the lesion (eg, lower extremities)**
- **<u>preservation of the posterior columns</u>: sparing of proprioception, vibration, pressure, and fine touch.**

Anterior cord syndrome may occur after:
- <u>hyperflexion injuries</u> with bony instability, acute disc herniation, or hematoma formation.
- <u>direct or indirect injury to the anterior spinal cord</u>: crush injury or compression from a hematoma; indirect injury result from ischemia secondary to compression of the anterior spinal artery.

Choice A [Posterior cord syndrome] is associated with sensory ataxia: vibration and fine touch deficits and proprioception deficits – decreased coordination of voluntary movements, leading to poor balance, unsteady gait, and falls. It usually occurs in the setting of B12 deficiency, late Neurosyphilis, or Multiple sclerosis.

Central cord syndrome [choice C] usually occurs after a fall with neck hyperextension and is characterized by significant strength impairments more prominent in the upper extremities (especially the hands) in a shawl like distribution compared to the lower extremities.

Choice D [Brown Sequard syndrome] usually presents with ipsilateral motor, vibratory, and proprioception deficits and contralateral pain and temperature deficits. It usually occurs after a penetrating injury to the spinal cord.

Choice E [Middle cerebral artery stroke] presents with contralateral motor and sensory deficits of the face and upper extremity greater than the lower extremity.

11. ENDOCRINOLOGY – TYPE 1 DIABETES MELLITUS [HISTORY AND PHYSICAL EXAMINATION]

Weight loss [choice D] is more of a feature of Type 1 Diabetes mellitus due to
- hypovolemia and increased catabolism.
- Insulin deficiency impairs glucose utilization in skeletal muscle and increases fat and muscle breakdown.
- ketosis leads to nausea and anorexia, contributing to weight loss.

Ketonuria and weight loss are uncommon at time of diagnosis in patients with Type 2 Diabetes mellitus.

The 3 classic presentations of Type I Diabetes mellitus include:
- [1] <u>Hyperglycemia without acidosis</u>: most common initial presentation — polyuria, polydipsia, polyphagia; weight loss, paresthesias, blurred vision (lens exposed to hyperosmolar fluids).
- [2] <u>Diabetic ketoacidosis</u> second most common initial presentation — ketonemia & ketonuria.
- [3] <u>Silent (asymptomatic)</u> incidental discovery. Lethargy, weakness, or fatigue

Choice A [Fatigue], choice B [Polyuria], and choice C [polydipsia] can be seen in both.

Choice E [Vulvovaginal infection] is more common in Type 2 Diabetes mellitus compared to Type 1 Diabetes mellitus.

12. HEMATOLOGY – HEREDITARY SPHEROCYTOSIS [MOST LIKELY]

Hereditary spherocytosis (HS) [choice D] should be suspected in patients with:
- **splenomegaly** (due to increased hemolysis)
- <u>**spherocytes**</u> **and increased reticulocytes on peripheral blood smear**
- <u>**hyperchromic RBCs**</u> **[elevated mean corpuscular hemoglobin concentration (MCHC)]**
- mild or moderate hemolytic anemia
- <u>**negative Direct antiglobulin (Coombs) test**</u> (distinguishes HS from Autoimmune hemolytic anemia).

Choice A [Gilbert syndrome] is associated with an isolated indirect bilirubinemia without hemolysis.

Choice B [Glucose-6-phosphate dehydrogenase deficiency] is associated with episodic hemolytic anemia without a predominance of spherocytes.

Choice C [Warm autoimmune hemolytic anemia] is also associated with hemolytic anemia and spherocytes on peripheral smear, but Warm AIHA is associated with Direct antiglobulin test positivity for IgG.

Choice E [Cold agglutinin disease] is also associated with hemolytic anemia but CAD is also associated with Direct antiglobulin test positivity for complement (C3).

13. ENDOCRINOLOGY – DIABETIC KETOACIDOSIS [CLINICAL INTERVENTION]

Treatment should be switched to 5% Dextrose in saline [choice C] when the serum glucose approaches 200 mg/dL in Diabetic ketoacidosis (DKA) or 250-300 mg/dL in Hyperglycemic hyperosmolar syndrome (HHS).

Dextrose is added to prevent Hypoglycemia from continued Insulin therapy and keeping the glucose >200 mg/dL to reduce the incidence of cerebral edema.

Choice A [IV 0.9% sodium chloride, IV regular Insulin, IV Potassium chloride] is used in the management of DKA with a serum glucose >250 mg/dL.
Choice B [Hemodialysis] is not routinely used in the management of DKA and HHS.

Treatment adjustments of Insulin and potassium based on serum K+:
- If Hypokalemia (<3.3 mEq/L): replace potassium and hold insulin.
- If Hyperkalemia (>5.5 mEq/dL): hold the potassium, give insulin [choice D]
- Normal potassium (3.3 and 5.5 mEq/dL): give both potassium and insulin and adjust based on labs monitored every 1-2 hours [choice A].

14. GENITOURINARY – ACUTE PYELONEPHRITIS [PHARMACOLOGY]

Fluoroquinolones, such as Ciprofloxacin or Levofloxacin [choice C] are first-line outpatient management for Acute pyelonephritis if resistance rate is <10%.
Patients with acute complicated UTI of mild to moderate severity who can tolerate oral medications reliably can be treated in the outpatient setting.

In patients who cannot tolerate Fluoroquinolones or if resistance >10%, initiate with a long-acting parenteral agent (eg, IV or IM Ceftriaxone, Gentamicin, Tobramycin, Ertapenem) followed by an oral Fluoroquinolone.
Alternatives for oral follow-up after LA parenteral agents include TMP-SMX [choice E], Ampicillin-sulbactam, Cefpodoxime, Cefdinir, or Cefadroxil.

Indications for admission include:
- older age
- signs of obstruction
- comorbid conditions
- inability to tolerate oral antibiotics or maintain oral hydration
- persistently high fever (eg, >38.4°C/>101°F) or persistent pain.

15. GASTROINTESTINAL/NUTRITION – ACHALASIA [MOST LIKELY]

Key features of Achalasia [choice E] include:
- gradual dysphagia for both solids and liquids
- regurgitation of bland undigested food
- **Barium esophagram: dilation of the distal esophagus with a narrowed esophagogastric junction with "bird-beak" appearance.**
- **Esophageal manometry confirms diagnosis — aperistalsis in the distal two-thirds of the esophagus and incomplete lower esophageal sphincter relaxation (increased LES pressure).**

Choice A [Distal esophageal spasm] is associated with a "corkscrew" or "rosary bead" appearance on Barium esophagram.

Choice B [Hypercontractile esophagus] is associated with increased pressure during peristalsis >180 mmHg or duration of contraction >7.5 seconds but normally sequential contractions on manometry.

Choice C [Gastroesophageal reflux disease] is associated with decreased lower esophageal pressure on manometry.

Choice E [Zenker diverticulum] is associated with outpouching of the esophagus at the cricopharyngeal junction on Barium swallow with fluoroscopy.

16. PSYCHIATRY/BEHAVIORAL – NEUROLEPTICS/ANTIPSYCHOTICS (OLANZAPINE) [PHARMACOLOGY]

Compared to the other second-generation antipsychotics, Olanzapine has a higher incidence of weight gain [choice D], Dyslipidemia, and Diabetes mellitus.

Other adverse effects include
- Orthostatic hypotension
- prolonged QT interval
- Hyperglycemia
- transaminase elevation.

Olanzapine is not associated with Serotonin syndrome [choice C] because it is a serotonin (5-HT2A and 5-HT1A) antagonist & dopamine antagonist (D4 & D3 > D2 receptors).

17. PULMONARY - RESPIRATORY DISTRESS SYNDROME IN THE NEWBORN [MOST LIKELY]

Respiratory distress syndrome in the newborn [choice C] should be suspected in:
- **preterm infants <34 weeks especially between 26-28 weeks**
- **respiratory distress**: eg, tachypnea, tachycardia, cyanosis, nasal flaring, expiratory grunting, and chest wall retractions.
- radiographs: air-bronchograms, ground-glass appearance, and decreased lung volume.

Hyaline membrane disease [Infant (neonatal) respiratory distress syndrome] occurs due to inadequate production of surfactant resulting in alveolar collapse shortly after birth.

Management includes oxygen, continuous positive airway pressure, exogenous surfactant, and in severe or refractory cases, intubation and extracorporeal membrane oxygenation.

Choice A [Congenital cyanotic heart disease] is usually associated with milder respiratory distress and is not associated with ground-glass appearance characteristic of Neonatal respiratory distress syndrome.

Choice D [Persistent pulmonary hypertension of the neonate] is more common in near- or at-term infants and is associated with mostly clear lungs; it is often a result of meconium aspiration [choice B].

Choice E [Transient tachypnea of the newborn] more commonly occurs in term or late preterm infants and is associated with milder respiratory distress.

18. PSYCHIATRY/BEHAVIORAL – NEUROLEPTIC MALIGNANT SYNDROME [PHARMACOLOGY]

Dantrolene [choice E] &/or Bromocriptine may be added to Benzodiazepines in patients with Neuroleptic malignant syndrome (NMS).

Dantrolene is a direct-acting skeletal muscle relaxant that is effective in reducing the fever and muscle rigidity not fully relieved with Benzodiazepines.

Bromocriptine is a dopamine agonist used to increase dopamine.

Neuroleptic malignant syndrome (NMS) most commonly occurs on initiation of or changing the dose of an antipsychotic medication. **Key features of NMS include:**
- **altered mental status, "lead-pipe" muscle rigidity, autonomic instability** (tachycardia, tachypnea, hyperthermia, fever, blood pressure changes, diaphoresis),
- **incontinence, leukocytosis** & Rhabdomyolysis (increased CPK, LDH, & LFTs).

19. GASTROINTESTINAL/NUTRITION – INTUSSUSCEPTION [LABS AND DIAGNOSTIC STUDIES]

Pneumatic pressure by enema [choice A] is both diagnostic and therapeutic (pneumatic decompression to push back the Intussusception) for suspected Intussusception.

Air enema is preferred over contrast-based enemas due to lower risk of perforation and reduced radiation exposure.

Intussusception, invagination (telescoping) of the bowel into itself, classically presents in **children 3 months-36 months of age with the classic triad of:**
- **(1) vomiting +**
- **(2) abdominal pain** (recurring paroxysms) +
- **(3) passage of blood per rectum** – **"currant jelly" stools (stool mixed with blood & mucus)** only seen in 1/3 of patients.

Choice B [Rectal suction biopsy followed by transanal mucosal biopsy if negative] is indicated for suspected Hirschsprung disease, which classically presents as a meconium ileus and megacolon on imaging.

Choice C [Barium swallow] is not indicated to establish the diagnosis or for therapy of Intussusception.

Choice D [99m technetium pertechnetate (Meckel) scan] is used to diagnose Meckel diverticulum, which presents with painless gastrointestinal bleeding.

Choice E [Rehydration and electrolyte replacement, followed by Pyloromyotomy] is used in the diagnosis and management of Infantile hypertrophic pyloric stenosis. It usually presents in younger children 3-12 weeks with projectile vomiting and an olive shaped mass after vomiting.

20. CARDIOLOGY – HEART FAILURE [HISTORY AND PHYSICAL]

An S3 (third heart sound) [choice D] is associated with ventricular systolic dysfunction, such as Heart failure with reduced ejection fraction (HFrEF), ischemic heart disease, Dilated cardiomyopathy, Myocarditis, and Cor pulmonale.

An S3 heart sound represents rapid filling of a dilated ventricle.

The presence of an S3 is the most sensitive indicator of ventricular dysfunction.

Choice A [Diastolic knock] is associated with Constrictive pericarditis.

Choice B [Pulsus bisferiens] may be seen with Hypertrophic cardiomyopathy.
Choice C [Weak delayed carotid pulses] is hallmark of Aortic stenosis.
Choice E [Fourth heart sound], or S4 gallop, is associated with ventricular diastolic dysfunction.

21. PULMONOLOGY – COMMUNITY-ACQUIRED PNEUMONIA [PHARMACOLOGY]

Combination therapy with an antipneumococcal beta-lactam (eg, Ceftriaxone, Cefotaxime, Ceftaroline, Ampicillin sulbactam) plus a Macrolide (eg, Azithromycin or Clarithromycin XL) [choice C] is the treatment of choice for patients with Community-acquired pneumonia (CAP) treated as an inpatient not requiring intensive care unit (ICU) admission.

Doxycycline may be used as an alternative to a Macrolide, especially in patients at high risk of QT interval prolongation.

For patients who cannot take a beta-lactam plus a macrolide, monotherapy with a respiratory fluoroquinolone (eg, Levofloxacin, Moxifloxacin) is an alternative.

Choice A [Vancomycin] can be added to therapy if there is an increased risk for Methicillin resistant Staphylococcus aureus (MRSA).

Choice B [Piperacillin/tazobactam] can be used in patients with increased risk for *Pseudomonas aeruginosa* infection.

Choice D [Doxycycline] monotherapy is used for the outpatient management of CAP.

Choice E [Amoxicillin plus clavulanic acid] can be used in the outpatient management of Aspiration pneumonia.

22. REPRODUCTIVE – PRIMARY OVARIAN INSUFFICIENCY [MOST LIKELY]

Primary ovarian insufficiency [choice C] is seen in women <40 years of age, associated with:
- **decreased serum estradiol (ovarian dysfunction)**
- **elevated follicle-stimulating hormone (FSH) and Luteinizing hormone (LH)** as the pituitary gland attempts to stimulate the hypofunctioning ovaries.

Patients may present with menopausal symptoms (eg, hot flushes, vaginal atrophy and dryness).

Choice B [Functional hypothalamic amenorrhea], choice D [Pituitary adenoma], and choice E [Pituitary infarction (Sheehan syndrome)] are associated with decreased estrogen, FSH, and LH.

23. MUSCULOSKELETAL – GOUT ARTHROPATHY [APPLYING FOUNDATIONAL CONCEPTS]

The classic radiograph findings of Gout arthropathy due to Monosodium urate crystal deposition [choice E] include the "mouse" or "rat" bite lesions, characterized by punched out bone erosions with sclerosis and overhanging edges.
Periarticular hyperdense soft tissue swelling "tophi" may also be seen, as in this patient (arrowhead).

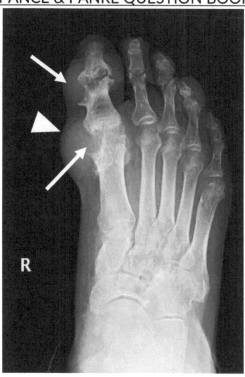

Choice A [Calcium pyrophosphate crystal deposition] can result in calcification of the cartilage (chondrocalcinosis) and Pseudogout.

Choice B [Bony destructive changes due to chronic bacterial infection of the bone] is associated with Chronic osteomyelitis, which is associated with involucrum and sequestrum on radiographs.

Choice C [Localized inflammation of the joint due peripheral neuropathy from Diabetes mellitus] is associated with Charcot arthropathy.

Choice D [The presence of a pannus resulting in joint destruction] occurs in Rheumatoid arthritis, which is associated with symmetric joint narrowing, joint destruction, and osteopenia.

24. REPRODUCTIVE – PLACENTA PREVIA [MOST LIKELY]

Placenta previa [choice C] should be suspected in women who present with painless vaginal bleeding in the third trimester with a nontender uterus.

Placenta previa is the leading cause of third-trimester bleeding, complicating 4 in 1,000 pregnancies over 20 weeks.

Placenta previa occurs when all or part of the placenta traverses the cervical os.

Management is similar to Abruptio placentae and consists of:
- Hemodynamic status of the mother should be immediately evaluated, and stabilization established if needed.
- Continual monitoring of the fetal heart rate.

Choice A [Uterine rupture] is associated with extreme abdominal pain, decreased or absent uterine contractions, abnormal bump in the abdomen, & possible regression of fetal parts.

Choice B [Vasa previa] is associated with painless vaginal bleeding but with fetal distress (eg, fetal bradycardia or heart rate changes).

Choice D [Abruptio placenta] is associated with painful vaginal bleeding and a tender uterus.

Choice E [Threatened abortion] is a cause of vaginal bleeding in pregnancies <20 weeks.

25. PULMONOLOGY – EMPYEMA [CLINICAL INTERVENTION]
In addition to antibiotic therapy, drainage of pleural fluid, either with single tube or catheter thoracostomy [choice C] is the management of choice of a complicated Pleural effusion and Empyema (with or without a course of tPA/DNase to break up any loculations).
Empyema should be suspected if chest radiographs reveal an effusion with an obtuse angle with the chest wall, marked asymmetry, or biconvex in shape.

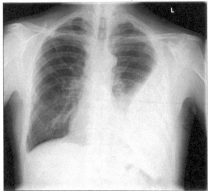

Pleural fluid analysis suggestive of Empyema include:
- pH <7.2
- pleural fluid glucose <60 mg/dL
- WBC >50,000/mm^3
- LDH >1,000 units/L
- Positive gram stain

Video assisted thoracoscopy [choice D] may be indicated in symptomatic patients with parapneumonic effusion or Empyema that fails to resolve with antibiotics, tube thoracostomy, and a course of tPA/DNase.

Choice A [Thoracotomy] is an invasive procedure that is not usually used for Empyema.
Choice B [Prednisone] is not used in the management of Empyema; Systemic corticosteroids may be used in the management of Acute bacterial exacerbations of Chronic bronchitis.
Choice E [Bronchoscopy] is not used in the management of Empyema.

26. MUSCULOSKELETAL – ACHILLES TENDON RUPTURE [HISTORY AND PHYSICAL]
A positive Thompson test, absence of plantar flexion when squeezing the gastrocnemius muscle [choice C], marks a positive test, is indicative of an Achilles tendon rupture.
The Thompson test has a sensitivity of 96% and a specificity of 93%.
Achilles tendon rupture occurs when sudden forces are exerted upon the Achilles tendon during strenuous physical activities that involve sudden pivoting on a foot or rapid acceleration.
The classic presentation is sensation as if the patient were struck violently in the back of the ankle. Some hear a "pop" and experience severe, acute pain.

Choice D [Tenderness along the base of the fifth metatarsal] is hallmark of a Jones fracture.

27. GASTROINTESTINAL/NUTRITION – ACUTE DIVERTICULITIS [LABS AND DIAGNOSTIC STUDIES]

Abdominal CT scan with oral and intravenous (IV) contrast [choice D] is the imaging test of choice to establish the diagnosis of Acute diverticulitis because it has a high sensitivity and specificity for Acute diverticulitis and is useful to rule other causes of abdominal pain.

Acute Diverticulitis classically presents with lower abdominal pain (especially left lower quadrant).

Constipation and Western diet increases the risk for Acute diverticulitis.

Choice A [Amylase and lipase levels] are useful to establish the diagnosis of Acute pancreatitis, which classically presents with epigastric pain radiating to the back.

Choice B [Barium enema] is contraindicated during Acute diverticulitis due to increased risk of bowel perforation during the procedure.

Choice C [Colonoscopy] is contraindicated during Acute diverticulitis due to increased risk of bowel perforation during the procedure. However, colonoscopy is recommended 4-6 weeks after an episode of Acute diverticulitis to rule out Colorectal cancer.

Choice E [Abdominal ultrasound] is not sensitive in detecting Acute diverticulitis.

28. CARDIOLOGY – PERICARDIAL EFFUSION [LABS AND DIAGNOSTIC STUDIES]

A pericardial effusion is generally diagnosed by echocardiography [choice C], with additional cardiac imaging performed only in selected cases.

Decreased heart sounds and enlarged cardiac silhouette suggest Pericardial effusion, which should be evaluated with an echocardiogram.

Echocardiography provides a dynamic assessment of the Pericardial effusion, permitting for quantification of the effusion's size and to assess for evidence of hemodynamic instability (eg, cardiac tamponade physiology).

Pericardial effusion is identified as anechoic fluid surrounding the heart.

Choice A [Stress test] is used to evaluate for Coronary artery disease.

Although an ECG [choice B] should be performed in patients with suspected pericardial disease, findings suggestive of Pericarditis or effusion should be followed up by Echocardiogram.

Choice D [Pericardiocentesis] is used for patients to treat pericardial tamponade or recurrent effusions.

Choice E [Cardiac catheterization] is usually reserved for patients (usually with suspected cardiac tamponade) undergoing pericardial fluid drainage.

29. GASTROINTESTINAL/NUTRITION – CHOLEDOCHOLITHIASIS [MOST LIKELY]

Choledocholithiasis [choice B] refers to the presence of gallstones within the common bile duct without evidence of infection.

Although most patients are asymptomatic, symptoms include right upper quadrant or epigastric pain, nausea, and vomiting.

Physical examination may reveal right upper quadrant or epigastric tenderness and jaundice (due to cholestasis).

Labs may reveal a cholestatic pattern of marked increase in alkaline phosphatase (ALP) and gamma-glutamyl transpeptidase (GGT) more pronounced than elevations in ALT and AST.

Because there is no infection, patients are afebrile with a normal white cell count.

Choice A [Acute Hepatitis] is associated with lymphocytosis, fever, & right upper quadrant pain.

PANCE & PANRE QUESTION BOOK

Choice C [Acute Cholecystitis] is classically associated with the triad of fever, right upper quadrant pain, and leukocytosis without jaundice since the stone is in the cystic duct and not the common bile duct.

Choice D [Acute Cholangitis] is associated with Charcot triad: fever, right upper quadrant pain, and jaundice. It is often associated with a leukocytosis due to infection. Choledocholithiasis is a precursor to the development of Acute ascending cholangitis.

Choice E [Cholelithiasis] is associated with intermittent right upper quadrant lasting <4 hours, normal examination, and normal labs.

30. CARDIOLOGY – GIANT CELL ARTERITIS [HEALTH MAINTENANCE]

In patients with Giant cell arteritis (GCA), 85% of vision loss occurs due to Arteritic anterior ischemic optic neuropathy [choice D]; other less common causes include central or branch retinal artery occlusion (CRAO/BRAO), posterior ischemic optic neuropathy (PION).

The prompt use of glucocorticoids improve the symptoms and prevent visual loss, which is the most common significant complication of GCA.

Cerebral ischemia [choice E] is a rare complication of GCA.

Other less common complications of GCA include Stroke [choice C], Aortic dissection [choice A], and Aortic aneurysm [choice B].

31. GASTROINTESTINAL/NUTRITION – CHRONIC PANCREATITIS [MOST LIKELY]

Chronic alcohol consumption [choice C] is the most common cause of Chronic pancreatitis in the United States.

Most patients with Chronic pancreatitis have more than one underlying etiology (all the other choices listed can cause or contribute to Chronic pancreatitis).

The classic triad of Chronic pancreatitis includes:
- abdominal pain
- steatorrhea (due to malabsorption)
- calcified pancreas on imaging.

32. REPRODUCTIVE – BREAST ABSCESS [CLINICAL INTERVENTION]

The management of a Primary breast abscess consists of [1] breast drainage (eg needle aspiration or surgical drainage) and [2] antibiotic therapy [choice B].

Breast abscess classically presents with painful inflammation of the breast associated with fever and malaise, in addition to a fluctuant, tender, palpable mass on physical examination.

Choice A [Warm compresses, use of supportive bra, and Cephalexin] is the treatment of choice for Infective mastitis.

Choice C [Warm compresses and use of a breast pump or manual pump] is an alternative management for Infective mastitis.

Choice D [Mammogram] is indicated for evaluation of Breast masses in women >40 years of age.

Choice E [Core needle biopsy] is used in the workup of a patient with a breast mass suspicious for Breast cancer.

33. DERMATOLOGY – PEMPHIGUS VULGARIS [MOST LIKELY]

Pemphigus vulgaris [choice C] is a generalized, mucocutaneous, autoimmune, blistering eruption characterized by:

- <u>**Mucosal involvement:**</u> the oral cavity is the most common site of panful mucosal lesions
- <u>**Cutaneous vesicles or bullae:**</u> **flaccid blisters that rupture easily,** leaving behind painful erosions that bleed easily
- <u>**Positive Nikolsky sign:**</u> induction of blistering via mechanical pressure at the edge of a blister or on normal skin.

Drugs that may induce Pemphigus vulgaris include Thiol medications, such as Captopril (as in this patient), and Penicillamine.

Choice A [Toxic epidermal necrolysis] may also develop flaccid bullae and a positive Nikolsky sign, but they are also associated with erythematous macules, dusky erythema, purpuric areas, and atypical target lesions (flat lesions with 2 rings instead of the 3 rings seen in Erythema multiforme) and involvement of >30% body surface area.

Choice B [Bullous pemphigoid] is associated with tense blisters that do not rupture easily and a Negative Nikolsky sign.

Choice D [Stevens-Johnson syndrome] may also develop flaccid bullae and a positive Nikolsky sign, but they are also associated with erythematous macules, dusky erythema, purpuric areas, and atypical target lesions (flat lesions with 2 rings instead of the 3 rings seen in Erythema multiforme) and involvement of <10% body surface area.

Choice E [Type IV hypersensitivity drug reaction] classically presents with a generalized erythematous maculopapular rash and Negative Nikolsky sign.

34. CARDIOLOGY – LEFT VENTRICULAR HYPERTROPHY (LVH) [MOST LIKELY]

The criteria for Left ventricular hypertrophy [choice C] include:
- **Sokolow-Lyon criteria: S in V1 + R in V5 (or V6)** >35 mm in men and >30 mm in women.
- **Cornell Criteria: R in aVL + S in V3** >28 mm in men and >20 mm in women.

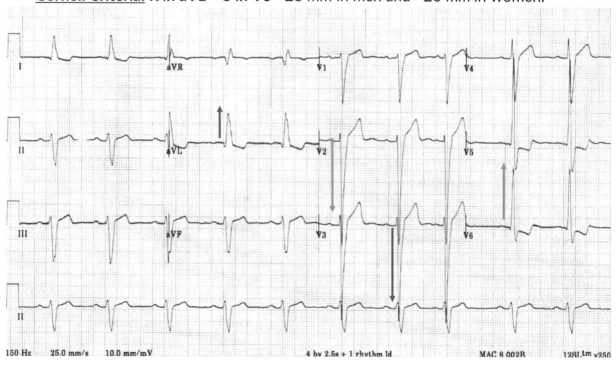

150 Hz   25.0 mm/s   10.0 mm/mV   4 by 2.5s + 1 rhythm ld   MAC 8 002B   12SI.tm v250

Causes of LVH include Aortic stenosis (as in this patient), Hypertension, and Hypertrophic cardiomyopathy.

Choice A [Right bundle branch block] is associated with an Rr' in leads V1 and V2, a wide QRS complex, and an S wave in V6.

Choice B [Right axis deviation] is associated with predominantly negative QRS complexes in I and predominantly positive QRS complexes in aVF. This patient has positive QRS complexes in lead I and negative QRS complexes in leads II and AVF, consistent with Left axis deviation.

Choice D [Acute pericarditis] is associated with PR depressions and ST elevations in the precordial leads.

Choice E [Brugada syndrome] is associated with a right bundle branch pattern in V1 and V2.

35. DERMATOLOGY – ATOPIC DERMATITIS [MOST LIKELY]

The atopic triad consists of [1] Atopic dermatitis (Eczema) [choice B], [2] Asthma, and [3] Allergic rhinitis. This patient has a transverse crease on his nasal bridge, often known as the "allergic salute" from constant nose rubbing.

Atopic dermatitis is characterized by:

- Acute phase: Intensely pruritic, erythematous papules and vesicles with crusting
- Subacute or chronic phase: dry, scaly, or excoriated, erythematous papules with or without skin thickening from chronic scratching.

In older children and adults, common areas involved are flexural creases (eg, antecubital and popliteal fossae), volar aspect of the wrists, ankles, and neck.

In infants and young children, common areas of involvement include the extensor surfaces, the scalp, and the face (eg, cheeks).

Choice A [Nonbullous impetigo] are associated with golden-colored crusting, especially on the face.

Choice C [Psoriasis] is associated with well-defined erythematous plaques covered by a thick silvery-white scale.

Choice D [Scabies] is associated with vesicopustules.

Choice E [Irritant contact dermatitis] is associated with geometrically shaped vesicles on specific areas exposed to an irritant.

36. ENDOCRINOLOGY – HYPOPARATHYROIDISM [LABS AND DIAGNOSTIC STUDIES]

Primary hypoparathyroidism is associated with increased serum phosphate levels [choice B] because low PTH levels cause the kidney to lose their signal to excrete phosphate in the urine (lack of inhibition of renal tubule phosphate reabsorption).

Primary hypoparathyroidism is associated with the classic triad of:
- **[1] Hypocalcemia**
- **[2] Elevated serum phosphorus level**
- **[3] low or inappropriately normal serum intact PTH level**
- **Normal or low serum 25-hydroxyvitamin D (25[OH]D)**
- Normal magnesium
- Normal creatinine
- Elevated fractional urinary excretion of calcium

37. GASTROINTESTINAL/NUTRITION – PSEUDOMEMBRANOUS COLITIS & CLOSTRIDIOIDES DIFFICILE [HISTORY AND PHYSICAL EXAMINATION]

Pseudomembranous colitis, a severe inflammation of the inner lining of the colon may occur as an antibiotic-associated colonic inflammatory complication [choice E].

Pseudomembranous colitis most commonly results from a serious *Clostridium difficile* infection. Antibiotics disrupt the natural colonic flora, allowing for *C. difficile* colonization.

C. difficile induces colitis via exotoxin production, toxin A, and toxin B that result in inflammation, and immune system activation, resulting in the pseudomembranous appearance of the colon.

Severe Pseudomembranous colitis can manifest with profound leukocytosis, with white blood cell counts up to 100,000/mm^3.

Choice A [Use of Ibuprofen for back pain] may result in Gastric ulcer formation.

Choice B [Drinking untreated water] may result in Traveler's diarrhea.

Choice C [Consuming undercooked pork] can result gastroenteritis due to *Yersinia enterocolitica*.

Choice D [Consuming raw oysters] can result in gastroenteritis due to *Vibrio vulnificus*.

38. PULMONARY - LARYNGOTRACHEITIS (CROUP) [PHARMACOLOGY]

Nebulized Epinephrine (Racemic or L-Epinephrine) [choice C] is added to glucocorticoid therapy in patients with moderate to severe Croup as Epinephrine provides rapid relief within 1 hour of administration and decreases airway edema [choice C].

The management of moderate to severe Croup include:
- **Nebulized Epinephrine**
- **Single dose of a glucocorticoid (eg, Dexamethasone)**
- **Supportive care:** eg, oxygen or humidified air as needed, antipyretics, and encouragement of fluid intake.

Choice A [Supplemental oxygen via face mask] can be used as adjunctive therapy in patients as needed. This patient is not hypoxic and although adjunctive therapy is needed, oxygen does not reduce subglottal narrowing.

Choice B [Intubation and mechanical ventilation] is reserved for refractory cases of Croup.

Choice D [Nebulized Albuterol] does not reduce subglottic narrowing and is not a first line agent of Croup.

Choice E [Chest radiograph] may be indicated to confirm the diagnosis of Croup and rule out other etiologies.

39. CARDIOLOGY – NON-ST ELEVATION MYOCARDIAL INFARCTION (NSTEMI) [PHARMACOLOGY]

Dual antiplatelet therapy P2Y12 receptor antagonist (eg, Ticagrelor, Prasugrel, Clopidogrel) [choice D] in addition to Aspirin is used in all patients with Unstable angina or Non-ST elevation myocardial infarction (NSTEMI).

Dual antiplatelet therapy (Aspirin + P2Y12 receptor blocker) results in a substantial decrease in cardiovascular death and recurrent Myocardial infarction compared to Aspirin monotherapy.

Dual antiplatelet therapy (DAPT) also diminishes the risk of stent thrombosis, so DAPT recommended for at least 6-12 months in all patients following drug-eluting stent placement. This patient had a Non-ST-elevation MI (positive cardiac biomarkers + ST depression and T wave changes on ECG).

Choice A [Rivaroxaban] is not indicated in the routine management of NSTEMI.

Choice B [Nifedipine] has no mortality benefit post myocardial infarction.

Thrombolytics, such as Alteplase [choice C] are not used in the management of Unstable angina and Non-ST elevation MI.

Choice E [Verapamil] has no mortality benefit and may possibly cause harm post Myocardial infarction due to a reduction in myocardial contraction.

40. PSYCHIATRY/BEHAVIORAL – POSTTRAUMATIC STRESS DISORDER [HEALTH MAINTENANCE]

For most adults newly treated for PTSD, first-line treatment with a Trauma-focused psychotherapy that includes exposure [choice E] rather than a serotonergic reuptake inhibitor (SRI) is often recommended.

Trauma-focused psychotherapy is considered as the first-line treatment in adults as well as children, and it includes Trauma-focused CBT (cognitive-behavioral therapy), Eye movement desensitization and reprocessing (EMDR), Cognitive processing therapy, and Imaginal exposure.

41. INFECTIOUS DISEASE – METHICILLIN RESISTANT STAPHYLOCOCCUS AUREUS (MRSA)/CUTANEOUS ABSCESS [PHARMACOLOGY]

<u>Oral antibiotics</u> with Methicillin resistant *Staphylococcus aureus* (MRSA) coverage include:
- **Trimethoprim-sulfamethoxazole [choice B].**
- **Clindamycin**
- **Linezolid**

<u>IV antibiotics</u> with Methicillin resistant *Staphylococcus aureus* (MRSA) coverage include:
- **Vancomycin**
- **Daptomycin**
- **Linezolid**
- **Ceftaroline.**

For Cellulitis with MRSA risk factors, Trimethoprim-sulfamethoxazole is given in addition to Cephalexin (TMP-SMX good for Staphylococcus spp. but does not cover Streptococcus).

42. INFECTIOUS DISEASE – SHIGELLA [HISTORY AND PHYSICAL]

Seizures are the most common neurologic complication associated with *Shigella* infection [choice B] in children especially children <15 years of age.

It is classically associated with diarrhea that is initially watery before coming bloody.

HUS has been described most commonly in the context of infection due to Shiga toxin-producing *Escherichia coli* (STEC) infections; less frequently, it has also been associated with *Shigella dysenteriae*.

Choice A [Rotavirus] causes a noninvasive watery diarrhea.

Choice C [Vibrio cholerae] causes a noninvasive watery diarrhea.

Choice D [Intussusception] causes intermittent abdominal pain and passage of stools that contain blood and mucous but is not classically associated with causing febrile seizures.
Choice E [Enterotoxigenic Escherichia coli] causes a noninvasive watery diarrhea.

43. HEMATOLOGY – TRANSFUSION-RELATED ACUTE LUNG INJURY (TRALI) [MOST LIKELY]

Transfusion-related acute lung injury (TRALI) [choice B] should be suspected if within minutes to 6 hours after a transfusion, a patient develops:

- **fever, chills**
- **acute respiratory distress (dyspnea, tachypnea, hypoxia)**
- **hypotension**
- **new infiltrates (whiting out of the lungs) on chest radiography (similar to ARDS) with a normal capillary wedge pressure.**

Transfusion-related acute lung injury (TRALI) occurs when the recipient's immune system responds by the release of mediators that increase capillary permeability, leading to leakage of protein & fluid, resulting in Noncardiogenic pulmonary edema (similar to ARDS).
TRALI is the #1 cause of transfusion-related deaths.
Management is largely supportive and may include supplemental oxygen, intubation, mechanical ventilation, and vasopressor support.

Choice A [Acute transfusion-related hemolytic reaction] presents with fever, chills, flank pain, and oozing from intravenous sites.
Choice C [Transfusion-associated circulatory overload/TACO] is associated with hypertension, S3 gallop, evidence of congestion &/or pulmonary edema on imaging similar to CHF; Fever is not a classic feature of TACO.
Choice D [Acute febrile nonhemolytic transfusion reaction]
Choice E [Anaphylactic transfusion reaction] presents with angioedema, wheezing, stridor, pruritus, &/or hypotension.

44. EENT - VESTIBULAR SCHWANNOMA (ACOUSTIC NEUROMA) [MOST LIKELY]

Vestibular schwannoma (Acoustic neuroma) [choice B] should be suspected in any individual presenting with unexplained unilateral or asymmetric sensorineural hearing loss on audiometry.
Vestibular schwannomas (Acoustic neuromas) are Schwann cell-derived, histologically benign tumors of the eighth cranial nerve, arising within the internal auditory canal and gradually grow to involve the cerebellopontine angle.

Features of sensorineural hearing loss include:
- **Webber test: lateralization to the normal ear**
- **Rinne test: air conduction > bone conduction**

Choice A [Cerumen impaction] is a cause of conductive hearing loss, resulting in [1] lateralization to the affected ear on Webber test and [2] bone conduction greater than air conduction in the affected ear on Rinne testing.

Choice C [Cholesteatoma] is a cause of conductive hearing loss, resulting in [1] lateralization to the affected ear on Webber test and [2] bone conduction greater than air conduction in the affected ear on Rinne testing.

Choice D [Benign paroxysmal positional vertigo] causes episodic vertigo lasting a few seconds up to 1 minute and no hearing loss.

Choice E [Otosclerosis] is a cause of conductive hearing loss, resulting in [1] lateralization to the affected ear on Webber test and [2] bone conduction greater than air conduction in the affected ear on Rinne testing.

45. DERMATOLOGY – HERPES ZOSTER [PHARMACOLOGY]

Oral Valacyclovir (1,000 mg tid) [choice B], Famciclovir (500 mg tid), or Acyclovir (800 mg five times daily) are used in the management of Herpes zoster in immunocompetent patients, especially within 72 hours of symptom onset and with lesions that are not crusted over.

Antivirals promote healing of skin lesions, lessen the severity and duration of acute neuritis, and reduce the incidence or severity of chronic pain (eg, postherpetic neuralgia).

Herpes zoster is secondary reactivation of Varicella zoster virus (VZV) that classically presents with a prodrome, followed by the development of grouped vesicles on an erythematous base before crusting over.

Choice A [Topical Betamethasone] is not used in the management of VZV.

Choice C [Oral Fluconazole] is an agent used in systemic fungal infections.

Choice D [Topical Butenafine] is an agent used on dermatophytic fungal infections.

Choice E [Topical Mupirocin] is an agent used in bacterial infections (eg, Impetigo).

46. GASTROINTESTINAL/NUTRITION – FOLATE DEFICIENCY [LABS AND DIAGNOSTIC STUDIES]

Normal methylmalonic acid with increased homocysteine [choice C] are most consistent with Folate deficiency.

Medications that interfere with Folate metabolism include Trimethoprim-sulfamethoxazole and Phenytoin (this patient is on both); other medications include Methotrexate and Sulfasalazine.

Choice A [Megakaryocytes and decreased platelet count] is associated Immune thrombocytopenic purpura (ITP).

Choice B [Increased methylmalonic acid, increased homocysteine] is associated with B12 deficiency.

Choice E [Elevated prothrombin time, decreased platelets] may be seen in Disseminated intravascular coagulation.

47. DERMATOLOGY – ERYSIPELAS [APPLYING FOUNDATIONAL CONCEPTS]

Erysipelas involving the face is most commonly caused by *Streptococcus pyogenes* (Group A beta-hemolytic streptococcus) [choice A], seen in 60-68% of cases.

Less commonly G group streptococci (14–25%) or Group B streptococci (3–9%) are causative agents.

Erysipelas is a superficial form of Cellulitis that begins with skin breaks resulting in a portal of entry for the infection.

Although it presents similar to Cellulitis with erythema, tenderness, and warmth, key features that distinguish Erysipelas from Cellulitis include sharply demarcated borders, and bright erythema (often called "St. Anthony's fire"), as well as prominent systemic symptoms (eg, malaise, myalgia, fever, chills).

48. PROFESSIONAL PRACTICE – HYPOSPADIAS [HEALTH MAINTENANCE]

Hypospadias repair usually performed in healthy full-term infants most commonly 6 months-1 year of age [choice D].

Routine newborn circumcision is contraindicated in patients with Hypospadias because:
- [1] there are increased complication with early neonatal circumcision with the standard methods and use of devices
- [2] the foreskin needs to be preserved for possible reconstruction and repair of the defect in cases of standard and severe Hypospadias.

Elective surgical correction (arthroplasty) may include penile straightening.

Infants with Hypospadias only are not usually at greater risk for other anomalies.

Hypospadias is a congenital anomaly in males that results in abnormal placement of the urethral opening on the ventral surface of the penis.

Choice A [Perform an echocardiogram] is not usually indicated in isolated distal Hypospadias as they are not classically associated with congenital cardiac anomalies.

Choice B [Ultrasound of the kidneys] is not usually indicated as isolated Hypospadias are not usually associated with congenital renal abnormalities since external genital development occurs post the key stages of renal development.

Choice C [Proceed with circumcision] is usually contraindicated in early infancy as it is usually deferred until 6 months-1 year of age for better outcomes.

Choice E [Perform karyotype analysis] is indicated in patients with Hypospadias also associated with other congenital anomalies.

49. EENT – ACUTE MASTOIDITIS [CLINICAL INTERVENTION]

In patients with Acute mastoiditis with a history of recurrent Acute otitis media (AOM) or recent antibiotic use, Piperacillin-tazobactam [choice E] is an appropriate initial broad-spectrum antibiotic in addition to middle ear drainage with or without a tympanostomy tube. Imaging with CT scan may be indicated to confirm the diagnosis, determine the extent of infection, and to evaluate for potential complications.

Acute mastoiditis is a complication of AOM and is associated with fever, ear pain, postauricular erythema, tenderness, and swelling; displacement of the auricle.

Choice A [Tympanostomy tube placement] may be adjunctive treatment to the standard therapy.

Choice B [Otolaryngology consult] is not needed in uncomplicated Mastoiditis as the best next step.

Choice C [Ciprofloxacin otic and placement of an ear wick for better absorption] is used in the management of Acute otitis externa. The treatment of Acute mastoiditis requires parenteral antimicrobial therapy.

Choice D [Switch oral Cefdinir to Amoxicillin-clavulanate] is inappropriate as the treatment of Acute mastoiditis requires parenteral antimicrobial therapy.

50. PULMONOLOGY – COR PULMONALE [MOST LIKELY]

Cor Pulmonale (Right-Sided Heart Failure) [choice B] is an enlarged right ventricle resulting from an underlying lung condition.

Pulmonary hypertension resulting from chronic hypoxemia can lead to right ventricular hypertrophy and eventually right-sided Heart failure, which manifests as peripheral edema, jugular venous distension, hepatojugular reflux.

Chronic bronchitis may result in Group 3 Pulmonary hypertension (due to hypoxemia).

In Pulmonary hypertension, a fixed split S2 may be seen due to elevated pulmonary artery pressure.

The classic ECG findings of cor pulmonale include:
- <u>Right ventricular hypertrophy</u>: positive QRS complex >7 mm in height in lead V1
- <u>Right axis deviation</u>: QRS predominantly negative in lead I and positive in lead aVF
- <u>P pulmonale (right atrial enlargement)</u>: P wave >3 mm in height

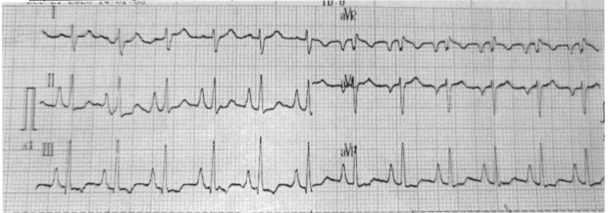

Choice A [Left atrial enlargement] or P mitrale is associated with a bifid (m-shaped) P wave in lead II.

Choice C [Wolff-Parkinson white] is associated with a delta wave, a short PR interval, and a wide QRS complex.

Choice D [Multifocal atrial tachycardia] is associated with at least 3 different discernable P wave morphologies with a heart rate >100 bpm.

Choice E [Wandering atrial pacemaker] is associated with at least 3 different discernable P wave morphologies with a heart rate <100 bpm.

51. ENDOCRINOLOGY – DIABETES INSIPIDUS [LABS AND DIAGNOSTIC STUDIES]
A Desmopressin stimulation test [choice E] is used to differentiate between AVP (ADH) deficiency (Central Diabetes insipidus) or AVP resistance (Nephrogenic Diabetes insipidus).
- Increase in serum osmolality after ADH/AVP administration is consistent with AVP deficiency
- Continued production of dilute urine (no significant increase in urine osmolality) is consistent with AVP resistance.

The classic triad of the presentation of Diabetes insipidus include increased thirst, polyuria, and nocturia.

Choice A (Dexamethasone suppression test) is used in the diagnosis of Cushing syndrome.

Choice B [Glucose suppression test] is used to confirm the diagnosis of Acromegaly.

Choice C [Fasting plasma glucose test] is used to diagnose Diabetes mellitus.

Choice D [Cosyntropin stimulation test] is used to establish the diagnosis of Adrenal insufficiency.

52. HEMATOLOGY – ALPHA THALASSEMIA INTERMEDIA (HEMOGLOBIN H DISEASE) [MOST LIKELY]

Most individuals with Hemoglobin H disease [choice E] are symptomatic at birth (neonatal jaundice often present).

~70 percent of individuals with Hb H disease develop complications associated with ineffective erythropoiesis and extramedullary hematopoiesis [eg, bone deformities (eg, frontal bossing), hepatosplenomegaly, and iron overload by adulthood, even with minimal to no transfusion history].

Classic findings on peripheral smear include hypochromia, microcytosis, target cells, increased reticulocytes, and normal or increased RBC count.

Hemoglobin electrophoresis may reveal 10-40% of hemoglobin H.

Choice A [Iron deficiency anemia] is associated with a microcytic anemia without evidence of hemolysis.

Choice B [Alpha thalassemia minor] is usually asymptomatic or associated with a mild anemia. It is not associated with evidence of extramedullary hematopoiesis.

Choice C [Hemoglobin Barts disease] is usually not compatible with life so individuals

Choice D [Beta thalassemia major (Cooley anemia)] individuals are normal at birth, but after 6 months (when hemoglobin synthesis switches from HbF to HbA), severe anemia occurs, often requiring periodic transfusion.

53. NEUROLOGY – MULTIPLE SCLEROSIS [LABS AND DIAGNOSTIC STUDIES]

MRI/MRA of the brain with and without contrast [choice C] is recommended in patients at higher risk for secondary Trigeminal neuralgia (TGN) in patients:
- **<40 years of age to rule out TGN as a presenting manifestation of Multiple sclerosis**
- those with bilateral symptoms, and
- those in whom physical examination reveals sensory loss are at a higher risk of secondary Trigeminal neuralgia.

Choice A [Noncontrast CT head] is not routinely indicated in the workup of TGN.

Choice B [Temporal artery biopsy] is the definitive diagnostic test to rule out Giant cell arteritis, which presents usually >50 years of age with headache, jaw claudication, and vision changes.

Choice D [Trigeminal reflex testing] is not routinely used in the workup of TGN.

Choice E [Lumbar puncture] may be useful to establish the diagnosis of Multiple sclerosis when clinical and MRI imaging is unable to establish the diagnosis of MS.

54. PULMONOLOGY – HYPERSENSITIVITY PNEUMONITIS/BIRD FANCIER'S LUNG [HEALTH MAINTENANCE]

In addition to identification and avoidance of inciting antigens (in this case avian proteins and excrements), a course of oral glucocorticoids [choice A] may be indicated for symptomatic subacute Hypersensitivity pneumonitis with reduced lung function.

Glucocorticoids have been shown to reduce symptoms. By reducing inflammation, glucocorticoids may delay lung fibrosis.

Bird fancier's lung (Bird breeder disease) is a type of Hypersensitivity pneumonitis associated with chronic exposure to avian proteins.

It can present with acute, subacute, or chronic symptoms.

Choice A [Azithromycin] may be used in the management of Acute infection with Chlamydophila psittaci associated with recent bird exposure. This patient presents with chronic symptoms.

Choice B [Albuterol] has not been shown to reduce fibrosis in Bird fancier's lung.

Choice D [Lung transplantation] may be an option in the management of advanced lung disease due to HP.

Choice E [Montelukast] has not been shown to reduce fibrosis in Bird fancier's lung.

55. ENDOCRINOLOGY - GOITER/THYROID NODULE [MOST LIKELY]

Toxic adenoma [choice E] should be suspected when labs show:

- **<u>Primary hyperthyroid profile</u>: decreased TSH and increased serum free T4 &/or T3**
- **<u>Thyroid radioactive iodine uptake scan</u>: increased focal uptake (hot nodule).**

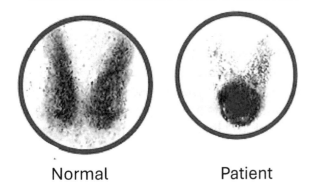

Normal   Patient

Toxic adenoma and Toxic multinodular goiter (MNG) are common causes of hyperthyroidism, second in prevalence only to Graves' disease.

In Toxic adenoma and Toxic multinodular goiter, somatic mutations result in focal and/or diffuse hyperplasia of thyroid follicular cells that function independent of regulation by TSH.

Choice A [Hashimoto thyroiditis] is associated with diffuse decreased uptake on thyroid scintigraphy.

Choice B [Toxic multinodular goiter] is associated with multiple areas of increased and decreased uptake on thyroid scintigraphy.

Choice C [Graves' disease] is associated with diffuse increased uptake on thyroid scintigraphy.

Choice E [Papillary thyroid carcinoma] is associated with no focal uptake (cold nodule) on thyroid scintigraphy.

56. CARDIOLOGY – PULMONIC REGURGITATION [HISTORY AND PHYSICAL]

Hallmark features of Pulmonic regurgitation [choice E] include:

- **high-pitched "blowing" diastolic murmur begins with an accentuated second heart sound (P2 component) best heard in the left upper sternal border.**
- **the intensity of the murmur may increase during inspiration (right-sided murmur).**

Pulmonary hypertension (in this patient due to COPD) and congenital heart defects, especially Tetralogy of Fallot, are the leading causes of Pulmonic regurgitation.

Choice A [Aortic regurgitation] sounds just like Pulmonic regurgitation but would decrease in intensity with inspiration as it is a left-sided murmur.

Choice B [Aortic stenosis] is characterized by a harsh systolic crescendo-decrescendo murmur best heard at the right upper sternal border.

Choice C [Pulmonic stenosis] is a harsh diastolic murmur best heard at the left upper sternal border.

Choice D [Mitral stenosis] is a diastolic rumbling murmur best heard at the apex.

57. PULMONOLOGY – PERTUSSIS [PHARMACOLOGY]

Macrolides (eg, Azithromycin) [choice B] is the first line antibiotic management of Pertussis. Trimethoprim-sulfamethoxazole is an alternative for patients with a contraindication to or who cannot tolerate Macrolide antibiotics.

Pertussis occurs in 3 stages:
- [1] catarrhal stage symptoms similar to an upper respiratory infection; lasts 1-2 weeks.
- [2] paroxysmal stage characterized by paroxysms of coughing, an inspiratory whoop, and post tussive vomiting or cyanosis; lasts 2-8 weeks.
- [3] convalescent stage: resolution of cough; subsides over several weeks to months.

58. CARDIOLOGY – INFERIOR WALL ST ELEVATION MYOCARDIAL INFARCTION (STEMI) [CLINICAL INTERVENTION]

The primary goal in the management of ST elevation MI (STEMI) is rapid restoration of blood flow to the acutely occluded coronary artery via reperfusion therapy with either:
- **[1] Percutaneous coronary intervention (PCI) [choice A] preferred ideally within 90 minutes from door to catheterization lab OR 120 minutes for transfer** to hospital with a cath lab. **PCI is the preferred method of reperfusion.**
- [2] Fibrinolytics (thrombolytics) [choice B] if PCI cannot be performed.

Reperfusion ideally performed as soon as possible and within 12 hours of chest pain onset.

Acute ST-Elevation Myocardial Infarction (STEMI) Inferior

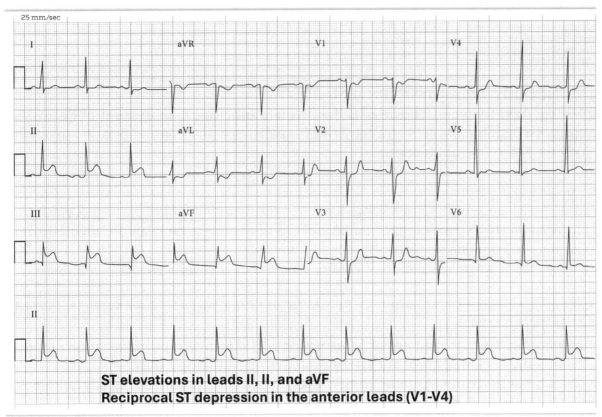

25 mm/sec

ST elevations in leads II, II, and aVF
Reciprocal ST depression in the anterior leads (V1-V4)

Choice E [Add Verapamil] is not used in the acute management of STEMI as it can worsen cardiac contractility.

Choice D [TIMI risk factor assessment] is used as part of the diagnostic algorithm in patients with Unstable angina or NSTEMI to assess the need for early catheterization.

Choice E [Add IV Morphine] is not indicated as it can reduce preload; Posterior wall MIs are often dependent on preload to maintain cardiac output.

59. INFECTIOUS DISEASE – INFLUENZA [CLINICAL INTERVENTION]

Oseltamivir [choice E] is indicated in the management of individuals with Influenza
- **[1] in high-risk patients (eg, Asthma) regardless of symptom duration and**
- **[2] in individuals not at high risk who present within 48 hours or in all high-risk patients regardless of symptom duration.**

Choice A [Influenza vaccination] is not administered in patients who are ill with symptoms of an acute infection.

Choice B [Amantadine] is not routinely used in the management of Influenza due to increased resistance.

Choice C [Doxycycline] is used in the management of Bacterial infections.

Choice D [Ibuprofen] and supportive management is indicated for the management of Influenza for outpatients with uncomplicated illness who are not at high risk with symptoms ≥48 hours due to lack of any significant benefit of Oseltamivir.

60. PULMONOLOGY – CYSTIC FIBROSIS [LABS AND DIAGNOSTICS]

The sweat chloride test [choice E] is the primary initial test for the diagnosis of Cystic fibrosis (CF).

Sweat chloride ≥60 mmol/L is abnormal. If confirmed on a second occasion, this is sufficient to confirm the diagnosis of CF in patients with clinical symptoms of CF.

If the test is abnormal, DNA testing is indicated.

Cystic fibrosis may be suspected in children with:
- meconium ileus
- failure to thrive
- pancreatic insufficiency, which may include deficiencies in fat-soluble vitamins A, D, E, and K
- respiratory tract involvement
- sinus and nasopharyngeal disease.

Choice A [Transglutaminase antibodies] are helpful in establishing the diagnosis of Celiac disease.

Choice B [Anti-mitochondrial antibodies] are useful in establishing the diagnosis of Primary biliary cirrhosis.

Choice C [Bronchial provocation testing] may be used in the diagnosis of Asthma.

Choice D [Parietal cell antibodies] are useful in the diagnosis of Pernicious anemia.

61. CARDIOLOGY – PULSELESS VENTRICULAR TACHYCARDIA [CLINICAL INTERVENTION]

Defibrillation (Unsynchronized cardioversion) [choice B] is the management of choice for Pulseless Monomorphic Ventricular tachycardia, in addition to cardiopulmonary resuscitation (CPR) as per the ACLS protocol.

Pulseless VT should be treated immediately with electrical cardioversion with high-energy defibrillator (150-200 J if biphasic and 360 J if monophasic).

Delaying defibrillation for ≥2 minutes decreases survival rate compared to patients receive immediate defibrillation.

Choice A [Urgent synchronized cardioversion] (following administration of sedation) is recommended for patients with monomorphic Ventricular tachycardia who are hemodynamically unstable (eg, systolic blood pressure in the double digits, altered mental status) with a discernible blood pressure and pulse.

Choice C [Amiodarone] is used in the management of Ventricular tachycardia in patients who are hemodynamically stable.

Choice D [Magnesium sulfate] is used as first-line management of Polymorphic Ventricular tachycardia (Torsades de pointes).

Choice E [Verapamil] is not the management of Ventricular tachycardia.

62. CARDIOLOGY – ABDOMINAL AORTIC ANEURYSM (AAA) [HEALTH MAINTENANCE]

Immediate surgical repair [choice D] is recommended in the management of Abdominal aortic aneurysm in men with aortic diameter ≥5.5 cm or > 0.5 cm expansion in 6 months, even if asymptomatic.

Aneurysm diameter is the strongest predictor of aneurysm rupture, with risk increasing markedly at aneurysm diameters >5.5 cm.

Larger aneurysm diameter and faster rate of aneurysm expansion are associated with an increased likelihood of symptoms and complications.

Ultrasonography every 3-6 months [choice B] is recommended if the diameter is 5-5.4 cm.
Ultrasonography every 6-12 months [choice C] is recommended if the diameter is 4.0-4.9 cm.
Ultrasonography every 3 years [choice E] is recommended if the diameter is 3.0-3.9 cm.

63. MUSCULOSKELETAL – FELTY SYNDROME/RHEUMATOID ARTHRITIS [APPLYING FOUNDATIONAL CONCEPTS]

Felty syndrome is a rare extra-articular manifestation of seropositive Rheumatoid arthritis characterized by the triad of:

- **[1] Rheumatoid arthritis**
- **[2] Neutropenia (ANC<1500 mm^3) [choice B], and**
- **[3] splenomegaly.**

Neutropenia occurs due to insufficient production due to infiltration of bone marrow by cytotoxic lymphocytes and increased sequestration due to splenomegaly.

Choice A [Arthrocentesis] is not necessary to establish the diagnosis of Felty syndrome.

Choice C [Chest radiograph revealing pulmonary nodules] and choice D [Pulmonary function testing showing a restrictive pattern] may result from Caplan syndrome, which is associated with the triad of [1] Rheumatoid arthritis, [2] pneumoconiosis, and [3] pulmonary nodules.

Choice E [Liver function testing showing AST:ALT ratio >2:1] is associated with Alcoholic hepatitis.

64. PULMONOLOGY – PULMONARY EMBOLISM [LABS AND DIAGNOSTIC STUDIES]

Ventilation/perfusion scan (V/Q scan) [choice A] remains the test of choice for diagnosing Pulmonary embolism (PE) in pregnancy for those with a normal chest radiograph.
V/Q scanning is mostly performed for patients in whom CTPA is contraindicated [eg, pregnancy (due to radiation exposure), elevated creatinine (due to increased risk of contrast-induced kidney injury)], if CTPA is inconclusive, or when additional testing is needed.
A normal chest radiograph is usually required before V/Q scanning.

Choice B [D dimer] is used to diagnose PE in low-risk patients when negative. If positive, CT scan (or VQ scan if CT is contraindicated) may be required.

Choice C [CT pulmonary angiography (High resolution CT scan)] is the test of choice in nonpregnant individuals with PE.

Choice D [Ultrasound of the lower extremities] may be used in patients with suspected PE in whom chest imaging is indeterminate or contraindicated.

Choice E [Pulmonary function testing] is not indicated for evaluation of Pulmonary embolism in most patients.

65. MUSCULOSKELETAL – OSTEOARTHRITIS [CLINICAL INTERVENTION]

Topical Nonsteroidal anti-inflammatory drugs (NSAIDs) such as Topical Diclofenac [choice C] is the first line pharmacotherapy for Osteoarthritis involving 1 or a few joints, especially

knee and/or hand OA, due to their similar efficacy compared with oral NSAIDs and their better safety profile.

The 3 classic findings of OA on radiographs include

- osteophyte formation,
- subchondral sclerosis, and
- asymmetric joint narrowing.

Oral NSAIDs [choice E] may be used in patients with inadequate symptom relief from topical NSAIDs, symptomatic OA in multiple joints, and/or patients with hip OA.

Choice A [Duloxetine] may be used in patients with OA in multiple joints and concomitant comorbidities that may contraindicate oral NSAIDs and for patients with knee OA who have not responded to other management.

Choice B [Intraarticular Triamcinolone] is not routinely used because of its short duration of action (~4 weeks), it may accelerate OA progression, and it may have negative effects on the hyaline cartilage.

Choice D [Topical Capsaicin] is a treatment option when one or a few joints are involved and other interventions are ineffective or contraindicated; however, its use may be limited by common local adverse effects.

66. PROFESSIONAL PRACTICE – INFORMED CONSENT

A written consent [choice C] is necessary in case of extensive intervention involving risks where anesthesia or sedation is used, restorative procedures, any invasive or surgical procedures, administering of medications with known high risks.
Expressed consent is typically done in writing.

Implied consent [choice E] is typically conveyed through a patient's actions or conduct passively cooperates in a process without discussion or formal consent. Implied consent does not need to be documented in the clinical record.

Verbal consent is where a patient states their consent to a procedure verbally but does not sign any written form. This is adequate for routine treatment such for diagnostic procedures and prophylaxis, as long as full records are documented.

67. NEUROLOGY – AMYOTROPHIC LATERAL SCLEROSIS (ALS) [MOST LIKELY]

Amyotrophic lateral sclerosis (ALS) [choice A] presents with combined upper and lower motor neuron findings in the absence of an alternative explanation, asymmetric limb weakness, bulbar involvement, and autonomic symptoms.
This patient presents with:

- [1] Upper motor neuron findings: hyperreflexia on the right with right upgoing plantar responses, spastic gait with spontaneous ankle clonus.
- [2] Lower motor neuron findings: flaccid weakness in right arm, left forearm muscle atrophy, fasciculations of the muscles of his tongue, and right biceps atrophy.

Motor neuron degeneration and death with gliosis replacing lost neurons are hallmark of Amyotrophic lateral sclerosis (ALS).

Choice B [Guillain-Barre syndrome] is a demyelinating   lower motor neuron disease characterized by symmetric ascending muscle weakness, flaccid paralysis, decreased or absent tendon reflexes, and sensory symptoms.

Choice C [Multiple sclerosis] can also present with upper motor neuron signs but usually also present with motor and sensory symptoms (eg, sensory loss in limbs or one side of the face, optic neuritis, trigeminal neuralgia, and internuclear ophthalmoplegia).

Choice D [Myasthenia gravis] presents with muscle weakness that is worse with repeated muscle use. The absence of upper or lower motor neuron bulbar signs, the presence of ocular findings, and diurnal variation is more characteristic of Myasthenia gravis.

Choice E [Inflammatory myopathies], such as Polymyositis and Dermatomyositis classically present with symmetric proximal muscle weakness without upper motor neuron signs.

68. REPRODUCTIVE – UTERINE FIBROIDS [HEALTH MAINTENANCE]
Options for the management of Uterine fibroids in women who desire fertility include:
- **Myomectomy [choice E] or**
- **Nonsurgical treatment (eg, NSAIDs).**

Submucosal fibroids are often amenable to hysteroscopic resection (myomectomy) and are efficacy in treating heavy menstrual bleeding in women who desire fertility.

Choice A [Endometrial ablation] is associated with a greater risk of infertility compared to myomectomy.

Choice B [Uterine artery embolization] is associated with a greater risk of infertility compared to myomectomy.

Choice C [Combination oral contraceptive pills] are an alternative to myomectomy but are counterproductive in women who desire to become pregnant.

Choice D [Copper-containing intrauterine device] would prevent her from getting pregnant.

69.   GASTROINTESTINAL/NUTRITION   –   ESOPHAGEAL   RUPTURE/BOERHAAVE SYNDROME [MOST LIKELY]
Effort rupture of the esophagus (Boerhaave syndrome) [choice D], is a spontaneous perforation of the esophagus that results from a sudden increase in intraesophageal pressure combined with negative intrathoracic pressure.
Inciting factors can include retching and vomiting (as in this patient).

The classic findings of Boerhaave syndrome include:
- excruciating retrosternal chest, neck, or back pain
- dysphagia, odynophagia, dyspnea
- **subcutaneous emphysema**: crepitus on palpation of the chest wall
- **Hamman's crunch**: mediastinal crackling with each heartbeat due to mediastinal emphysema.

The diagnosis can be established by water-soluble contrast esophagram (will show extravasation of contrast) or Computed tomography scan.

Choice A [Peptic ulcer perforation] classically presents with abdominal pain and peritoneal signs (guarding, rigidity, rebound tenderness) without Hamman's crunch.

Choice B [Mallory-Weiss tear] can also present after retching and/or vomiting with hematemesis and little to no pain without Hamman's crunch. MWT is due to a superficial longitudinal laceration of the esophagus without a full thickness rupture.

Choice C [Acute pancreatitis due to alcohol] can also present with epigastric pain radiating to the back but without subcutaneous and/or mediastinal emphysema.

Choice E [Aortic dissection] can present with chest, abdominal, and back pain but without subcutaneous and/or mediastinal emphysema.

70. CARDIOLOGY – CONGENITAL LONG QT SYNDROME [PHARMACOLOGY]

Beta blockers, such as Propranolol [choice C] and Nadolol are first line pharmacotherapy for patients with congenital long QT syndrome (LQTS) with a history of syncope or seizures, due their superior efficacy. They are also recommended for asymptomatic patients with LQTS.

The protective effect of Beta blockers is related to their adrenergic blockade, which diminishes the risk of cardiac arrhythmias.

Patients with LQTS-associated sudden cardiac arrest (SCA), while compliant with Beta-blocker therapy, should generally receive an Implantable cardioverter defibrillator (AICD).

Long QT syndrome (LQTS) is defined by a QT interval of >460 msec for women and >440 msec for men on ECG.

Antiarrhythmics that can induce arrhythmias, including Torsades de pointes, in patients with congenital long QT syndrome (LQTS) and should be avoided when possible in include:
- Sotalol (class II and III agent)
- Dofetilide (class III agent)
- Ibutilide (class III agent)
- Amiodarone (class III agent). In contrast to other class III agents, Amiodarone is rarely associated with TdP.
- Quinidine (class IA agent)
- Disopyramide
- Procainamide (class IA agent)

71. PSYCHIATRY/BEHAVIORAL – ALCOHOL USE DISORDER [HEALTH MAINTENANCE]

Naltrexone [choice A] is the preferred initial pharmacotherapy for newly diagnosed patients with Alcohol use disorder.

Naltrexone is a preferred agent due to its preferable dosing schedule and the ability to begin treatment for alcohol use disorder while the individual is still drinking.

Naloxone blocks the mu-opioid receptor, reducing the reinforcing effect of endogenous opioids.

Naloxone also suppresses alcohol consumption via modification of the hypothalamic-pituitary-adrenal axis.

In patients who cannot tolerate or have no response to Naltrexone, alternative options include Topiramate and Disulfiram.

Choice A [Flumazenil] is an antidote for Benzodiazepine toxicity.

Choice C [Naloxone] is an antidote for Opioid toxicity.

Choice D [Methadone] is used in the management of Opioid dependence.

Choice E [Chlordiazepoxide] is used for tapering in patients with alcohol withdrawal.

72. RENAL – NEPHROBLASTOMA (WILM TUMOR) [MOST LIKELY]

Nephroblastoma (Wilm tumor) [choice A] is the most common renal malignancy in children, peaking at ages 2-5 years.

Wilms tumor may occur as a part of a multiple malformation syndrome including WAGR syndrome (Wilms tumor, Aniridia, Genitourinary malformations, & mental Retardation).

The most common presentation is detection of an abdominal mass or swelling without other signs or symptoms or abdominal pain, hematuria, and hypertension.

Choice B [Neuroblastoma] is not as common as Nephroblastoma but can present with an abdominal mass that can cross the midline.

Choice C [Pheochromocytoma] presents with palpitations, headache, and excessive sweating.

Choice D [Ewing sarcoma] usually presents with bone pain.

Choice E [Renal cell carcinoma] is more common in older adults.

73. HEMATOLOGY – HODGKIN LYMPHOMA [MOST LIKELY]

Nodular sclerosis Hodgkin lymphoma [choice B] is the most common form of Hodgkin lymphoma (HL), accounting for ~70% of HL.

Hodgkin lymphoma is characterized on histology by Reed-Sternberg (RS) cells, seen by at least two nucleoli in separate nuclear lobes (bilobed or multilobed) and present a characteristic "owl's eyes" appearance.

Other histological types of HL include:
- Mixed cellularity
- Lymphocyte rich
- Lymphocyte depleted.

Choice C [Diffuse large B cell] is the most common cause of Non-Hodgkin lymphoma.

74. RENAL – RENOVASCULAR HYPERTENSION/RENAL ARTERY STENOSIS [PHARMACOLOGY]

Angiotensin-converting enzyme (ACE) inhibitors, such as Lisinopril [choice A] and angiotensin II receptor blockers (ARBs) are effective in patients with bilateral renal artery stenosis.

Antihypertensive therapy is recommended to control Hypertension in all patients with bilateral renal artery stenosis (or unilateral stenosis in a single viable kidney).

Indications for surgical intervention for definitive management (choices B, C, or D) include:
- severe disease or inadequate response to medical therapy
- recurrent unexplained CHF or pulmonary edema
- creatinine >4.0 mg/dL
- increased creatinine with ACE inhibitor treatment
- >80% stenosis, or
- bilateral disease.

75. HEMATOLOGY – MYELODYSPLASTIC SYNDROMES (MDS) [MOST LIKELY]

In Myelodysplastic syndromes (MDS) [choice A] granulocytes may reduce segmentation, decreased or absent granulation (pseudo-Pelger-Huet abnormality), and/or bilobed nuclei.

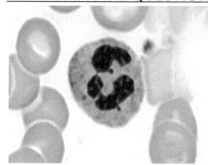 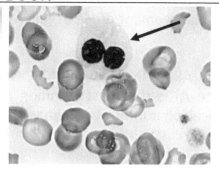

Normal neutrophil   **Pseudo Pelger-Huet**

MDS are a group of acquired clonal disorders of the hematopoietic stem cell.
They are characterized by the constellation of
- cytopenias
- hypercellular marrow is often seen
- morphologic abnormalities in ≥1 hematopoietic stem cell lines
- genetic abnormalities.

MDS are usually idiopathic, but etiologies include prior exposure to cytotoxic chemotherapy, radiation (as in this patient), or due to genetic variants.

Choice B [Primary myelofibrosis] is also associated with pancytopenia but would show dacrocytes (teardrop-shaped red cells).
Choice C [Polycythemia vera] is a myeloproliferative disorder associated with increased red cell mass (increased hemoglobin and a hematocrit).
Choice D [Chronic myelogenous leukemia] is also associated with pancytopenia without pseudo-Pelger-Huet abnormality.
Choice E [Hodgkin lymphoma] is associated with the Reed-Sternberg cell.

76. CARDIOLOGY – PRINZMETAL (VARIANT ANGINA] [PHARMACOLOGY]
Calcium channel blockers such as Diltiazem [choice B] and Amlodipine are the mainstay of therapy for Vasospastic (Prinzmetal) angina.
Calcium channel blockers alleviate symptoms in Variant angina by preventing vasoconstriction and promoting vasodilation in the coronary vasculature.
Initial therapy consists of sublingual Nitroglycerin as needed for symptoms, smoking cessation, risk factor reduction, and Calcium channel blockers.
Vasospastic angina occurs due to coronary artery vasospasm, resulting in transient myocardial ischemia, often occurring at rest as it is a supply problem (vasospasm) not a demand problem.

Medications to avoid in Vasospastic (Prinzmetal) angina include:
- Nonselective beta blockers, such as Propranolol [choice A] as is can exacerbate vasospasm.
- Aspirin [choice C] should be used with caution and at low doses, due to its inhibition of prostacyclin at high doses (prostacyclin is a vasodilator that relaxes smooth muscle and inhibits platelet aggregation).

Choice D [Cilostazol] is used in the management of claudication for patients with Peripheral arterial disease.

Choice E [Digoxin] is used in the management of Heart failure with reduced ejection fraction [HFrEF].

77. PULMONARY - PNEUMONIA [APPLYING FOUNDATIONAL CONCEPTS]
Streptococcus pneumoniae [choice A] is the most common cause of Community acquired pneumonia especially with a typical lobar infiltrate on imaging.
Although *S. pneumoniae* (pneumococcus) is the most commonly detected bacterial cause of CAP in most studies, the overall incidence of pneumococcal pneumonia is decreasing.
This decline in the US is due to widespread use of pneumococcal vaccination, reducing individual rates of pneumococcal pneumonia and herd immunity in the population.

78. MUSCULOSKELETAL – MEDIAL COLLATERAL LIGAMENT [MOST LIKELY]
Valgus stress testing is the best way to test the integrity of the Medial collateral ligament (MCL) directly [choice D]. The MCL resists vaLgus force (Lateral trauma) to the knee.
The knee should be brought into 30 degrees of flexion. The examiner should grasp the ankle with one hand and push the ankle laterally while applying a valgus force to the knee with the other hand.
Pain and laxity is considered to be a positive test.

Choice A (Patellofemoral syndrome) is associated with anterior knee pain in runners and is associated with a positive apprehension test.
Choice B [Lateral collateral ligament injury] is associated with a positive Varus stress test.
Choice C [Anterior cruciate ligament injury] is associated with positive Anterior drawer and Lachman tests.
Choice E [Posterior cruciate ligament injury] is associated with a Posterior drawer test.

79. ENDOCRINOLOGY – THYROID NODULE [LABS AND DIAGNOSTIC STUDIES]
Thyroid ultrasound [choice C] is part of the initial evaluation of a thyroid nodule to confirm the presence of the nodule, assess sonographic features (risk of benign vs. malignant), and assess for lymphadenopathy as well as adjacent neck structures.
The initial evaluation of a thyroid nodule includes:
  - [1] history and physical examination
  - [2] measurement of serum thyroid-stimulating hormone (TSH), and
  - [3] thyroid Ultrasound.

Choice A [Serum free T4 and Total T3] has little diagnostic utility in patients with a thyroid nodule and normal TSH.
Choice B [Iodine 131 nuclear medicine scan (scintigraphy)] is the next most appropriate step to evaluate thyroid nodules with a low serum TSH to assess for a Toxic thyroid adenoma (focal increased area of uptake).
Choice D [Fine needle aspiration] is indicated if [1] physical examination is concerning for malignancy, [2] large nodules (eg, >1.5 cm), or [3] if there are malignant characteristics seen on ultrasound.
Choice E [Basal calcitonin measurements] is not usually warranted in nodular thyroid disease unless Medullary thyroid cancer is suspected.

80. NEUROLOGY – ALZHEIMER DISEASE [PHARMACOLOGY]

Memantine [choice C] can be used in combination with a cholinesterase inhibitor, such as Donepezil, in the management of Moderate to severe Alzheimer disease (MME ≤18).

A combination capsule of Donepezil-Memantine is available.

Memantine is an N-methyl-D-aspartate (NMDA) receptor antagonist, slowing calcium influx & nerve damage.

Glutamate is an excitatory neurotransmitter of the NDMA receptor; excitotoxicity causes cell death.

NMDA antagonists, such as memantine, reduce glutamate excitotoxicity.

Choice A [Bromocriptine] is a dopamine agonist used in Parkinson disease.

Choice B [Levodopa-Carbidopa] is a precursor of dopamine used in Parkinson disease.

Choice D [Deutetrabenazine] may be used for Tardive dyskinesia and for Huntington disease.

Choice E [Aducanumab] has been FDA-approved for Alzheimer disease but is not routinely used because there is uncertainty about whether patients with AD benefit clinically from Aducanumab.

81. MUSCULOSKELETAL – MARFAN SYNDROME [HISTORY AND PHYSICAL]

Hallmark features of Marfan syndrome include:
- **Ectopia lentis (dislocation of the lens) [choice A]**
- **tall stature**
- **arachnodactyly abnormally long fingers**
- **long bones**
- **dislocation of the lens, retinal**
- **detachment, pectus carinatum &/or excavatum**
- **high incidence of progressive aortic dilation**

Marfan syndrome (MFS) is caused by a variety of mutations in the fibrillin (FBN1) gene.

Choice B [Skin hyperextensibility] is seen with Ehlers-Danlos syndrome.
Choice C [Macroorchidism] is seen with Fragile X syndrome.
Choice D [Multiple soft tissue bruises] is seen with Ehlers-Danlos syndrome.
Choice E [Hypertrophic scar formation] is seen with Ehlers-Danlos syndrome.

82. CARDIOLOGY – PERIPHERAL ARTERIAL DISEASE [HISTORY AND PHYSICAL]

Classic physical examination findings consistent with Peripheral arterial disease include:
- **Dependent rubor [choice E] and pallor with leg elevation**
- Decreased pulses
- <u>Atrophic skin changes</u>: dry, shiny, and hairless skin
- Skin cool to the touch and dry
- Lateral malleolar ulcers.

Classic physical examination findings consistent with Chronic venous insufficiency include:
- skin that is warm to the touch
- venous stasis dermatitis (eczematous patches or plaques with brownish discoloration)

- medial malleolar ulcers
- peripheral edema.

83. EENT – CHALAZION [CLINICAL INTERVENTION]

Referral to an ophthalmologist [choice B] for possible incision and curettage or glucocorticoid injection is recommended for Chalazia that do not resolve over 1-2 months.

Persistent or recurring lesions, especially if unilateral, may be an indication for biopsy to evaluate for possible malignancy.

Most Chalazia spontaneously clear after several weeks with frequent warm compresses applied to chalazia expedite spontaneous drainage.

A Chalazion is a chronic localized inflammation that results from the obstruction of the meibomian glands.

Choice A [Prescribe topical Methylprednisolone acetate] do not result in resolution of Chalazia.
Choice C [Prescribe Ciprofloxacin ophthalmic solution] is not indicated as topical antibiotics are not helpful in resolving Chalazia since they result from a granulomatous process.
Choice D [Continue warm compresses and follow up in 8 weeks] is not appropriate since the lesion has not healed within 2 months.
Choice E [Prescribe Amoxicillin-clavulanate] and other systemic antibiotics are unnecessary for Chalazia unless there is concurrent Preseptal cellulitis.

84. NEUROLOGY – SUBDURAL HEMATOMA/HEMORRHAGIC STROKE [APPLYING FOUNDATIONAL CONCEPTS]

Subdural hematomas (SDH) most commonly occur due tearing of the cortical bridging veins [choice A], located between the arachnoid membranes and the dura in most cases.

SDH forms between the dural and the arachnoid membranes overlying the brain.

Because the bleeding occurs in the subdural space, the bleeding can cross the suture lines and appears as a convex shaped bleed on neuroimaging.

Less common causes of SDH include rupture of the small cortical arteries [choice C].

Choice B [Rupture of a Berry aneurysm] most commonly results in Subarachnoid hemorrhage.
Choice D [Arteriovenous malformations] are uncommon causes of nontraumatic EDH.
Choice E [Rupture of the middle meningeal artery] may result in an Epidural hematoma.

85. NEUROLOGY – MEDIAN NEUROPATHY/COLLE'S FRACTURE [HISTORY AND PHYSICAL]

Median nerve compression can occur with a distal radius fracture with dorsal displacement (Colle's fracture) resulting in:
- **motor deficits: decreased thumb abduction and opposition [choice B]**
- **sensory deficits: sensory deficits of the lateral 3 and lateral aspect of the fourth fingers.**

Other early complications include Extensor pollicis longus tendon rupture (the most common complication) and rarely, compartment syndrome, and vascular compromise.

Choice A [Loss of two-point discrimination over the fifth finger] occurs with ulnar nerve injuries.

Choice C [Decreased extension of the wrist against resistance] occurs with radial nerve injuries, resulting in a wrist drop. Radial nerve injuries are more common in elbow dislocations, humeral shaft fractures, and supracondylar fracture.

Choice D [Adduction of the index and fourth digit] occurs with injury to the ulnar nerve, affecting the palmar interossei.

Choice E [Inability to make the O.K. sign by touching the tips of the index finger and the thumb together] is a positive Froment sign, indicative of an ulnar nerve injury.

86. EENT – EPISTAXIS [APPLYING FOUNDATION CONCEPTS]

Posterior epistaxis arises most commonly from the posterolateral branches of the sphenopalatine artery [choice C] & may also arise from branches of the carotid artery.

Posterior bleed may be suggested by bleeding emanating from both nares or in the posterior oropharynx or if measures to control anterior epistaxis have failed.

Anterior nosebleeds, which is by far more common, occur within the vascular watershed area of the nasal septum (Kiesselbach's plexus) [choice A] with consist of anastomosis of the septal branch of the anterior ethmoidal artery; the lateral nasal branch of the sphenopalatine artery; and the septal branch of the superior labial branch of the facial artery.

87. PSYCHIATRY/BEHAVIORAL – ANTIPSYCHOTICS [PHARMACOLOGY]

Of the second-generation antipsychotics, Aripiprazole [choice B] & Ziprasidone are associated with the LOWEST amount of weight gain & dyslipidemia.

Aripiprazole has little or no tendency to cause hyperglycemia, hyperprolactinemia, or weight gain.

Choice A [Olanzapine] and choice C [Clozapine] are associated with the highest risk of weight gain.

Choice D [Haloperidol] is more likely to cause further worsening of his Parkinsonism symptoms.

Choice E [Chlorpromazine] has a moderate to high risk of weight gain.

88. RENAL – HYPERCALCEMIA/PRIMARY HYPERPARATHYROIDISM [HISTORY AND PHYSICAL EXAMINATION]

Hypercalcemia increases the excitation threshold, resulting in decreased GI contractions, manifested by decreased or absent bowel sounds [choice E].

The classic findings of Hypercalcemia include:
- stones: nephrolithiasis
- bones: bone pain
- groans: decreased bowel sounds or ileus
- psychic moans: irritability
- thrones: polyuria due to Nephrogenic Diabetes insipidus
- increased tones: Hypertension.

All of the other choices listed are hallmark of Hypocalcemia.

89. RENAL – HORSESHOE KIDNEY [APPLYING FOUNDATIONAL CONCEPTS]

Ureteropelvic junction obstruction [choice B] is the most common congenital urologic abnormality in patients with Horseshoe kidney.

Ureteropelvic junction obstruction occurs in 30% of patients which may result in obstruction of the ureters.

Renal stones are also common in patients with horseshoe kidneys and are related to ureteropelvic junction obstruction.

Urinary stasis also predisposes to infection, resulting in recurrent urinary tract infections.

Horseshoe kidney may be associated with
- other congenital urologic abnormalities eg, ureteropelvic junction obstruction most common, vesicourethral reflux) or
- other genital abnormalities: eg, bicornuate or septate uterus in girls as well as Cryptorchidism & Hypospadias in boys.

Choice A [Aniridia] is associated with Nephroblastoma.

90. REPRODUCTIVE – PRETERM LABOR [CLINICAL INTERVENTION]

The management of moderate Preterm labor (32-34 weeks) include [choice B]:
- **Antenatal corticosteroids** to enhance fetal lung maturity
- **Tocolysis: eg, Nifedipine** to delay labor to maximize the effects of the corticosteroids,
- **Penicillin G if Group B streptococcus (GBS) positive or unknown.**

Preterm labor presents with regular contractions causing cervical change at <37 weeks with intact membranes.

Choice A [Continue progression of labor] is an alternative to first line management of Preterm labor.

Choice C [Indomethacin and Betamethasone] can be used in the management of very Preterm labor (<32 weeks of gestation). Use of Indomethacin after 32 weeks may result in premature closure of the ductus arteriosus.

Choice D [Observation and watchful waiting] is not the best management of Preterm labor.

Choice E [Cesarean section] may be indicated if maternal instability, intrauterine infection, or fetal distress/demise.

91. EENT – CHEMICAL OCULAR INJURY [CLINICAL INTERVENTION]

After rapid determination of pH with pH paper, immediate continuous irrigation for at least 30 minutes with 2-3L of Lactated ringers or Normal saline [choice A] until a neutral pH (7.0–7.4) is achieved is recommended in patients with Ocular chemical injury.

A topical anesthetic may be applied prior to irrigation but nothing should delay irrigation.

LR ideal because it is closer to a normal pH & is less irritating.

Unless there is a strong suspicion for Globe rupture, do not delay irrigation.

Once the pH is normal, the eye can safely be examined via a comprehensive ocular assessment [choices B, C, and D].

92. GENITOURINARY – OVERFLOW INCONTINENCE [MOST LIKELY]

Overflow urinary incontinence [choice B] typically presents with continuous urinary leakage or dribbling in the setting of incomplete bladder emptying due to either [1] bladder underactivity or [2] bladder outlet obstruction.

Associated symptoms can include weak or intermittent urinary stream, hesitancy, frequency, and nocturia.

Overflow UI is more common in men and most often associated with bladder outlet obstruction due to benign prostatic hyperplasia (BPH).

Women can develop Overflow incontinence as a result of a neurogenic bladder secondary to peripheral neuropathy (eg, diabetic neuropathy as in this patient), prolapsed uterus, or urogenital malignancies.

Choice A [Urge incontinence] is associated with an abrupt onset of an urge to urinate without warning.

Choice C [Genitourinary syndrome of menopause] may present with urinary symptoms in the setting of atrophy, pelvic organ prolapse, or dyspareunia from vaginal dryness (this patient has none of those additional symptoms).

Choice D [Stress incontinence] is associated with leakage of urine when intrabdominal pressure exceeds urethral pressure (eg, with coughing, laughing, sneezing, Valsalva).

Choice E [Urethral hypomobility] is a cause of Stress incontinence (see choice D).

93. INFECTIOUS DISEASE – LUDWIG ANGINA [LABS AND DIAGNOSTIC STUDIES]

Computed tomography (CT) of the neck with intravenous contrast [choice A] is the imaging modality of choice for the diagnosis of Ludwig angina and other deep neck space infections.
Suggestive findings include soft tissue thickening, increased attenuation of the subcutaneous fat, loss of fat planes in the submandibular space, gas bubbles within soft tissues, focal fluid collections, and muscle edema.

CT has a sensitivity of 95% and a specificity of 53%, but when combined with suggestive clinical findings, the specificity increases to 80%.

Ludwig angina is a bilateral infection of the floor of the mouth which classically presents on physical examination with a tender, symmetric, and "woody" induration, sometimes with palpable crepitus, in the submandibular area ("bull neck").

Choice B [Magnetic resonance imaging (MRI) of the neck] is an alternative to CT, it should not be performed if there is any question of airway compromise and/or challenges with controlling respiratory sections (this patient is drooling), due to the length of time it takes to obtain the test.

Choice C [Needle aspiration] is indicated in abscesses not Ludwig angina. This patient has no fluctuance.

Choice D [Early surgical decompression] is usually not needed because there isn't usually a drainable collection when patients present. Surgical drainage may be indicated if an abscess is seen on imaging.

Choice E [IV Methylprednisolone] is not indicated in the routine management of Ludwig angina.

94. RENAL – RENAL OSTEODYSTROPHY [APPLYING FOUNDATIONAL CONCEPTS]

Renal osteodystrophy due to Chronic kidney disease [choice C] is associated with the classic triad of Secondary hyperparathyroidism:
- [1] Hypocalcemia +
- [2] increased serum phosphate +
- [3] increased serum intact PTH.

Calcium levels may be normal early on in the disease.

The classic radiograph findings of Osteitis Fibrosa Cystica include subperiosteal erosions, bony cysts with thin trabeculum & cortex, as well as a "salt & pepper" appearance of the skull (punctate trabecular bone resorption in the skull).

Choice A [Parathyroid adenoma] and choice B [Parathyroid hyperplasia] are associated with Primary hyperparathyroidism, which is associated with the triad of Hypercalcemia, increased PTH, and decreased phosphate.

Choice D [Multiple myeloma] is associated with Hypercalcemia and punched out lytic lesions on imaging.

95. MUSCULOSKELETAL – POLYMYOSITIS [LABS AND DIAGNOSTIC STUDIES]

Muscle biopsy [choice D] is the test of choice to make the definitive diagnosis of Polymyositis and distinguish it from Dermatomyositis.
- [1] <u>Polymyositis (PM):</u> CD8+ cells infiltrating the endomysium layer of the muscle with degeneration and regenerating muscle fibers.
- [2] <u>Dermatomyositis (DM):</u> CD4+ cells infiltrating the perimysium layer of the muscle with degeneration and regenerating muscle fibers.

Choice A [Electromyography] is part of the workup of PM but findings suggestive of PM are not specific.

Supportive labs of Polymyositis include anti-Jo-1 antibodies, anti-signal recognition particle (SRP) antibodies, and elevated muscle enzymes (eg, creatine kinase and aldolase). [choice B] but aldolase is not specific for PM.

Both PM and DM present with gradual onset of symmetric proximal muscle weakness.

Choice C [Acetylcholine receptor antibodies] are elevated in Myasthenia gravis, which is associated with generalized muscle weakness that worsens with repeated muscle use.

Choice E [Erythrocyte sedimentation rate] is often elevated in PM but ESR is a nonspecific marker of inflammation.

96. NEUROLOGY – CARPAL TUNNEL SYNDROME [CLINICAL INTERVENTION]

Nocturnal wrist splinting in the neutral position [choice A] or a glucocorticoid injection are initial nonsurgical therapies for Carpal tunnel syndrome (CTS).

Either approach can reduce CTS symptoms and may delay or eliminate need for surgery in mildly symptomatic patients.

Choice B [Place the patient in an ulnar gutter splint with orthopedic follow-up] is used in the management of fifth metacarpal (Boxer's) fractures.

Choice C [Surgical decompression] is usually reserved for severe or refractory CTS.

Choice D [Oral Prednisone] is an alternative to glucocorticoid injection, especially in combination with splinting if inadequate response to initial nonsurgical therapy.

NSAIDs [choice E] are not recommended in the management of CTS because there is no significant benefit for nonsteroidal anti-inflammatory drugs (NSAIDs) for improving CTS symptoms.

97. EENT – PERIODONTAL ABSCESS [CLINICAL INTERVENTION]

First-line outpatient treatment of Dental abscess include Penicillin VK [choice E] and Amoxicillin or other regimens that cover mouth flora streptococci and anaerobes.

Amoxicillin-clavulanate, Clindamycin, Cefuroxime, and Levofloxacin are second-line alternatives.

Patients with deep neck infections require IV antibiotics (eg, Ampicillin-sulbactam in immunocompetent patients).

Treatment of odontogenic infections includes appropriate antibiotic therapy (aerobic and anaerobic coverage) and surgical drainage of abscesses if needed.

98. CARDIOLOGY – FIRST-DEGREE AV BLOCK [HEALTH MAINTENANCE]

Asymptomatic patients with First-degree AV block do not require any specific therapy [choice B].

First-degree atrioventricular (AV) block, defined as a prolonged PR interval (>200 ms at resting heart rates), is not a true block but is rather delayed or slowed AV conduction.

Choice A [Atropine] is a first line agent for many symptomatic or unstable bradycardia, This patient is hemodynamically stable and has no symptoms.

Choice C [Transcutaneous pacing] can be used for patients with Third-degree (complete) heart block.

Choice D [Epinephrine] can be an alternative to Atropine in some patients with symptomatic or unstable bradycardia.

Choice E [Permanent pacemaker placement] is rarely used in the management of First-degree AV block, except in the rare occurrence of First-degree AV block and symptoms consistent with the loss of atrioventricular synchrony ("pseudopacemaker syndrome,") is a potential candidate for a pacemaker.

99. REPRODUCTIVE – PAGET DISEASE OF THE NIPPLE [MOST LIKELY]

A history of longstanding eczematous pruritic scaly or vesicular lesion on the breast (nipple then spreads to the areola) should increase the suspicion of Paget disease of the breast (PDB) [choice B].

PDB is usually unilateral.

After a careful history and physical exam, workup should be initiated with either a mammography or a biopsy of the lesion.

Choice A [Intraductal papilloma] can present with a bloody discharge and a palpable lump.

Choice C [Contact dermatitis] usually presents with vesicles.

Choice D [Candida mastitis] present with a beefy red erythematous plaque with satellite lesions.

Choice E [Inflammatory breast cancer] presents similar to Cellulitis with breast erythema, warmth, and tenderness; the skin may have a peau d'orange appearance (orange peel) due to lymphedema.

100. PROFESSIONAL PRACTICE – PATIENT AND PROVIDER RELATIONSHIPS

Expectant management is an option for women with otherwise uncomplicated pregnancies who choose this option after weighing the risks and benefits of induction vs. expectant management [choice B].

This allows her to make an informed consent about her decision and respects patient autonomy.

Although prompt induction of labor is the preferred treatment for Prelabor rupture of membranes (PROM) and waiting for spontaneous delivery increases risk for fetal and neonatal complications, expectant management is also an option.

1. A 49-year-old man with a history of Alcohol use disorder presents to emergency department with generalized muscle weakness, nervousness, diarrhea, and a fine hand tremor. His last drink was 72 hours ago. Initial labs are significant for a serum potassium level of 2.7 mEq/L (3.5-5). He is treated with Lorazepam and IV potassium chloride, followed by oral potassium supplementation. On his follow-up visit to the clinic, his serum potassium is 3.0 mEq/L. Which of the following is the most likely the reason for the lack of potassium repletion?
a. Hypomagnesemia
b. Vitamin B1 (Thiamine) deficiency
c. Hypoalbuminemia
d. Hypercalcemia
e. Alcohol withdrawal syndrome

2. A 33-year-old man presents to the emergency department for difficulty with walking. He has noticed some lightheadedness when standing up from a seated position and some numbness and burning in the bilateral lower extremities. He recently recovered from a diarrheal illness that was nonbloody, then became bloody and self-resolved. Physical examination is notable for 3/5 strength, decreased sensation to light touch and pinprick in the bilateral lower extremities, and absent patellar and ankle reflexes. Based on the most likely diagnosis, consumption of which of the following would most likely be in this patient's history?
a. Undercooked hamburgers
b. Undercooked chicken skewers
c. Raw shellfish
d. Undercooked pork chops
e. Untreated water from a remote stream

3. A 30-year-old G4P3 woman at 24 weeks gestation presents to the clinic for a routine prenatal visit. She has no complaints. Fundal height measures 24 cm. Vitals are stable. She is asked to ingest 50 mg glucose and have her blood glucose checked in 1 hour; it returns as 147 mg/dL. Which of the following is the best next step in the management of this patient?
a. Initiate Insulin therapy
b. Perform oral glucose tolerance test
c. Encourage the patient to diet to lose weight
d. Initiate Glyburide therapy
e. Do a fasting blood glucose level

4. A 27-year-old female presents to the clinic complaining of decreased libido, irregular menstrual cycle for the past 3 months, fatigue, and an occasional milky white discharge from both nipples. Physical examination is unremarkable. Initial labs reveal a negative urine beta-hCG. An MRI is performed, revealing a pituitary microadenoma. Based on the most likely diagnosis, which of the following is the recommended first-line management of choice?
a. Transsphenoidal resection of the tumor
b. Octreotide
c. Radiation therapy
d. Cabergoline
e. Estradiol and progestin therapy

5. A 65-year-old female presents with worsening cough. She recently began coughing up blood and has lost 10 pounds in the last 3 months. She has a 40 pack-year smoking history. Physical examination and laboratory evaluation are within normal limits. The following is seen on chest radiograph.

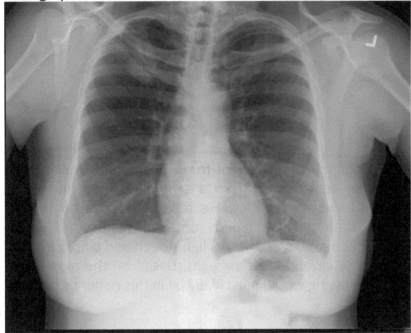

Which of the following is the most likely diagnosis?
a. Bronchioloalveolar carcinoma
b. Squamous cell lung cancer
c. Small cell lung cancer
d. Adenocarcinoma
e. Large cell carcinoma

Photo credit:
Yale Rosen from USA, CC BY-SA 2.0 <https://creativecommons.org/licenses/by-sa/2.0>, via Wikimedia Commons

6. A 32-year-old female presents with delirium, agitation, nausea, and vomiting. Vitals are temperature 102°F (38.89°C), blood pressure 160/92 mmHg, pulse 130/minute, and respirations 25/minute. Warm and moist skin, fine hand tremor, exophthalmos, and lid lag are noted. ECG shows sinus tachycardia. In addition to IV Normal saline, administration of which of the following is the most important next step?
a. Dantrolene
b. Propylthiouracil
c. IV Hydrocortisone
d. Propranolol
e. Potassium iodide

7. A 20-year-old male presents to the ED after being hit in the face with a fast-moving baseball. He is complaining of pain and decreased vision to his left eye. Physical examination reveals a right pupil that is round and vigorously responsive to light. The left pupil is teardrop-shaped and sluggishly reactive to light. Which of the following is the most appropriate next step in the management of this patient?
a. Topical Ciprofloxacin ophthalmic and topical Cyclopentolate
b. Globe tonometry
c. Slit lamp examination with Fluorescein
d. CT scan of the orbits
e. Rigid eye shield and emergency ophthalmology consult

8. A 26-year-old woman with Systemic lupus erythematosus presents for evaluation of recurrent pregnancy losses. She has experienced 3 spontaneous abortions at <10 weeks gestation and 1 fetal death at 12 weeks. Her past medical history is positive for a DVT 2 years ago after being placed on combined oral contraceptives. Physical examination shows mottled lace-like purplish discoloration of the legs. Which of the following is the best initial test to diagnose the underlying condition?
a. Anti Histone antibodies
b. Anti double-stranded DNA antibodies
c. Antinuclear antibodies
d. Anti cyclic citrullinated peptide antibodies
e. Anticardiolipin antibodies

9. A 45-year-old male presents with chest pain and palpitations. He is found to have a narrow complex tachycardia. During evaluation, the patient becomes unresponsive. There are no palpable femoral, carotid, or radial pulses. The following is seen on the cardiac monitor (see photo).

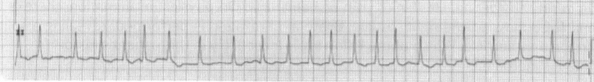

In addition to performing chest compressions, which of the following is the most appropriate next step?
a. IV Metoprolol
b. Rapid synchronized cardioversion
c. Rapid unsynchronized cardioversion
d. IV Epinephrine
e. IV Adenosine

Photo credit:
Shutterstock (used with permission)

10. A 32-year-old female with no past medical history presents for a 1-month postpartum follow-up. She has been experiencing fatigue and increased sweating. Physical examination is notable for a nontender goiter without nodularity. Initial labs reveal:
- TSH: 0.04 mIU/L (0.5-5.0)
- Free T4: 4.8 ng/dL (0.9-2.4)
- T3: 204 ng/dL (60-171).

Thyroid scintigraphy is performed (see photo).

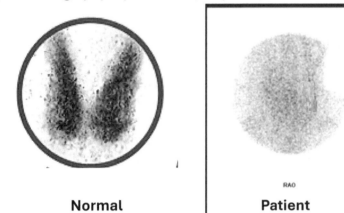

| Normal | Patient |

Which of the following is the most likely diagnosis?
a. Sheehan syndrome
b. Graves' disease
c. Toxic adenoma
d. TSH-secreting pituitary adenoma
e. Postpartum thyroiditis

11. A 30-year-old male presents to his primary care provider after noticing swelling of his right testicle during showering. He denies pain or hematuria. On physical examination, there is a firm and fixed mass on the right testicle. Bilateral ultrasound is performed, revealing a solid mass in the right testicle. Which of the following is most likely in this patient's history?
a. Fragile X syndrome
b. Cryptorchidism
c. Epispadias
d. Spermatocele
e. Vasectomy

12. A 33-year-old man comes to the office reporting mild exertional dyspnea and a "thumping" heart over the past five months. He is uncomfortably aware of his heart beating strongly. Vital signs include a blood pressure of 154/42 mmHg and a pounding pulse at a heart rate of 80 bpm. Which of the following is most likely responsible for his presentation?
a. Aortic regurgitation
b. Mitral valve prolapse
c. Hypertrophic cardiomyopathy
d. Aortic stenosis
e. Ventral septal defect

13. A 40-year-old male with a history of Polycystic kidney disease presents to the emergency department with a history of a 10/10 headache of sudden onset. Physical examination is notable for nuchal rigidity. The following is seen on CT scan of the head (see photo).

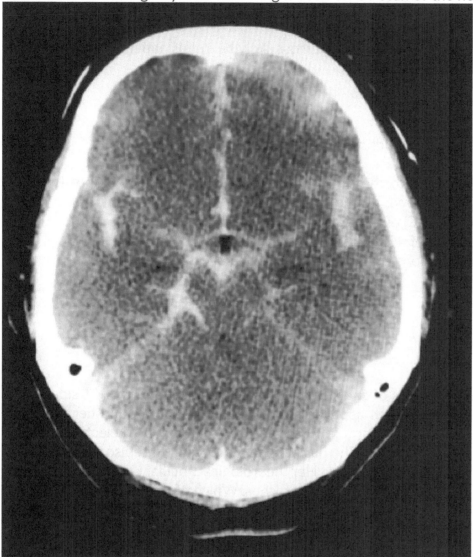

Which of the following medications is a first-line agent to reduce cerebral vasospasms in this patient?

a. Diltiazem
b. Propranolol
c. Nitroglycerin
d. Nimodipine
e. Enalapril

Photo credit:
Shutterstock (used with permission)

14. A 10-month-old boy is brought to the clinic after developing a "goose-egg" swelling to his forehead that occurred while crawling and bumping his head. Physical examination is notable for a forehead hematoma. Initial labs are significant for:
- activated partial thromboplastin time (aPTT) 42 seconds [<35]
- Factor VIII titer 0.01 U/mL [0.5–1.5].

Which of the following types of bleeding would most likely be in this patient's history?
a. Small ecchymosis to the skin
b. Petechiae
c. Excessive bleeding after minor cuts
d. Immediate bleeding after surgery
e. Bleeding into the muscles after childhood vaccinations

15. A 34-year-old male presents to the clinic with fever, mouth ulcers, and sore throat. A complete blood count (CBC) showed:
- white blood cell count (WBC) of 720 cells/mm^3 (5,000-10,000)
- absolute neutrophil count of 450 (2,500-6,000).

Which of the following medications is the most likely cause for his presentation?
a. Bupropion
b. Sertraline
c. Clozapine
d. Mirtazapine
e. Aripiprazole

16. A 57-year-old woman complains of an extremely severe, sharp, shooting right-sided facial pain that began initially when she was applying foundational makeup around her forehead, cheeks, and eyebrows. The pain lasts for a few seconds, feels like a jolt of electricity, and is triggered by drafts of wind and chewing. She has been experiencing 3-4 episodes a week but has now increased to 8-10 episodes daily. Her neurological, ocular, auricular, and oral examinations are within normal limits. There are no rashes. Which of the following is the initial management of choice?
a. Prednisone
b. Gabapentin
c. 100% Oxygen via nonrebreather
d. Oxcarbazepine
e. Sumatriptan

17. A 29-year-old woman presents to an urgent care center for dyspnea on exertion over the last 8 months. She denies any other symptoms and denies having ever smoked or been exposed chronically to second-hand smoke. Physical examination is notable for decreased breath sounds with diffuse wheezing bilaterally and hepatomegaly. Labs reveal
- Alanine aminotransferase (SGPT) 79 U/L (4-36)
- Aspartate aminotransferase (SGOT) 68 U/L (5-40).

A chest radiograph is obtained (see photo).

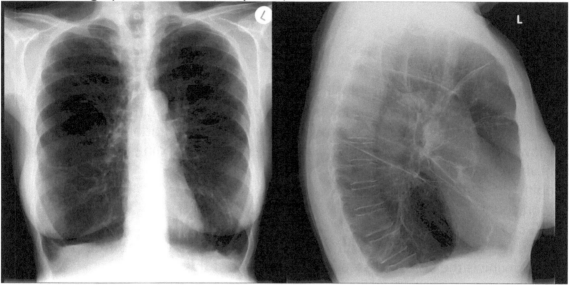

Which of the following is the most likely diagnosis?
a. Cystic fibrosis
b. Asthma
c. Alpha-1 antitrypsin deficiency
d. Bronchiectasis
e. Acute bronchitis

Photo credit:
Case courtesy of Andrew Dixon, Radiopaedia.org, rID: 9674

18. A 40-year-old male presents with increasing midline swelling for the last 3 months. Physical examination reveals a 2 cm x 3 cm swelling on the left side of the neck. Initial labs reveal
- Serum TSH: 4.2 µIU/mL (0.4–4.8).
- Serum free T4: 1.64 ng/dL (0.8–1.71)
- serum calcitonin 1,393 pg/mL (≤185)

Thyroid ultrasound reveals a hypoechoic lesion with microcalcifications. Which of the following is the most likely diagnosis?
a. Follicular adenoma
b. Medullary thyroid cancer
c. Papillary thyroid cancer
d. Anaplastic thyroid cancer
e. Follicular thyroid cancer

19. A 53-year-old female presents to the emergency department for low back pain radiating down the buttock and the back of both legs. He has been having issues with initiating urination. Physical examination reveals decreased pinprick sensation in the perianal region, absent ankle reflexes, and bilateral leg weakness. Straight leg raise results in increase pain in the legs and posterior thighs. Which of the following is the recommended next step?

a. Plain radiographs of the lumbar spine

b. CT myelography

c. Lumbar puncture

d. Electromyography

e. MRI of the lumbar spine

20. A 19-year-old, nulliparous woman with no significant medical history presented to the emergency department (ED) complaining of progressive lower abdominal pain and vaginal spotting. Her last menstrual period was seven weeks prior to presentation. Vitals are stable. She has right lower quadrant and adnexal tenderness. Moderate bleeding is noted on vaginal examination. Labs reveal:

- Hemoglobin 12.5 g/dL (12-15)
- White blood count 5,300 mm^3 (5,000-10,000)
- Serum hCG 5,200 mIU/mL

Pelvic ultrasound revealed a 4 cm x 4.5 cm complex adnexal mass with no free pelvic fluid. Which of the following is the best next step in management of this patient?

a. Methotrexate

b. Repeat quantitative serum hCG and Ultrasound in 48 hours

c. Laparoscopy

d. Dilation followed by suction curettage

e. Misoprostol

21. A 24-year-old male presents with scrotal swelling associated with a dull heaviness sensation that is worse with standing. Physical examination reveals a nontender left-sided scrotal fullness and a large, soft, left-sided scrotal mass with a "wormy" consistency. The swelling decompresses when the patient is placed into a supine position and does not transilluminate with penlight application to the scrotum. There is no evidence of hernia. He is explained that most cases of his condition are treated conservative. Surgical repair of this condition is performed primarily to prevent which of the following complications?

a. Incarcerated indirect hernia

b. Testicular torsion

c. Epididymitis

d. Infertility

e. Testicular cancer

22. A 22-year-old man presents to the emergency department after a motor vehicle accident. He sustained a brief loss of consciousness. He has a Glasgow score of 15. Physical examination is notable for a maximally dilated right pupil nonreactive to light. He undergoes a head CT without contrast (see photo).

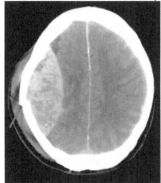

Which of the following cranial nerves is most likely responsible for these findings
a. II
b. III
c. IV
d. VI
e. VII

Photo credit:
Hellerhoff, CC BY-SA 3.0 <https://creativecommons.org/licenses/by-sa/3.0>, via Wikimedia Commons

23. A 33-year-old male presents to the clinic to establish care. He denies any GI symptoms but explains his sister was diagnosed with colorectal cancer at age 45, treated with surgical resection. His examination is unremarkable, and his blood work is within normal limits. Which of the following is the recommended colorectal cancer screening in this patient?
a. Colonoscopy at 40 years; then every 5 years thereafter
b. Colonoscopy at 35 years; then every 5 years thereafter
c. Colonoscopy at age 45; then every 5 years thereafter
d. Colonoscopy at 50 years; then every 10 years thereafter
e. Colonoscopy at 40 years; then every 10 years thereafter

24. A 6-year-old boy presents with a history Rhinosinusitis present to the pediatric emergency department for left eye pain, redness, swelling, and increased tearing. Physical examination is notable for periorbital warmth, swelling, and erythema that is tender to palpation. Extraocular muscle eye movements are intact and not associated with pain; there is no associated horizontal or vertical diplopia, proptosis, or visual changes. CT scan confirms the most likely diagnosis. Based on the most likely diagnosis, which of the following is the treatment of choice?
a. Oral Cephalexin
b. IV Vancomycin plus Ceftriaxone
c. Oral Amoxicillin-clavulanate
d. Warm compresses and eyelid hygiene
e. Ciprofloxacin ophthalmic ointment 0.3%

25. A 21-year-old female presents with a rash that is worsening. Initially, she developed a single oval-shaped lesion on her right thigh that was mildly pruritic. About 10 days later, she developed multiple smaller oval-shaped salmon-colored patches and papules up to 1.5 cm in diameter, surrounded by light white scales on her back, thighs, upper arms, and chest area along the skin lines. Which of the following is the most appropriate management in this patient?
a. Oral Acyclovir
b. Topical Ketoconazole
c. RPR, education, reassurance, and topical Fluocinonide
d. Oral Erythromycin
e. UV light phototherapy

26. A 20-year-old female migrant presents to the clinic for fatigue. She is 20 weeks pregnant. She was recently treated for Rocky Mountain spotted fever with Chloramphenicol. Physical examination is notable for extremity petechiae and pallor. Labs reveal
   • Hemoglobin: 9.1 g/dL (13.5-17.5)
   • Hematocrit: 28% (40-54)
   • Platelet count 20,200 cells/mm^3 (150,000-450,000)
   • Mean corpuscular volume (MCV): 99 fL (80-100)
   • White cell count 2,200/mm^3 (5,000-10,000)
   • Reticulocyte count 0.1% (0.5-2.5)
Which of the following would most likely be seen on bone marrow aspiration?
a. Hypocellularity with increased fat cells and marrow stroma
b. Absent iron stores
c. Ringed sideroblasts
d. Increased myeloblasts but <20%
e. Increased number of megakaryocytes with normal morphology

27. A 40-year-old male presents to establish care. As part of the routine screening, the Hepatitis B panel results are:
   • Hepatitis B core antibody (anti-HBc): positive for IgG
   • HB surface antibody (anti-HBs): negative
   • Hepatitis B surface antigen (HBsAg): positive
   • Hepatitis B e antigen (HBeAg): negative
   • Hepatitis B e antibody (anti-HBe): negative.
Which of the following is the most likely status of the blood donor?
a. Resolved infection (recovery)
b. Successfully vaccination
c. Chronic carrier
d. Acute hepatitis
e. Window period

28. A 19-year-old female presents with crampy lower abdominal pain and cramping in her thighs occurring on the first day of her menstrual cycle for the last 5 months. The pain gradually subsides on the second or third day of menstruation. She denies heavy menstruation. Her cycle is regular occurring every 28 days and lasting for 5-6 days. Physical examination is unremarkable. Urine beta-hCG is negative. Which of the following is the first line management of this patient?

a. Levonorgestrel-releasing intrauterine device (IUD)

b. Naproxen

c. Norethindrone

d. Leuprolide acetate depot

e. Transcutaneous electrical nerve stimulation

29. A 41-year-old woman presents to the physician's office for joint stiffness in her hands and hip. She experiences stiffness every morning in hands and right foot. On examination, there is tenderness, warmth, and erythema to the MCP, PIP, and DIP joints with fusiform swelling of some of the fingers. There is tenderness along the plantar fascia of the right foot. Radiographs are obtained (see photo).

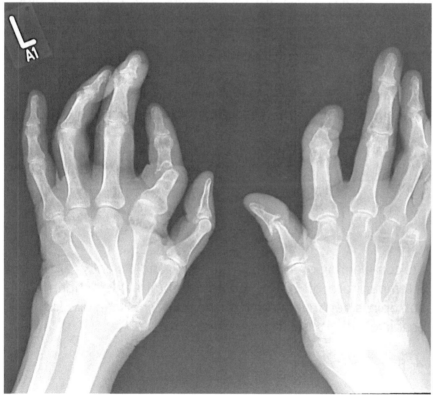

Which of the following is the most likely diagnosis?

a. Osteoarthritis

b. Psoriatic arthritis

c. Acute calcium pyrophosphate crystal arthritis

d. Rheumatoid arthritis

e. Gouty arthritis

Photo credit

Case courtesy of Ahmed Elowaidy, Radiopaedia.org, rID: 25019

30. An 18-year-old female presents with lower abdominal pain, dyspareunia, and vaginal discharge. She is sexually active with 2 male partners. Vital signs are blood pressure 110/73 mmHg, respiratory rate 18 breaths/min, temperature 98.8°F (37.11°C), and heart rate 80 bpm. Pelvic examination is notable for a mucopurulent discharge in the endocervical canal and cervical motion tenderness. Laboratory investigations show a white cell count of 17,000 per microliter (5,000-10,000) and negative urine hCG. Which of the following is the first line management?
a. Intramuscular Ceftriaxone, oral Metronidazole, and oral Doxycycline with outpatient follow-up
b. Exploratory laparoscopy
c. Oral Metronidazole and Doxycycline with outpatient follow-up
d. Oral Vancomycin with outpatient follow-up
e. Hospitalization, IV Cefotetan + IV Doxycycline + Metronidazole

31. A 9-year-old boy is brought the emergency department for difficulty walking. Over the last 5 days, he has been complaining of left hip and thigh pain. This morning, he refused to ambulate due to pain. He has no past medical history. Vitals are temperature 102°F (38.9°C), blood pressure 110/72 mmHg, pulse 114/min, respirations 18/min, and oxygen saturation 99% on room air. Initial labs reveal:
   • WBC count 12,600/mm^3 (5,000-10,000) with normal differential
   • ESR 80 mm/hr (0-15)
Radiographs are unremarkable. An MRI of the thigh and knee reveals periosteal reaction and cortical destruction of the distal femur. Which of the following is the most likely infectious agent in this patient?
a. *Pseudomonas aeruginosa*
b. *Staphylococcus aureus*
c. Salmonella species
d. Group B streptococcus
e. *Staphylococcus epidermidis*

32. A 25-year-old woman presents complaining of dysuria, frequency, and urgency for the last 2 days. Vitals are notable for a temperature of 101°F. Costovertebral angle tenderness is positive. Human chorionic gonadotropin is negative. Which of the following seen on Urinalysis most reliably distinguishes the most likely diagnosis from Acute cystitis?
a. Pyuria
b. >10 red blood cells/high power field
c. Positive Nitrites
d. White blood cell casts
e. Bacteriuria

33. Which of the following most strongly suggests abnormal grief?
a. Simple hallucinations of the deceased that the patient understands is not real
b. Appetite or sleep disturbances
c. Intense emotions
d. Weight loss
e. Symptoms lasting >1 year

34. A 10-year-old boy presents to his pediatrician for left ear pain, pruritus, and discharge. He has been having difficulty hearing from his left ear. He has no significant past medical history. He recently joined a diving team. Physical examination is notable for otalgia with auricle is pulled and manipulation of the pinna. There is auricular discharge and external auditory canal edema and erythema with poor visualization of the tympanic membrane. Which of the following organisms is most likely responsible for his presentation?
a. *Staphylococcus aureus*
b. *Candida albicans*
c. *Bacteroides* species
d. *Streptococcus pyogenes*
e. *Pseudomonas aeruginosa*

35. A 50-year-old male presents with fever, chills, productive cough with foul-smelling sputum, dyspnea, and right-sided pleuritic chest pain. He has a history of Hypertension and Amyotrophic lateral sclerosis. Vitals reveal tachypnea and tachycardia. Physical examination is notable for increased fremitus in the right upper lobe. A chest radiograph is performed (see photo).

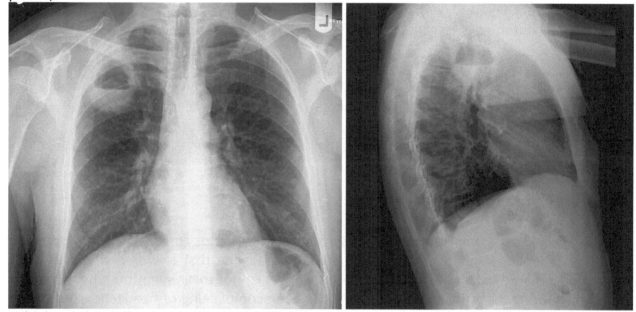

Which of the following is the most likely predisposing factor for the development of this condition?
a. Gastroesophageal reflux
b. Inhalation of pathogens via respiratory droplets
c. Impaired swallowing
d. Hematogenous spread
e. Reduced mucociliary escalator clearance

Photo credit:
Case courtesy of Abu-Rahmeh Zuhair, Radiopaedia.org, rID: 30554

36. A 9-year-old male presents to the clinic with painful left scrotal swelling. 11 days ago, he had low-grade fever, jaw swelling, earache, and difficulty swallowing, which resolved on its own. He denies abdominal pain, nausea, or vomiting. On examination, there is scrotal edema and tenderness with erythema and shininess of the overlying skin. Which of the following is the recommended management of this patient?
a. Perform testicular ultrasound to rule out a testicular mass
b. Ibuprofen, bed rest, scrotal support, & cold packs to the scrotum
c. Surgical referral for Orchiopexy
d. Initiate Trimethoprim-sulfamethoxazole
e. Refer to urology for urological workup

37. A 23-year-old female is being evaluated for heavier than usual menstrual bleeding. She has always had a history of menorrhagia but has recently had to change her pads more frequently. Review of systems is positive for easy bruising. She is otherwise healthy with no past medical history. Labs reveal:
- Hemoglobin 12 g/dL (11-16)
- Hematocrit 37% (36-46)
- Platelet count 190,000 cells/mm^3 (150,000-450,000)
- Prothrombin time of 12 seconds (11-13)
- INR of 1.2
- Activated partial thromboplastin time of PTT 44 seconds (25-35)
- White cell count of 6,000 cells/mm^3 (5,000-10,000).

Which of the following is the most likely etiology of this patient's menorrhagia?
a. Hemophilia A
b. Factor V Leiden mutation
c. Antiphospholipid syndrome
d. Von Willebrand disease
e. Hemophilia B

38. A 22-year-old male presents with a 12-day history of fever, loss of smell, and a productive cough that is worse at night. In addition, he has a headache that is worse when he leans forward and radiated to his left upper teeth. About 1 week prior to his symptoms, he had runny nose with sneezing that initially improved. He has been complaining of headache, sore throat and worsening of rhinorrhea. His past medical history is unremarkable, and he has no known drug allergies. Vitals reveal a temperature of 102°F (38.89°C), BP: 120/80 mmHg, and respirations 16/min. There is tenderness with palpation over the left cheek. Which of the following is the recommended next step?
a. Ibuprofen, intranasal sterile saline spray, and reassess in 48-72 hours
b. Trimethoprim-sulfamethoxazole
c. Clindamycin
d. Water's view radiographs
e. Amoxicillin/clavulanic acid

39. A 67-year-old male undergoes prostatectomy. Day 3 postoperatively, he complains of abdominal pain and nausea. On examination the abdomen is distended and hyper-tympanic with the absence of bowel sounds. There is mild voluntary guarding. Abdominal imaging is performed (see photo).

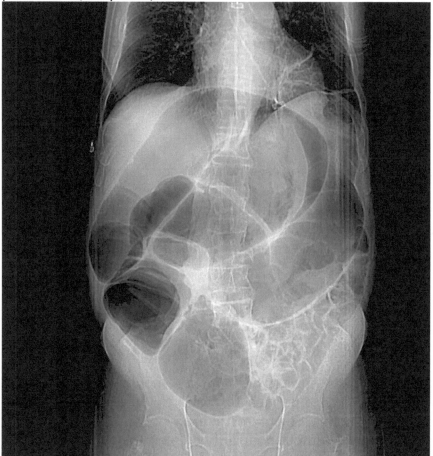

Which of the following tests, if abnormal, would significantly alter the management of this patient's condition?
a. White blood cell count
b. Lactate
c. Urinalysis
d. Amylase and lipase
e. AST and ALT

Photo credit:
Case courtesy of The Radswiki, Radiopaedia.org, rID: 11684

40. Which of the following vaccines is contraindicated in pregnancy?
a. Influenza
b. Meningococcal
c. SARS-CoV-2
d. Tetanus
e. Varicella

41. A 40-year-old female presents with anorexia, weakness, fatigue, nausea, and vomiting. She has a history of Sarcoidosis and Raynaud phenomenon. Physical examination is unremarkable. Initial labs reveal:
- Serum cortisol 1 microg/dL (4-22)
- Baseline ACTH 2 pg/mL (7-69)

Which of the following is the most likely etiology of her presentation?
a. Waterhouse-Friderichsen syndrome
b. Tuberculosis
c. Autoimmune adrenalitis
d. Prior history of long-term therapy with glucocorticoids
e. Cushing disease

42. A 32-year-old male presented to his primary care provider complaining of recurrent headaches that typically last 2 days. He has a headache currently. The pain he is experiencing now is located on the right side of the head and is accompanied by nausea and light sensitivity. The headache is pulsatile, worse with routine activity, and is triggered by eating chocolates. Which of the following is the recommended management for this patient at this time?
a. Verapamil and Ubrogepant
b. Sumatriptan and Prochlorperazine
c. 100% oxygen via nonrebreather and Ibuprofen
d. Carbamazepine
e. Ethosuximide

43. A 57-year-old man is being evaluated by the urologist for a 4-month history of lower abdominal pain, dysuria, frequency, urgency, and perineal discomfort worse with ejaculation. He denies fevers, chills, or erectile dysfunction. Digital rectal examination is notable for an enlarged, mildly tender, edematous prostate without nodularity or warmth. Urinalysis reveals pyuria and hematuria. Which of the following is the most likely diagnosis?
a. Prostate cancer
b. Acute cystitis
c. Acute prostatitis
d. Benign prostatic hyperplasia
e. Chronic prostatitis

44. A 35-year-old male presents to the clinic complaining of fatigue, facial swelling, and frothy urine. Physical examination is notable for periorbital and dependent pedal edema. Initial labs reveal HCV RNA 1,224,890 IU/mL and decreased serum complement. Urinalysis reveals 4+ proteinuria, dysmorphic red cells, and red cell casts. Renal biopsy shows mesangial interposition into the capillary wall with a double-contour appearance on light microscopy. Which of the following is the most likely diagnosis?
a. Membranoproliferative glomerulonephritis
b. Postinfectious glomerulonephritis
c. IgA Glomerulonephritis
d. Minimal change disease
e. Focal segmental glomerulosclerosis

45. A 44-year-old male presents with right mid flank pain and hematuria. Physical examination is remarkable for mid abdominal tenderness and right costovertebral angle tenderness on palpation.

Urinalysis reveals:

- Red blood cells: 50/hpf (<5)
- Nitrites; negative
- Leukocyte esterase: negative
- urine pH: 9
- multiple magnesium ammonium phosphate crystals in the urine sediment.

An ultrasound is performed (see photo).

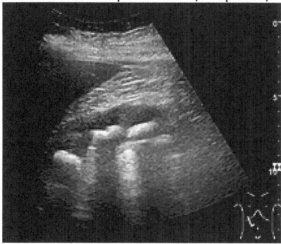

Which of the following is the preferred next step in the management of this patient?

a. Percutaneous nephrostomy tube insertion

b. Extracorporeal shock wave lithotripsy

c. Obtain urology consultation for emergent decompression

d. Discharge home with Ibuprofen, increased fluid intake, and Tamsulosin to facilitate stone passage

e. Perform a CT scan of the abdomen and pelvis with intravenous contrast

Photo credit:

Kristoffer Lindskov Hansen, Michael Bachmann Nielsen and Caroline Ewertsen, CC BY 4.0 <https://creativecommons.org/licenses/by/4.0>, via Wikimedia Commons

46. A 29-year-old male presents with abrupt episodes of "panic attacks" consisting of severe pounding headache, heart racing, profuse perspiration and pallor before spontaneously going away. Vitals are notable for blood pressure 178/102 mmHg and pulse 116 bpm. The abdomen is soft and non-distended with no palpable masses. Which of the following is the most likely etiology of his presentation?

a. Disease of the adrenal cortex

b. Disease of the adrenal medulla

c. Narrowing of the renal artery

d. Aldosterone-producing adenoma

e. Coarctation of the aorta

47. A 43-year-old male presents to the Emergency department with dizziness and dyspnea. The following is seen on ECG.

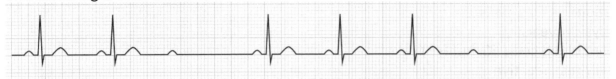

Which of the following is the initial management of choice in this patient?
a. IV Amiodarone
b. IV Adenosine
c. IV Dobutamine
d. Transcutaneous pacing
e. Observation and reassurance it is self-limiting

Photo credit:
Shutterstock (used with permission)

48. A 66-year-old man presents to the emergency department with cough and dyspnea that woke him up in the middle of the night. He has a history of poorly controlled Hypertension. Vitals are temperature 99.0°F (37.2°C), blood pressure 174/98 mmHg, pulse 128/min, respirations 24/min, and oxygen saturation 90% on room air. Bibasilar crackles and increased jugular venous pressure are noted. Which of the following is the most appropriate next step in the management of this patient?
a. Nitroglycerin
b. Digoxin
c. Furosemide
d. Sacubitril-Valsartan
e. Carvedilol

49. A 16-year-old male presents to the ED after being ejected unhelmeted from an all-terrain vehicle while on vacation. He presents 3 days later complaining of a salty sensation in the back of his throat, clear fluid coming from his right nostril, headache, and facial pain. Physical examination is notable for tenderness to the nasal septum, mastoid ecchymosis, and bilateral periorbital ecchymosis. Which of the following would most likely be present on physical examination?
a. Diplopia with upward gaze
b. Upward Babinski
c. Irregular tear-shaped pupil
d. Blue to purple hue of the tympanic membrane
e. Papilledema

50. Which of the following is not associated with increased risk of Endometrial cancer?
a. Tamoxifen use
b. Obesity
c. Early menarche
d. Nulliparity
e. Raloxifene use

51. A 52-year-old male presents to the clinic with a 1-year history of progressive dyspnea on exertion. Physical examination is notable for diffuse fine crackles without wheezing. Chest radiographs are obtained (see photo).

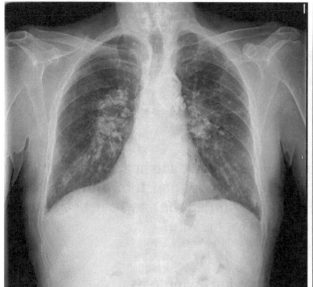 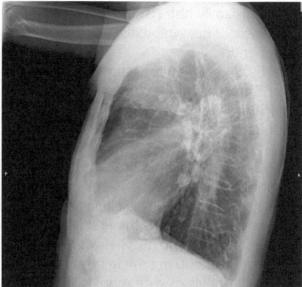

PFTs reveal increased FEV1/FVC and decreased residual volume (RV). Which of the following would most likely be in this patient's history?
a. 30 pack-year smoking history
b. Cystic fibrosis
c. Occupation as a plumber and pipefitter
d. Working in a fluorescent light bulb and electronics manufacturing plant
e. Occupation as a stonecutter

Photo credit:
Case courtesy of Albert Prat Matifoll, Radiopaedia.org, rID: 32491

52. A 25-year-old male suffered a spinal cord injury from a traumatic fall from height. The presence of which of the following findings is most consistent with an upper motor neuron finding?
a. Muscle atrophy
b. Muscle twitching (fasciculations)
c. Increased deep tendon reflexes
d. Flaccid paralysis
e. Downward Babinski sign

53. In which of the following situations is Informed consent not required?
a. Radiation therapy for a 20-year-old male with Hodgkin lymphoma
b. A 50-year-old male in which a liver biopsy is required
c. A 42-year-old female undergoing an upper endoscopy
d. A 40-year-old female undergoing a laparoscopic cholecystectomy
e. A 50-year-old male who becomes unconscious with pulseless ventricular tachycardia

54. A 55-year-old female presents to the clinic for worsening hot flushes associated with profuse sweating that sometimes wakes her up in the middle of the night. She also experiences dyspareunia. Her last menstrual period was 3 years ago. She has no past medical or surgical history. She has no personal or family history of Breast or Endometrial cancer. Which of the following is the first line management of her symptoms?
a. Gabapentin
b. Oral Estrogen and Progestin
c. Oral Tamoxifen
d. Oral Sertraline
e. Oral Estrogen

55. A 60-year-old male is brought to the ED for confusion, fever, and headache. Examination is significant for a positive Kernig sign. He undergoes a lumbar puncture, and CSF analysis reveals gram-negative intracellular diplococci. His wife is worried she may have been exposed. Which of the following is the first line recommendation for his wife?
a. Reassurance that no prophylaxis is warranted
b. Azithromycin 500 mg single dose
c. Initiate prophylaxis with Amoxicillin 2 grams if she develops symptoms
d. Initiate Rifampin 600 mg every 12 hours 2 days (4 doses) of oral therapy
e. Initiate Clindamycin 600 mg single dose

56. A 10-year-old boy presents to the ED complaining of a 7-hour history of abdominal pain associated with nausea and vomiting. The pain originated in the periumbilical area but, since this morning, has migrated to the right lower quadrant. On examination, there is tenderness to the right lower quadrant with moderate guarding. Palpation of the left lower quadrant elicits pain in the right lower quadrant. Labs are remarkable for a white cell count of 14,000. Which of the following signs is positive in this patient?
a. Murphy
b. Rovsing
c. Obturator
d. McBurney
e. Psoas

57. A 42-year-old woman comes to the office for a routine health examination. She is sexually active with 1 male partner and underwent a tubal ligation for contraception. She has not experienced abnormal bleeding or recent changes in weight. Menses are regular and last 3-5 days; her last menstrual period was 3 weeks ago. Pap tests have been normal to date. Pelvic examination shows a normal cervix without any visible lesions. The Pap test shows atypical glandular cells. Which of the following is the next best step in management of this patient?
a. Serum CA-125
b. Colposcopy and endometrial biopsy
c. Loop electrosurgical excision procedure
d. Return to routine Pap screening
e. Colposcopy

58. A 19-year-old otherwise healthy college student presents with a dry nonproductive cough for 2 weeks, sore throat, rhinorrhea, coryza, and new-onset pleuritic chest pain. Vital signs are normal. Physical examination is notable for scattered wheezing. CBC with peripheral smear shows RBC clumping and Direct antiglobulin test positivity for complement (C3) only. A chest radiograph is obtained (see photo).

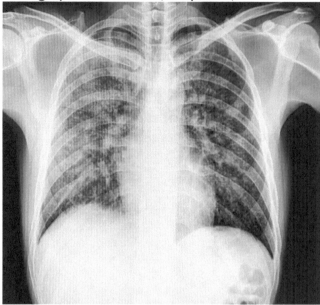

Which of the following is the first-line management of this patient?
a. Amoxicillin and supportive care
b. Supportive care only
c. Azithromycin and supportive care
d. Piperacillin-tazobactam
e. Doxycycline and Ceftriaxone

Photo credit:
Shutterstock (used with permission)

59. A 20-year-old woman delivered a girl, at 37 weeks of gestation after a prolonged vaginal delivery. She develops significant postpartum hemorrhage, requires a transfusion of 4 units of blood. She recovered fully and was discharged on the fourth day. After 2 weeks, she presents with fatigue, weakness, and decreased milk secretion. Vital signs are heart rate 70 bpm and blood pressure 90/60 mmHg. Initial labs reveal:
  • Hemoglobin 10.2 g/dL (12-16)
  • TSH 0.1 mIU/L (0.5-5.0)
  • Serum free T4 0.2 (0.8-1.8)
  • Serum sodium 130 mEq/L (135-145)
Which of the following is the most likely diagnosis in this patient?
a. Waterhouse-Friderichsen syndrome
b. Prolactinoma
c. Postpartum thyroiditis
d. Sheehan syndrome
e. Addison disease

60. A 41-year-old male presents to the clinic with his wife, who is concerned with personality changes. Over the past 6 months, he has become sexually promiscuous, impulsive, very easily agitated, and recently has difficulty with organizing, multitasking, and planning. Physical examination is notable for brief, irregular flailing movements of his arms and head thrusts. Neuroimaging is performed (see photo).

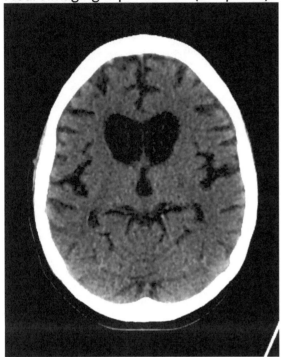

Which of the following is the most likely diagnosis?
a. Parkinson disease
b. Wilson disease
c. Huntington disease
d. Tourette syndrome
e. Alzheimer dementia

Photo credit
Case courtesy of Ian Bickle, Radiopaedia.org, rID: 82690

61. A 22-year-old male college student has become increasingly bizarre over the course of the last 4 months and is referred by his academic advisor to the student health clinic. He will not leave his room for 2 weeks at a time because he believes that voices in his head are telling him to continue searching the internet for hidden alien messages. He believes he is the only one on earth with this special ability. He is paranoid that the FBI knows this secret and is trying to prevent him from receiving these messages. What is the most likely diagnosis?
a. Schizophreniform disorder
b. Schizophrenia
c. Schizoaffective disorder
d. Schizotypal disorder
e. Brief psychotic disorder

62. A 35-year-old male presents to the ED complaining of knee pain for 3 hours. He was going down a flight of stairs when he suddenly felt his knee "give out." On examination, a large knee joint effusion and an inability to perform a straight leg raise are noted. Radiographs are obtained (see photo).

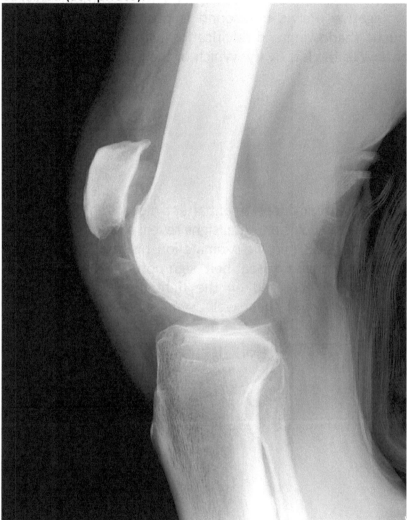

Which of the following is the most likely diagnosis?
a. Patellar tendon rupture
b. Patella dislocation
c. Quadriceps tendon rupture
d. ACL injury
e. Knee dislocation

Photo credit:
Case courtesy of Frank Gaillard, Radiopaedia.org, rID: 7514

63. A 22-year-old female presents with abdominal pain mostly in the left lower quadrant. The pain was sudden in onset, 10/10 in severity, dull, gradually worsening, and began while exercising in the gym. The pain is accompanied by nausea and vomiting. Vitals are stable Physical examination is positive for left adnexal mass and LLQ tenderness without cervical motion tenderness. Urine hCG is negative. Pelvic ultrasound is positive for a markedly hyperechoic nodule with distal acoustic shadowing and calcification within a 5.5 cm ovarian mass in the left and absent Doppler flow to the left ovary. Which of the following is the most likely etiology of her presentation?
a. Polycystic ovary syndrome
b. Tubo-ovarian abscess
c. Follicular cyst
d. Mature cystic teratoma (Dermoid cyst)
e. Corpus luteal cyst

64. A 22-year-old male is brought to the emergency department after a motor vehicle accident. He was wearing his seatbelt at the time of the collision. Vital signs reveal a blood pressure of 86/52 mmHg, pulse 148/min, and respirations 38/min. On examination, his neck veins are flat, and the trachea is slightly deviated to the left with a "seat belt' sign noted on the chest. On pulmonary examination, breath sounds are decreased on the right, there is dullness to percussion, decreased fremitus on the right, and chest wall asymmetry are noted. Chest radiographs are obtained (see photo).

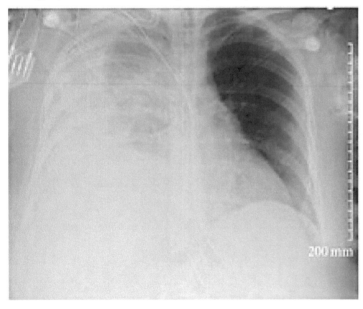

Which of the following is the most likely diagnosis?
a. Pleural effusion
b. Tension pneumothorax
c. Hemothorax
d. Pulmonary contusion
e. Cardiac tamponade

Photo credit:
Nidhi Sood, CC BY 4.0 <https://creativecommons.org/licenses/by/4.0>, via Wikimedia Commons

65. A 47-year-old male presents to the clinic with flu-like symptoms. He has been experiencing low-grade fever, chest pain, fatigue, myalgia, joint pains, and rash. He has spent the entire summer in Phoenix, Arizona on a construction project to build his own house. Physical examination is notable for erythematous tender plaques on his shins. A chest radiograph is positive for right infiltrate with right hilar adenopathy (see photo).

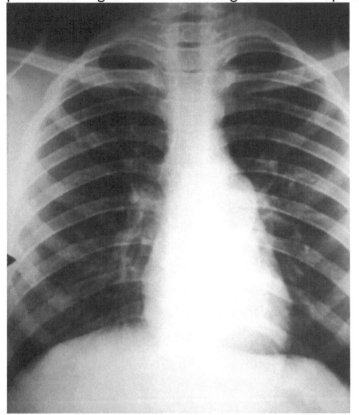

Which of the following organisms is most likely responsible for this patient's symptoms?
a. *Klebsiella pneumoniae*
b. *Pneumocystis jirovecii*
c. *Coccidioides immitis*
d. *Mycoplasma pneumoniae*
e. *Legionella pneumophilae*

Photo credit:
CDC/ Dr. Lucille K. Georg, Public domain, via Wikimedia Commons

66. A 23-year-old male presents to his primary care provider due to poor appetite and difficulty concentrating over the last 3 weeks. He no longer finds joy in his hobbies, has feelings of worthlessness, and experiences insomnias. He has experienced episodes in the past, but this one is particularly severe, interrupting his daily functioning. In addition to psychotherapy, which of the following is a first line agent?
a. Buspirone
b. Sertraline
c. Lorazepam
d. Phenelzine
e. Amitriptyline

67. A 55-year-old male is brought to the ED via ambulance for chest pain and acute onset dyspnea. Vitals reveal a blood pressure 80/60 mmHg, pulse 90, oxygen saturation 89% on 4L of oxygen via nasal cannula. He is pale with cold limbs and increased pressure in the jugular vein. An ECG is obtained (see photo).

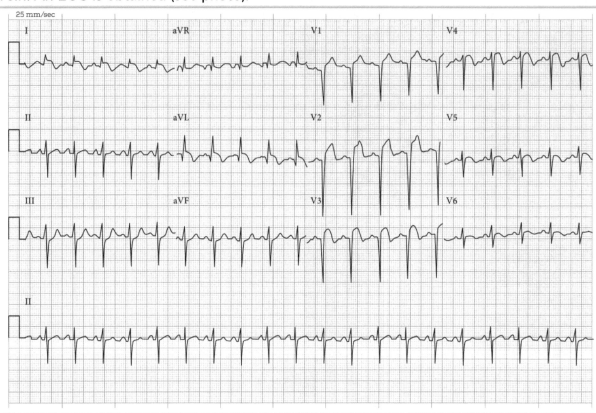

The patient is given IV Norepinephrine, Aspirin 325 mg, and an intravenous volume challenge of 250 mL of 0.9% sodium chloride. Which of the following is the most appropriate next step?
a. IV Nitroglycerin
b. IV Metoprolol
c. IV Furosemide
d. Emergent pericardiocentesis
e. Coronary angiography

Photo credit: Shutterstock (used with permission)

68. A 49-year-old male with a longstanding history of poorly controlled Type 2 Diabetes mellitus presents with a burning and tingling sensation to both feet. Physical examination is notable for hyperesthesia of both feet as well as decreased vibratory sensation and 2-point discrimination. In addition to strict glucose control, which of the following is a first line agent to relieve his symptoms?
a. Tramadol 50 mg
b. Capsaicin cream 0.075%
c. Duloxetine 20 mg
d. Lidocaine 5% patch
e. Electrical nerve stimulation

69. A 55-year-old male presents to the clinic complaining of pain in the upper two thirds of the calves when walking more than 10 blocks that is relieved with rest. He has a history of Hypertension and Dyslipidemia. On physical examination his calvers are dry and hairless with no leg ulcers. Based on his symptoms, narrowing which of the following arteries is most likely the etiology of his presentation?
a. Popliteal
b. Common femoral
c. Superficial femoral
d. Tibial
e. Peroneal

70. A 64-year-old male presents to the clinic with gradually progressive dyspnea on exertion, cough, hoarseness, and night sweats. He has a 40-year history as a plumber and shipbuilder in a shipyard. Physical examination is notable for decreased air movement on the left side and dullness to percussion at the left lung base. Chest radiograph reveals reduced lung volume of the left hemithorax, circumferential pleural thickening with calcification involving the left hemithorax and pleural rind (see photo).

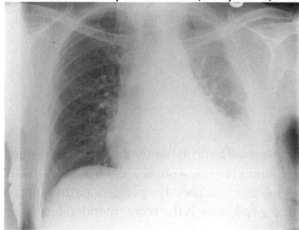

Which of the following is the most likely diagnosis?
a. Caplan syndrome
b. Loffler syndrome
c. Large cell carcinoma
d. Bronchial carcinoid tumor
e. Mesothelioma

Photo credit:
Case courtesy of Ian Bickle, Radiopaedia.org, rID: 63133

71. In a patient with Chronic obstructive pulmonary disease, which of the following physical examination findings is most consistent with Emphysema compared to Chronic bronchitis?
a. Obese habitus
b. Peripheral edema
c. Rhonchi
d. Distant breath sounds
e. Cyanotic lips

72. A 30-year-old male stockbroker presents with a 10-month history of intermittent headaches. He describes the headaches as a pressure on both sides of the head as if he had on a tight cap. The headache is not throbbing and worse when he is staring at his computer at work. The headache is not exacerbated with routine activity. He denies photophobia and phonophia. Neurological examination is within normal limits. Which of the following would most likely be seen in this patient's history or physical examination?
a. Pericranial muscle tenderness
b. Conjunctival erythema
c. Papilledema
d. Nausea and vomiting
e. Pain reproduced with stroking the face and chin

73. A 23-year-old sexually active woman presents to the clinic with complaints of a painful ulcer on the skin near her genitalia. On examination, there is a single, painful, non-indurated, and well demarcated 1 cm ulcer with an erythematous base on the skin immediately adjacent to her left labium major. There is tender right inguinal lymphadenopathy. Which of the following is the most likely organism responsible for her presentation?
a. Haemophilus ducreyi
b. Klebsiella granulomatis
c. Herpes simplex virus 2
d. Chlamydia trachomatis serovars
e. Treponema pallidum

74. A 42-year-old female presents to the clinic after feeling a small lump in her right breast. She denies breast pain, dimpling, or nipple discharge. Physical examination reveals a small 2 cm mass in the left breast that is soft and freely mobile. There is no evidence of axillary lymphadenopathy, nipple inversion, change in breast contour, or dimpling. Which of the following is the recommended next step in the evaluation of this patient?
a. Ultrasound of the breast
b. Core needle biopsy
c. Fine needle aspiration
d. Mammogram
e. MRI of the breast

75. A 30-year-old male has a 6-month history of abdominal bloating, cramping, pain, and diarrhea. He recently developed a pruritic rash. On examination, there are pruritic papules and vesicles that occur in grouped arrangements on the dorsal forearms and knees. There are very few intact papules and vesicles, with erosions and excoriations seen. Which of the following is the most appropriate next step in the evaluation of this patient?
a. Upper endoscopy with small bowel biopsy
b. Sweat chloride testing
c. Tissue transglutaminase IgA antibodies
d. Hydrogen breath testing
e. Skin scraping with KOH preparation

76. A 42-year-old male presents to the clinic to establish care. He has a history of Hypertension and Chronic Hepatitis B virus for 5 years. He has a 10 pack-year smoking history. Initial labs:
- Alanine aminotransferase (SGPT) 102 U/L (4-36)
- Aspartate aminotransferase (SGOT) 96 U/L (5-40).

Which of the following screening tests should be performed in this patient?
a. Colonoscopy
b. CT scan of the abdomen and pelvis
c. Abdominal ultrasound
d. Cancer antigen 19-9
e. Carcinoembryonic antigen

77. A 69-year-old male presents to the ED for sudden onset of left leg pain. He has a history of Atrial fibrillation, Dyslipidemia, and Hypertension. On examination, the left leg is cold and pale. There is 3/5 muscle strength in the left leg with significantly reduced sensation in the left leg from the toes up to the middle third of the leg with inaudible Doppler signal. Which of the following is the most appropriate next step in management of this patient?
a. Supervised graded exercise regimen and Aspirin
b. Surgical thrombectomy
c. CT angiogram of the left lower extremity
d. IV Alteplase
e. IV unfractionated Heparin drip

78. A 4-week-old infant is brought to the ED for persistent episodes of projectile vomiting after feedings over the last 48 hours. His is an avid feeder, even after he vomits. Vitals reveal a blood pressure of 106/62 mmHg. An olive-shaped mass in the epigastric region, flat neck veins, sunken fontanelles, and delayed capillary refill are noted. Labs show:
- blood pH 7.49 (7.35-7.45)
- serum potassium: 3.0 mEq/L (3.5-5)
- serum sodium: 157 mEq/L (135-145)
- urine sodium: 5 mEq/L

Which of the following is the first-line management of his Hypernatremia?
a. Dextrose 5% in water
b. 0.9% sodium chloride solution
c. 0.45% sodium chloride solution
d. 3% sodium chloride solution
e. Fluid restriction

79. A 6-year-old presents to the pediatric clinic for a painful nonpruritic rash on the face for the last 4 days. The rash began as a papulovesicular eruption before rupturing. Vitals are stable. Physical examination reveals erythematous pustules, papules, and golden-colored crusts around his mouth and chin. Which of the following is the first line management in this patient?
a. Oral Cephalexin
b. Oral Valacyclovir
c. Oral Dicloxacillin
d. Topical Mupirocin
e. Topical Neomycin

80. A 54-year-old left-hand dominant woman presents with insidious onset of right shoulder stiffness. It began as nagging shoulder pain worse at night. Over 3 months, as the pain subsided, the stiffness worsened. She denies any inciting trauma. On physical exam, there is substantial reduction in both active and passive range of motion. She is also unable to reach 90° with passive abduction. Which of the following is most likely in her history?
a. Rheumatoid arthritis
b. Repetitive shoulder microtrauma
c. Hypertension
d. Diabetes mellitus
e. Prior anterior glenohumeral dislocation

81. A 4-year-old boy presents to the clinic with high-grade fever, malaise, headache, cough, sore throat, and dysphagia for 2 days. He has been refusing to eat or drink due to pain. Vitals reveal a temperature of 103°F (39.44°C). Physical examination is notable for vesicles and yellow/grayish ulcerations with a rim of intense erythema on the anterior pillars of the fauces, uvula, soft palate, and tonsils. There are no lesions on the hard palate, tongue, or buccal mucosa. Which of the following is the most likely diagnosis?
a. Herpetic gingivostomatitis
b. Herpangina
c. Aphthous ulcers
d. Hand, foot, and mouth disease
e. Varicella

82. A 20-year-old male presents to the clinic with tea-colored urine. He has been training for a decathlon and denies any past medical history. Physical examination is notable for bilateral thigh tenderness without significant muscle weakness. Urine dipstick is positive for blood. Urinalysis with microscopy shows 2 RBCs/hpf (0-5). Which of the following would be most useful to establish the most likely diagnosis?
a. Serum myoglobin
b. Anti-Jo-1 and anti-signal recognition peptide antibodies
c. Serum creatine kinase
d. Serum potassium
e. Electromyography

83. A 67-year-old man presents to his primary care provider after noticing blood in his urine at the end of urination. He denies any abdominal pain, urinary hesitancy, dysuria, or urinary frequency or urgency. He has no significant past medical history. He has a 40 pack-year smoking history. Physical examination and routine blood testing are unremarkable. Urinalysis demonstrates a large red blood cell count with normal red blood cell morphology without casts. Which of the following would most likely confirm the most likely diagnosis?
a. Urine cytology
b. Intravenous pyelogram
c. Ultrasound
d. Cystoscopy
e. CT scan of the abdomen and pelvis

84. A 35-year-old female presents to the clinic for follow-up after recently being placed on a medication. Her baseline ECG was within all normal parameters. An ECG obtained on this visit reveals a corrected QT interval of 500 msec (<460). Which of the following medications is most likely responsible for these ECG changes?
a. Levofloxacin
b. Propranolol
c. Penicillin V potassium
d. Albuterol
e. Clonazepam

85. A 20-year-old male presents with left eye pain, excessive tearing, photophobia, and blurred vision since last night. He had trouble removing his left contact lens last night and went to sleep with the left one in. When he removed it this morning, he still felt a foreign body sensation. There is no foreign body noted with visual inspection or lid eversion. Slit lamp examination with fluorescein shows uptake in an epithelial defect with no corneal infiltrate. Which of the following is the most appropriate next step in the management of this patient?
a. Topical Prednisolone acetate suspension 1%
b. Topical Ofloxacin solution 0.3%
c. Placement of a black fabric eye patch for comfort
d. Topical Erythromycin ointment 0.5%
e. Topical Proparacaine 0.5%

86. A 17-year-old female presents to her primary care provider for daytime symptoms of shortness of breath and wheezing 3 times a week requiring use of her Albuterol nebulizer. She experiences nocturnal awakening 3 times a month. Her home medications include low-dose Fluticasone. PFT shows a Forced expiratory volume (FEV1) of 84% predicted. Which of the following is the most appropriate next step in her management?
a. Add Formoterol
b. Discontinue Fluticasone and switch to Salmeterol
c. Add Omalizumab
d. Add oral Prednisone
e. Add Cromolyn sodium

87. A 19-year-old G1P1 woman undergoes spontaneous vaginal delivery. She received Magnesium sulfate for Preeclampsia with severe features and underwent prolonged labor. After expulsion of the placenta, she experienced continued bleeding with an estimated blood loss of 1,300 mL. On examination, the uterus is enlarged, boggy, and 5 cm above the umbilicus. Ultrasound after expulsion revealed no placental tissue. Which of the following is the most likely etiology for the bleeding?
a. Uterine rupture
b. Retained placenta
c. Uterine trauma
d. Uterine inversion
e. Failure of uterine contraction

88. A 40-year-old male presents to the clinic complaining of tongue soreness and dry, cracked lips. He is also complaining of numbness and "pins and needles" sensation in his fingers and toes. He has recently diagnosed 1 month ago with Tuberculosis, for which he is taking Rifampin, Isoniazid, Ethambutol, and Streptomycin. Physical examination is notable for decreased 2-point discrimination of his fingertips and angular cheilitis. The rest of his examination is within normal limits. Coadministration of which of the following vitamins would have most likely prevented his presentation?
a. B1
b. B12
c. A
d. C
e. B6

89. A 31-year-old male presents to the clinic for follow-up after an incidental finding of a pulmonary nodule located in the periphery seen on an admission chest radiograph. He has never smoked and has no family history of lung cancer. CT scan of the chest shows a 6 mm (0.6 cm) well-circumscribed solid dense homogenous pulmonary nodule. Which of the following is the recommended next step in this patient?
a. No routine follow-up required
b. Active surveillance with CT scan
c. Bronchoscopy
d. Transthoracic needle aspiration
e. Resection with biopsy

90. A 42-year-old male with a history of HIV infection presents to the dermatology clinic with a facial rash associated with mild pruritus. Physical examination erythematous plaques and papules with overlying yellow greasy scales on his face, nose, glabella, and cheeks. Which of the following is the most likely diagnosis?
a. Psoriasis
b. Rosacea
c. Systemic lupus erythematosus
d. Seborrheic dermatitis
e. Tinea versicolor

91. A 25-year-old male presents to the office complaining of knee and ankle pain and stiffness and left heel pain. Over the last 2 days, he has developed burning during urination. He recovered from an acute episode of nonbloody diarrhea 10 days ago. Vital signs are stable. Physical examination is notable for right conjunctival erythema, normal visual acuity, no discharge from the urethral meatus, and tenderness along the Achilles tendon. The right knee is edematous, warm, and tender. Arthrocentesis is performed, reveal a white blood cell count of 28,000/μL. Which of the following is the most appropriate treatment for this patient's condition?
a. Naproxen
b. Colchicine
c. Ceftriaxone
d. Acetaminophen
e. Intraarticular Triamcinolone acetonide

92. A 59-year-old man presents to his primary care provider after noticing a suspicious lesion on the inside of his cheek. He denies any trauma to his oral mucosa. Physical examination is notable for white plaque with irregular borders on the buccal oral mucosa that cannot be scraped off or wiped off with a gauze. He is referred for biopsy. Which of the following is the most common risk factor for this condition?
a. Use of tobacco products
b. Uncontrolled Diabetes mellitus
c. Herpes simplex virus 1
d. Epstein-Barr virus
e. Inhaled glucocorticoids

93. A 21-year-old male is being evaluated in the clinic due to lack of ability to make friends in college. He has a sense that people are looking at him, making him mistrustful of others. He was so concerned that bad things were going to happen during the Solar eclipse earlier this week, so he brought wind chimes to protect himself. He feels certain frequencies of people when he enters a room. On examination, his speech is vague and contains odd phrases. He is unkempt and his emotional reactions do not match what is occurring during the interview. Which of the following is the most likely diagnosis?
a. Schizophreniform disorder
b. Schizophrenia
c. Schizoid personality disorder
d. Paranoid personality disorder
e. Schizotypal personality disorder

94. A 66-year-old female presents for a well check. Her last menstrual period was 12 years ago. A dual-energy x-ray absorptiometry (DEXA) scan is obtained. Her T-score is -2.7. Labs reveal a normal serum levels of vitamin D, calcium, phosphorus, PTH, and alkaline phosphatase. Which of the following is the best next step in the management of this patient?
a. Teriparatide
b. Raloxifene
c. Alendronate
d. Denosumab
e. Reassure the patient and repeat DEXA scan in 2 years

95. A 30-year-old female presents with right dull achy leg pain and swelling. The pain began a few days after returning to the US from China via plane. She denies any trauma. On examination, there are dilated superficial veins on the left calf. The left calf is warm, tender, and 34 cm. The right calf measures 30 cm and is nontender. There is left calf pain on passive dorsiflexion of the foot. Which of the following findings is most specific for the most likely diagnosis?
a. Pain and tenderness along the course of the involved veins
b. Calf warmth
c. Dilated superficial veins on the left calf
d. Difference in calf circumferences
e. Calf pain on passive dorsiflexion of the foot

96. A 51-year-old male presents to the clinic for a well visit. He received a Tetanus diphtheria, and pertussis vaccine 5 years ago, and a SARS-CoV-2 vaccine last year. He denies any complaints. In addition to SARS-CoV-2 and the inactivated Influenza vaccines, which of the following vaccines is recommended for him at this time?
a. Zoster vaccine recombinant, adjuvanted
b. Tetanus-diphtheria-pertussis toxoid booster
c. 20-valent pneumococcal conjugate vaccine
d. Pneumococcal polysaccharide vaccine (*PPSV23*)
e. Meningococcal B vaccine

97. A 21-year-old, previously healthy woman is complaining of fatigue, malaise, and arthralgias. Recently, she developed pleuritic chest pain. She is not on medications. Vital signs are normal. There is tenderness, warmth, and effusions of her wrist and knee joints. There is a scratching sound heard over the lung. Laboratory results reveal:
  • Hemoglobin 10.2 g/dL (12-16)
  • Creatinine 1.3 mg/dL (0.6-1.2)
  • Urinalysis: 2+ protein
  • 12 red blood cells/hpf (0-5)
Which of the following tests is most specific based upon the most likely diagnosis?
a. Anti-topoisomerase I antibodies
b. Antinuclear antibodies
c. Anti Smith antibody
d. Anti-Ro antibody
e. Anti cyclic citrullinated peptide antibody

98. A 23-year-old female presented to the emergency department with fever of 39°C (102.2°F), diffuse abdominal pain, and nonbloody diarrhea. She is currently on the sixth day of her menstrual period and has had to use both pads and tampons and pads due to menorrhagia. There is a diffuse, erythematous, macular rash resembling sunburn that involves her entire body, including her palms and soles. There is hyperemia of the vaginal and oropharyngeal mucosa. Which of the following would most likely be seen on physical examination of this patient?
a. Raised target lesions
b. Systolic blood pressure <90 mmHg
c. Pulse rate <60 beats per minute
d. Splinter hemorrhages on the nailbeds
e. Diffuse petechiae

99. A 25-year-old female with a past medical history of Hashimoto thyroiditis is being evaluated in the dermatology clinic for hair loss. On examination, there is a smooth, circular, discrete areas of complete hair loss. There is no scarring, erythema, scaling or inflammation. At the edge of the patch, there are short broken hairs where the proximal end of the hairs are narrower than the distal end. Which of the following interventions is most appropriate for the suspected diagnosis?
a. Topical Minoxidil
b. Refer for psychiatric counseling
c. Oral Baricitinib
d. Intralesional Triamcinolone
e. Topical Diphenylcyclopropenone (DPCP)

100. A 45-year-old woman presents with abdominal pain and early satiety. Workup is positive for Ovarian cancer. She is informed of the diagnosis and her treatment options. Her husband is her health care proxy and comes to the office a few days later. He is very concerned about his wife and believes she is not forthcoming on what her diagnosis is yet. Which of the following is the most appropriate next step?
a. Inform the husband that it is inappropriate to discuss his wife's medical condition
b. Inform the husband of the treatment options without giving him the actual diagnosis
c. Inform the husband if she does not tell him to have his input on decision making
d. Call the wife and teleconference so you can share the information in her presence
e. Inform the husband of her condition since he is her health care proxy

END OF EXAM 6

1.   RENAL   –   HYPOMAGNESEMIA/HYPOKALEMIA   [APPLYING   FOUNDATIONAL CONCEPTS]

Because patients with Hypokalemia may also have Hypomagnesemia [choice A] due to concurrent loss with diarrhea or diuretic therapy, measurement of serum magnesium should be considered in patients with hypokalemia, especially if Hypokalemia is refractory to repletion.

This is because hypomagnesemia can result in renal potassium wasting.

It may be difficult to replete potassium in patients with concurrent Hypomagnesemia without magnesium repletion.

If Hypomagnesemia is detected, it should be treated as well.

Choice C [Hypoalbuminemia] may result in decreased measured serum calcium as the serum total calcium concentration falls by 0.8 mg/dL for every 1-g/dL fall in serum albumin concentration.

Choice D [Hypercalcemia] is not associated with causing Hypokalemia. Hypocalcemia is usually the calcium derangement associated with Hypokalemia.

2. INFECTIOUS DISEASES – CAMPYLOBACTER GASTROENTERITIS/GUILLAIN BARRÉ SYNDROME [HISTORY AND PHYSICAL EXAMINATION]

In the United States, most infections of *Campylobacter jejuni* and *C. coli* are associated with eating raw or undercooked poultry [choice B] or from food contaminated by these items.

Although other meats (choices A and D) can be contaminated with Campylobacter, contamination of poultry occurs more frequently.

C. jejuni gastroenteritis is the most common antecedent infection and precipitant of Guillain-Barré Syndrome, identified in ~25% of cases.

GBS classically presents with ascending muscle weakness (lower motor neuron findings), sensory changes, and hyporeflexia.

Choice A [Undercooked hamburgers] is most commonly associated with Enterohemorrhagic *E. coli* O157:H7.

Choice C [Raw shellfish] consumption is associated with *Vibrio vulnificus*.

Choice D [Undercooked pork chops] consumption is associated with *Yersinia* infections.

Choice E [Untreated water from a remote stream] consumption is associated with *Giardia lamblia*.

3. ENDOCRINE – GESTATIONAL DIABETES MELLITUS [HEALTH MAINTENANCE]

Confirmatory testing with a 3-hour 100g oral Glucose Tolerance Test (GTT) [choice B] as the criterion standard test if serum glucose is ≥140 mg/dL after 1-hour 50g oral glucose challenge test (nonfasting).

If confirmatory testing is positive, Lifestyle modifications is recommended (eg, diabetic diet & exercise (eg, walking)]. Self-monitoring of glucose.

If glucose remains elevated after lifestyle modifications, second-line management includes Insulin (preferred) [choice A]. Glyburide [choice D] or Metformin are alternatives.

Pregnant patients should never be encouraged to lose weight [choice C].

4. ENDOCRINE - LACTOTROPH MACROADENOMAS (PROLACTINOMAS) [CLINICAL INTERVENTION]

For patients with lactotroph macroadenomas (Prolactinomas) Dopamine agonists, such as Cabergoline [choice D] or Bromocriptine are the initial treatment of choice, regardless of tumor size.

This is because Dopamine inhibits prolactin, which results in shrinkage of the tumor in most.
Cabergoline is usually preferred over Bromocriptine due to less adverse effects.
90% of lactotroph adenomas respond to medical management with dopamine agonists and the majority of the remainder can be managed successfully with surgery.

Although Transsphenoidal resection surgery (TSS) [choice A] is the treatment for most pituitary adenomas, Prolactinomas are the exception. TSS is a reasonable alternative for patients in whom dopamine agonist treatment has been unsuccessful in reducing the serum prolactin concentration or size of the macroadenoma, or when symptoms or signs due to hyperprolactinemia or adenoma size do not improve.

Choice B [Octreotide] is an alternative for Somatotroph adenomas that secrete growth hormone.
Choice C [Radiation therapy] can be used either [1] post-surgery to prevent regrowth of residual tumor or [2] in the rare occurrence the tumor is refractory to medical and surgical therapy.
Choice E [Estradiol and progestin therapy] is an option to prevent bone loss and for the management of hypogonadism in premenopausal women who cannot tolerate or do not respond to dopamine agonists and do not want to become pregnant.

5. PULMONARY – LUNG CANCER/LUNG ADENOCARCINOMA [MOST LIKELY]

Adenocarcinoma [choice D] is the most common type of lung cancer, accounting for ~50% of lung cancer cases in the United States.
Adenocarcinoma is the most common type of lung cancer in men, women, smokers, and nonsmokers in the US.
Lesions are classically seen peripherally, and biopsy findings include mucin production.

The breakdown of lung cancer in the US is:
Non-Small cell lung cancer (NSCLC) ~85%
- **Adenocarcinoma ~50%**
- Squamous cell lung cancer ~30%
- Bronchioloalveolar carcinoma (rare)

Small cell lung cancer (SCLC)
- Small cell lung cancer ~15%

6. ENDOCRINE – THYROID STORM [PHARMACOLOGY]

Unless contraindicated, Beta blocker (eg, Propranolol) [choice D] should be initiated immediately in Thyroid storm to control the symptoms and signs of increased adrenergic tone (eg, heart rate, blood pressure, tremors).
Propranolol is the first line therapy because it is nonselective and is also inhibits conversion of T4 to T3 via inhibition of type 1 deiodinase.
IV therapy has a rapid onset of action.

Beta blocker administration should be immediately, followed by administration of the thionamide propylthiouracil (PTU) [choice B] to further block the conversion of T4 to T3 as well as inhibit thyroid hormone synthesis; Corticosteroids [choice C] should also be administered.

Choice E [Potassium iodide] should be administered 1 hour after thionamide administration.

Choice A [Dantrolene] is a skeletal muscle relaxant used in the management of malignant hyperthermia and Neuroleptic malignant syndrome.

7. EENT – GLOBE RUPTURE [CLINICAL INTERVENTION]

Patients with an open globe require emergent evaluation by an ophthalmologist [choice E] as it is vision-threatening ophthalmologic emergency.

Whenever globe rupture is obvious or strongly suspected, cover the eye with a metal eye shield or make a shield from a paper cup, and consult ophthalmology immediately without further manipulation.

Physical examination findings consistent with globe rupture include teardrop-shaped pupil and subconjunctival hemorrhage.

Other initial measures include:
- Elevation of the head of the bed to 45 degrees
- Avoidance of any eye manipulation (place a rigid eye shield)
- Bed rest, place the patient NPO (no oral intake)
- IV antiemetic therapy
- Administer broad-spectrum IV antibiotics (eg, Vancomycin plus Ceftazidime)
- Tetanus toxoid as necessary.

Choice A [Topical Ciprofloxacin ophthalmic and topical Cyclopentolate] is incorrect as use of any topical solutions should be avoided in suspected Globe rupture.

Choice B [Globe tonometry] is inappropriate as avoidance of any eye manipulation should avoided in Globe rupture.

Choice C [Slit lamp examination with Fluorescein] is inappropriate as avoidance of any eye manipulation should avoided in Globe rupture.

Choice D [CT scan of the orbits] should also be performed after the initial Ophthalmology consult is established.

8. MUSCULOSKELETAL - ANTIPHOSPHOLIPID SYNDROME [LABS AND DIAGNOSTIC STUDIES]

In patients with suspected Antiphospholipid syndrome (APS), antiphospholipid antibodies should be ordered, including:
- **Cardiolipin antibodies [choice E]**
- **Lupus anticoagulant**
- **Anti-beta2 glycoprotein I antibodies; IgG and IgM by ELISA.**

Antiphospholipid syndrome should be suspected in patients with:
- Thrombotic events (especially in young patients): venous or arterial thromboses/thromboemboli

- Recurrent fetal losses
- Livedo reticularis &/or Systemic lupus erythematosus in these patients increase the suspicion of APS.

Choice A [Anti Histone antibodies] is useful to establish the diagnosis of Drug-induced lupus.
Choice B [Anti double-stranded DNA antibodies] is associated with disease activity of SLE.
Choice C [Antinuclear antibodies] is a nonspecific screening test for SLE. The patient already has the diagnosis of SLE.
Choice D [Anti cyclic citrullinated peptide antibodies] are specific for Rheumatoid arthritis.

9. CARDIOLOGY – PULSELESS ELECTRICAL ACTIVITY (PEA) [CLINICAL INTERVENTION]

In patients with Pulseless electrical activity (PEA), after initiating CPR, immediately consider and treat reversible causes as appropriate and administer Epinephrine [choice D] (1 mg IV every 3-5 minutes) as soon as feasible.
Pulseless electrical activity (PEA) is defined as any one of a heterogeneous group of organized ECG rhythms (except for Ventricular tachycardia and Ventricular fibrillation) without sufficient mechanical contraction of the heart to produce a palpable pulse or measurable blood pressure.

Asystole and PEA do not respond to defibrillation [choice C].

Choice A [IV Metoprolol] is used in the management of Atrial fibrillation that is hemodynamically stable.
Choice B [Rapid synchronized cardioversion] is recommended for patients with monomorphic Ventricular tachycardia who are hemodynamically unstable (eg, systolic blood pressure in the double digits, altered mental status) with **a discernible blood pressure and pulse.**
Choice E [IV Adenosine] can be used in hemodynamically stable narrow complex tachycardias, such as Supraventricular tachycardia.

10. ENDOCRINE – POSTPARTUM THYROIDITIS [MOST LIKELY]

Caused of diffuse decreased radioactive iodine uptake (decreased Hormone synthesis) is consistent with:
- **Postpartum thyroiditis [choice E]**
- **Chronic lymphocytic (Hashimoto) thyroiditis**
- **Silent lymphocytic thyroiditis**

In Thyroiditis, release of preformed hormone from the thyroid gland due to inflammation suppresses the production of new thyroid hormone via negative feedback, resulting in diffuse decreased uptake on RAIU scan.

Postpartum thyroiditis and Silent lymphocytic thyroiditis are considered variants of Hashimoto thyroiditis; all 3 are associated with a transient primary hyperthyroid phase (decreased TSH and increased T4), antithyroid antibodies (eg, thyroid peroxidase and thyroglobulin antibodies), and are associated with diffuse decreased uptake on scan, followed by a hypothyroid phase (increased TSH and free T4).
Unlike Hashimoto thyroiditis, which is associated with long-term permanent hypothyroidism, both Postpartum thyroiditis and Silent lymphocytic thyroiditis often go onto a third phase of return to a euthyroid state after months (resolution).

Choice A [Sheehan syndrome] is associated with a secondary hypothyroidism pattern (both decreased TSH and free T4).

Choice B [Graves' disease], the most common cause of Primary hyperthyroidism, is associated with diffuse Increased uptake on thyroid scan, reflecting synthesis of new hormone.

Choice C Toxic adenoma] is associated with a focal area of increased uptake (hot nodule) on thyroid scan.

Choice D [TSH-secreting pituitary adenoma] is associated a secondary hyperthyroid pattern (increased TSH and free T4); similar to Graves' disease, TSH adenoma is associated with diffuse Increased uptake on thyroid scan, reflecting synthesis of new hormone.

11. GENITOURINARY – TESTICULAR CANCER [HISTORY AND PHYSICAL]

Males with Cryptorchidism [choice B] are at increased risk for testicular cancer.

Males with Cryptorchidism (undescended testicle) are at increased risk for testicular cancer in both the undescended and the normal testicles.

~10% of all testicular cancers occur in the setting of Cryptorchidism.

Surgical repositioning of the testis (orchiopexy) may help to reduce the risk of Testicular cancer in these patients.

Testicular cancer is one of the most common cancers in men aged 15–35 years and is one of the most curable cancers.

Other risk factors for Testicular cancer include:
- Hypospadias
- Family or personal history of Testicular cancer
- Genetic conditions: Klinefelter, Trisomy 21, Peutz-Jeghers syndrome

12. CARDIOLOGY - AORTIC REGURGITATION [HISTORY AND PHYSICAL EXAMINATION]

Chronic Aortic regurgitation [choice A] is classically associated with a widened pulse pressure (>60 mmHg), which can manifest as brisk bounding pulses and a pounding heart sensation.

In Chronic AR, some of the regurgitant blood flow into the LV, resulting in a rapid fall in arterial pressure (decreasing diastolic pressure); the increased stroke volume causes a more forceful contraction based on Frank Starling's law, resulting in an increased systolic pressure; both contributing to the wide pulse pressure.

In Chronic AR, the wide pulse pressure manifests as:
- Corrigan pulse – A "water hammer" or "collapsing" pulse is characterized by a rapidly rising and falling arterial pulse with a wide pulse pressure.
- de Musset sign – A head bob occurring with each heartbeat.
- Traube sign – A pistol shot pulse (systolic and diastolic sounds) heard over the femoral arteries.
- Duroziez sign – A systolic and diastolic bruit heard when the femoral artery is partially compressed.
- Quincke pulses – Capillary pulsations in the fingertips or lips.
- Mueller sign – Systolic pulsations of the uvula.

Choice D [Aortic stenosis] is associated with a narrow pulse pressure.

13. NEUROLOGY – SUBARACHNOID HEMORRHAGE [PHARMACOLOGY]

Oral administration of the dihydropyridine-type calcium channel blocker Nimodipine [choice D] is the standard of care for aneurysmal Subarachnoid hemorrhage and the only treatment with consistent, high-quality evidence for decreasing abnormal vasospasms of cerebral vascular smooth muscle.

Nimodipine 60 mg every four hours is administered to all patients with aneurysmal SAH starting within 48 hours of symptom onset, or sooner once the patient is stabilized. Treatment is continued for 21 days.

If the patient is unable to swallow, Nimodipine should be crushed and given via nasogastric tube as there is no evidence of the efficacy of intravenous Nimodipine.

IV Nicardipine is an alternative.

14. HEMATOLOGY – HEMOPHILIA A [HISTORY AND PHYSICAL EXAMINATION]

Hemophilia A is classically associated with deep tissue bleeding into the muscles, joints, and soft tissue hematomas [choice E].

Hemophilia A is an X-linked recessive disorder resulting in deficiency of Factor VIII, which results in a bleeding abnormality affecting the secondary coagulation pathway.

Labs may reveal a prolonged aPTT and decreased Factor VIII (8) <40% — most sensitive test. Mild disease >5%; moderate: 1-5%; severe <1%.

	Thrombocytopenia & VWD:	Hemophilia:
Major bleeding sites:	• **Mucocutaneous:*** mouth, nose, GI tract, menorrhagia.	• **Deep tissue*** joints, muscles • **Soft tissue hematomas**
Petechiae:	• **Common**	• Uncommon (platelet function is normal)
Ecchymosis:	• Generally small & superficial	• May be large
Excessive bleeding after minor cuts:	• Yes	• Not usually
Bleeding time:	• **Bleeding time prolonged***	• **Normal Bleeding time***
Bleeding after surgery:	• Often immediate	• Often during the procedure. • Delayed bleeding may also be seen with Hemophilia A.

15. PSYCHIATRY/BEHAVIORAL MEDICINE – CLOZAPINE/AGRANULOCYTOSIS [PHARMACOLOGY]

A rare but important adverse effect of Clozapine [choice C] is neutropenia and agranulocytosis, which occurs in 0.8% of patients.

Although one of the most effective antipsychotic drugs, the risk of agranulocytosis reserves its used for treatment-resistant Schizophrenia, with mandatory blood count monitoring for the duration of treatment.

Choice B [Bupropion] is associated with increased CNS activity, making it contraindicated in individuals at increased risk for seizures.
Choice C [Sertraline] and other SSRIs can cause GI symptoms and weight gain.
Choice D [Mirtazapine] causes sedation and weight gain resulting from its strong antihistaminic activity.
Choice E [Aripiprazole] may cause blurred vision, constipation, and headache.

16. NEUROLOGY – TRIGEMINAL NEURALGIA [PHARMACOLOGY]
Carbamazepine or Oxcarbazepine [choice D] are the first line initial therapy of choice for Trigeminal neuralgia (TGN).
For patients with TGN who cannot tolerate or if have contraindications to Carbamazepine or Oxcarbazepine, alternative agents include Gabapentin [choice B], Lamotrigine, or Baclofen.

Trigeminal neuralgia should be suspected in patients with:
- sudden brief episodes of stabbing lancinating unilateral facial pain that is recurrent
- pain in the territory of the second and third division of the trigeminal nerve
- triggers include stimulation of the affected trigeminal division by touching, chewing, or drafts of wind.

Choice A [Prednisone] is not used in the routine management of TN.
Choice C [100% Oxygen via nonrebreather] is the first line management of Cluster headache.
Choice E [Sumatriptan] is the first line abortive management of Migraine headache.

17. PULMONARY – ALPHA-1 ANTITRYPSIN DEFICIENCY [MOST LIKELY]
Suspect Alpha-1 antitrypsin deficiency [choice C] in nonsmokers or minimal smokers who develop early onset Emphysema (<45 years), especially bibasilar panacinar (diffuse) Emphysema and liver disease (Cirrhosis).
AATD represents 1-2% of all cases of COPD.
Alpha-1 antitrypsin is a protective enzyme against proteolytic enzymes (eg, elastase produced by macrophages during inflammation).
AATD results in increase destructive changes in the lungs, liver, and the skin.
Measurement of Alpha-1 antitrypsin levels is essential in establishing the diagnosis.

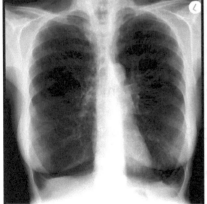 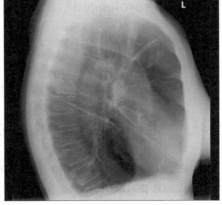

ALPHA 1 ANTITRYPSIN DEFICIENCY
- Marked hyperinflation of the lungs (note over 11 posterior ribs visible on PA projection, flattened hemidiaphragms, increased retrosternal air space) and hyperlucency of the lungs with distorted parenchymal architecture.

Choice A [Cystic fibrosis] is often associated with a chronic productive cough and chest radiographs classically show mucus plugging, atelectasis, interstitial lung markers, hyperinflation, and possibly tram track appearance consistent with Bronchiectasis [choice D]. Choice B [Asthma] can be associated with a normal chest radiograph (or less commonly, intermittent hyperinflation) on chest radiographs but is not associated with liver involvement. Choice E [Acute bronchitis] is usually associated with a normal physical examination and chest imaging.

18. ENDOCRINE – MEDULLARY THYROID CANCER [MOST LIKELY]
Serum calcitonin is frequently elevated in Medullary thyroid carcinoma [choice B] and is also a tumor marker used for metastatic disease.
Serum calcitonin >250 ng/L (73 pmol/L) or rising levels are best indications of recurrence or metastatic disease and may be beneficial as a postoperative marker for biochemical cure.
The serum calcitonin and carcinoembryonic antigen (CEA) concentrations should be measured in patients diagnosed with MTC during cytologic evaluation of a thyroid nodule.

Medullary thyroid cancer (MTC) is a neuroendocrine tumor of the parafollicular or C cells of the thyroid gland, the cells which normally produce calcitonin.

19. MUSCULOSKELETAL – CAUDA EQUINA SYNDROME [LABS AND DIAGNOSTIC STUDIES]
MRI of the lumbar spine [choice E] is the preferred study of choice to confirm the diagnosis of Cauda equina syndrome.
Early MRI and neurosurgical or orthopedic consultation (for surgical decompression) are necessary in the diagnosis and management of CES.

Cauda equina syndrome should be suspected in patients with sudden onset of back pain plus any one of the following:
- Radiculopathy: bilateral leg radiation of pain and weakness in multiple root distributions (L3-S1). May be unilateral.
- Involvement of S2-S4 spinal nerve roots
    - Saddle anesthesia — decreased sensation to the buttocks, perineum, and inner surfaces of the thigh. Erectile dysfunction in men.
    - New onset of urinary or bowel dysfunction
    - Decreased anal sphincter tone on physical examination

Choice A [Radiographs of the lumbar spine] can be used to assess for bony disorders, but they do not assess the spinal cord well.
Choice B [CT myelography] is an alternative to MRI for the evaluation of suspected Cauda equina syndrome if MRI is contraindicated (eg, pacemaker).
Choice C [Lumbar puncture] can be used if CNS infection is suspected.
Choice D [Electromyography] is used to assess nerve or muscle injuries.

20. REPRODUCTIVE – ECTOPIC PREGNANCY [CLINICAL INTERVENTION]
Indications for surgical (Laparoscopic) management of Ectopic pregnancy [choice C] include:
- **hCG >5,000 IU/mL**
- **gestational sac >3.5 cm**

- **embryonic cardiac activity**
- **Hemodynamically unstable patients**
- **evidence of rupture**
- anemia or thrombocytopenia
- liver disease
- immunosuppressed (eg, HIV).

Laparoscopic salpingostomy (with Ectopic pregnancy removal) is often the surgical procedure of choice when possible (may need reparative procedure to save reproductive organs) + IV fluids.
Salpingectomy is performed if salpingostomy cannot be performed.

Indications for medical management with Methotrexate [choice A] include satisfying the criterial of all the following 3:
- [1] hemodynamically stable patients with
- [2] early gestation (≤3.5 cm, hCG ≤5,000, no embryonic cardiac activity), & no evidence of rupture
- [3] patients who will be compliant to follow-up, are immunocompetent, & have normal liver and renal function tests.

Choice B [Repeat quantitative serum hCG and Ultrasound in 48 hours] is the management when patients present lower than the discriminatory zone (eg, hCG <1,500) with a pregnancy of unknown location on Ultrasound.
Choice D [Dilation followed by suction curettage] is inappropriate as ectopic pregnancies are outside the uterus.
Choice E [Misoprostol] is not used in the management of Ectopic pregnancy. Indications for Methotrexate include elective abortions and use as a cervical ripening agent.

21. GENITOURINARY – VARICOCELE [HEALTH MAINTENANCE]
Although most Varicoceles are asymptomatic, the 3 main complications of Varicoceles are:
- **decreased fertility [choice D]** due to the elevated scrotal temperature from the dilated veins
- **decreased production of sperm by the testis**
- **testicular pain or scrotal discomfort.**

For this reason, most Varicoceles do not require surgical intervention unless there is a concern for one of these 3 issues.

Varicoceles are often identified in infertile men. 40% of men with primary infertility are found to have a varicocele and in 75-81% of men with secondary infertility.
Varicocele repair may be offered to individuals with reduced ipsilateral testicular size (testicular hypertrophy) or abnormal semen parameters.
Surgical ligation or percutaneous venous embolization are the 2 most common surgical options.

All of the other choices are not classic complications of a Varicocele.

22. NEUROLOGY – EPIDURAL HEMATOMA/CRANIAL NERVE PALSY [HISTORY AND PHYSICAL]

Trauma or compression of the upper brain stem and third cranial nerve [choice B], which is responsible for eye muscles and movement (oculomotor function) can result in a "blown pupil" (dilated pupil with minimal to no light response).

An enlarging Epidural hematoma leads to eventual *elevation of* intracranial pressure, which may be detected in a clinical setting by observing ipsilateral pupil dilation (secondary to uncal herniation and oculomotor nerve compression).

Functions of the oculomotor nerve (cranial nerve III) [choice B] include:
- **Eye movement: all of the ocular muscles** except for the lateral rectus (CN VI) [LR6] and the superior oblique muscles (CN IV) [SO4].
- **Opens eyelid:** supplies the **levator palpebrae.** Damage can lead to **ptosis.**
- **Pupil constriction** (SLUDD-**C**) and accommodations: **efferent pupillary response** (CN III efferent; CN II afferent).

Pathology of CN III includes:
- unresponsive ipsilateral pupillary constriction on the affected side (the **pupil is fixed and dilated [blown pupil]**) when light is shined in either eye (**efferent pupillary defect**).
- **eye is "down and out"*.**
- **Diabetes can cause CN III palsy with pupil sparing.**

Choice A [II] is responsible for visual acuity and visual fields. It is also responsible for the afferent pupillary response.

Choice C [IV] innervates the Superior oblique muscle [SO4]. It depresses the eye when adducted in isolation (down and out).

Choice D [VI] is responsible for Lateral eye motion [LR6]: the lateral rectus muscle functions to abduct the ipsilateral eye (look away from the nose).

Choice E [VII] is responsible for motor innervation of the face, innervates the stapedius muscle, and is sensation of the anterior two-thirds of the tongue.

23. GASTROINTESTINAL/NUTRITIONAL – COLORECTAL CANCER SCREENING [HEALTH MAINTENANCE]

The USPST guidelines recommend screening Colonoscopy initially at 40-years of age OR 10 years before the age the relative was diagnosed (whichever is earlier, in this patient that would be 35 years of age), then colonoscopy every 5 years [choice B].

Choice A is only wrong because 10 years before the person was diagnose (35 in this case) is lower than age 40 years.

The USPSTF recommends Colonoscopy as a screening test is usually performed every 10 years for a patient at average risk of CRC, starting at age 50 years (Grade A) [choice D]
- Grade A recommendation: screening for colorectal cancer in all adults aged 50-70 years.
- Grade B recommendation: screening for colorectal cancer in all adults aged 45-49 years.

In patients with a first degree relative ≥60 years:
- start at age 40 years [OR 10 years earlier than age which the family member developed CR cancer, whichever is EARLIER] & every 10 years thereafter.

In patients with a first degree relative <60 years:
- start at age 40 years [OR 10 years earlier than age which the family member developed CR cancer, whichever is EARLIER] & every 5 years thereafter.

24. EENT – PRESEPTAL (PERIORBITAL) CELLULITIS [PHARMACOLOGY]

Empiric monotherapy with Amoxicillin-clavulanic acid [choice C] is the first line treatment for Periorbital cellulitis in the absence of trauma (eg, insect bite, skin abrasion, blunt trauma), to cover organisms colonizing the sinuses and nasopharynx are likely to be the cause of infection.

In patients with a history of trauma (eg, insect bite, skin abrasion, blunt trauma), *S. aureus* and *S. pyogenes* are the common causes of infection and coverage includes Either Trimethoprim-sulfamethoxazole or Linezolid plus one of the following agents: Amoxicillin-clavulanic acid, Cefdinir, Cefuroxime, or Cefpodoxime.

Choice A [Oral Cephalexin] does not cover all the organisms that are common causes of Preseptal cellulitis.

Choice B [IV Vancomycin plus Ceftriaxone] is the first line management of Postseptal (Orbital) cellulitis.

Choice D [Warm compresses and eyelid hygiene] are used in the management of Blepharitis.

Choice E [Ciprofloxacin ophthalmic ointment 0.3%] can be used for ocular infections in contact lens wearers.

25. DERMATOLOGY – PITYRIASIS ROSEA [CLINICAL INTERVENTION]

Most patients with Pityriasis rosea (PR) do not require specific therapy other than supportive measures [choice C], as PR is a self-limiting, exanthematous disease.

Medium-potency topical corticosteroids may be used for patients with mild itching who desire therapy.

The hallmark features of PR include the development of a slightly raised, oval-shaped scaly patch called a "herald patch," followed by the emergence of multiple clusters of similar scaly oval patches within 2 weeks following skin cleavage lines in a "Christmas tree" pattern.

In severe presentations:
- oral Acyclovir [choice A] or oral Erythromycin may result in faster resolution of the lesions.
- Phototherapy [choice E] is an alternative treatment option.

26. HEMATOLOGY – APLASTIC ANEMIA (APPLYING FOUNDATIONAL CONCEPTS)

The classic findings of Aplastic anemia and bone marrow biopsy are hypocellularity, morphologically normal residual hematopoietic cells, with the marrow space is mostly composed of fat cells and marrow stroma [choice A].

Aplastic anemia (AA) is a bone marrow failure (BMF) disorder characterized by pancytopenia with bone marrow hypoplasia/aplasia due to loss of hematopoietic stem cells (HSCs).

Chloramphenicol can result in either idiosyncratic or predictable bone marrow suppression.

Patients with AA generally present with clinical and lab findings related to pancytopenia: fatigue & dyspnea (anemia), fever &/or infections (neutropenia), or bleeding/bruising (thrombocytopenia).

Choice B [Absent iron stores] is associated with Iron deficiency anemia.

Choice C [Ringed sideroblasts] is associated with Sideroblastic anemia.
Choice D [Increased myeloblasts but <20%] is associated with Myelodysplastic syndrome.
Choice E [Increased number of megakaryocytes with normal morphology] is associated with Immune thrombocytopenic purpura.

27. GASTROINTESTINAL/NUTRITIONAL – HEPATITIS B INFECTION [HEALTH MAINTENANCE]

Hepatitis B serologies are suggestive of Chronic hepatitis B [choice C] if serologies reveal:
- **Positive Hepatitis B surface antigen (HBsAg) — HBsAg is a marker of infection**
- **Positive Hepatitis B core antibody (anti-HBc) IgG — marker of chronicity if HBSAg is positive.**

The presence of Hepatitis B core antibody IgG (IgG anti-HBc) signifies either:
- **[1] chronic Hepatitis B** — positive IgG anti-HBc + positive surface antigen (HBsAg) or
- **[2] recovery from Hepatitis B — positive** IgG anti-HBc + positive surface antibody (anti-HBs). [choice A]

A positive surface antibody (anti-HBs) is a marker of immunity and signifies either:
- positive surface antibody (anti-HBs). [choice A]
  - [1] successfully vaccination — positive surface antibody (anti-HBs) as the only positive serologic marker.
  - [2] recovery from Hepatitis B — positive IgG anti-HBc + positive surface antibody (anti-HBs). [choice A]

Simply put:
- Resolved infection (recovery): positive IgG anti-HBc + positive anti-HBs
- Successful vaccination: positive anti-HBs only
- Chronic hepatitis: positive IgG anti-HBc + positive HBsAg
- Acute hepatitis: positive IgM anti-HBc + positive HBsAg
- Window period towards recovery: positive IgM anti-HBc only.

28. REPRODUCTIVE – PRIMARY DYSMENORRHEA [PHARMACOLOGY]

Nonsteroidal anti-inflammatory drugs (NSAIDs) [choice B], Acetaminophen, and hormonal contraceptives are the mainstays of pharmacologic therapy for Primary dysmenorrhea.
For individuals who do not desire hormonal contraception or prefer/need to avoid hormonal therapy, NSAIDs are first line.

Because the progestin component of estrogen-progestin contraceptives induces the endometrial atrophy which improves dysmenorrhea, progestin-only contraceptives [choices A and C] may be an effective treatment, but they have not been studied as extensively as estrogen-progestin contraceptives.

Second-tier alternatives include Leuprolide acetate depot (choice D) or Transcutaneous electrical nerve stimulation [choice E].

29. MUSCULOSKELETAL – PSORIATIC ARTHRITIS [MOST LIKELY]

The classic radiograph findings of Psoriatic arthritis [choice B] is the "pencil in cup" deformity", which describes periarticular erosions and bone resorption giving the appearance of a pencil in a cup.

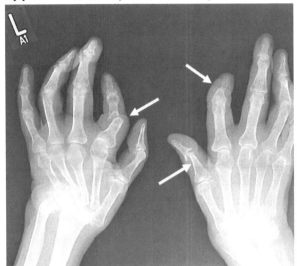 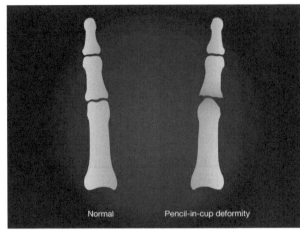

Psoriatic arthritis
· Multiple pencil in cup deformities, joint subluxation and sausage-shaped fingers in keeping with advanced psoriatic arthritis.

Photo credit:

Case courtesy of Ahmed Elowaidy, Radiopaedia.org, rID: 25019

Case courtesy of Sachi Hapugoda, Radiopaedia.org, rID: 54415

Psoriatic arthritis should be suspected in patients with:
- Asymmetric arthritis with distal joint involvement (eg, DIP joint)
- Enthesitis eg, Achilles tendon, plantar fasciitis (as in this patient)
- Dactylitis: fusiform "sausage-shaped" digit swelling
- Peripheral and axial joint involvement (this patient has hip pain)
- Psoriasis: rash of Psoriasis &/or nail pitting

Choice A [Osteoarthritis] is associated with osteophytes, asymmetric joint narrowing, and subchondral sclerosis on radiographs. OA is not associated with enthesitis or dactylitis.

Choice C [Acute CPP crystal arthritis] is associated with calcification of the cartilage (chondrocalcinosis) on radiographs.

Choice D [Rheumatoid arthritis] characteristically spares the DIP joint, has symmetric joint involvement, and is associated with periarticular osteopenia and joint erosions on radiographs.

Choice E [Gouty arthritis] is associated with punched out erosions with sclerosis and overhanging edges (mouse or rat bite lesions) on radiographs.

30. INFECTIOUS DISEASE - PELVIC INFLAMMATORY DISEASE [CLINICAL INTERVENTION]

IM Ceftriaxone, oral Doxycycline, Metronidazole, Naprosyn, follow-up in 2 days [choice A] is the first line outpatient management of Pelvic inflammatory disease (PID).

Most patients with PID can be managed as outpatients.

Indications for admission for Pelvic inflammatory disease (PID) [choice E] includes:
- severe clinical illness: fever ≥38.5°C [101°F]
- nausea and vomiting
- inability to take oral medications or lack of response to oral medications.
- complicated PID with pelvic abscess (including tubo-ovarian abscess)
- pregnancy.

Choice B [Laparoscopy] may be used to confirm the clinical diagnosis of PID but is not commonly performed in most uncomplicated cases.
Choice C [Oral Metronidazole and Doxycycline with outpatient follow-up] is incomplete as it does not include gonococcal coverage.
Choice D [Oral Vancomycin with outpatient follow-up] is not the management of PID.

31. MUSCULOSKELETAL – OSTEOMYELITIS [APPLYING FOUNDATIONAL CONCEPTS]
Staphylococcus aureus **[choice B] is the most common cause of Osteomyelitis in pediatric and adult patients.**
The femur and the tibia are the most common bones associated with Osteomyelitis in children.

Choice A [Pseudomonas aeruginosa] is associated with calcaneal Osteomyelitis associated with puncture wounds through tennis shoes.
Choice C [Salmonella species] infections in Osteomyelitis is pathognomonic for Sickle cell disease.
Choice D [Group B streptococcus] is seen in increased incidence in neonates with Osteomyelitis because GBS may be part of the vaginal flora.
Choice E [Staphylococcus epidermidis], also known as coagulase-negative staphylococci may cause osteomyelitis in neonates and children with indwelling vascular catheters (eg, for chronic hemodialysis) or in adults after recent prosthetic joint placement.

32. GENITOURINARY – ACUTE PYELONEPHRITIS [LABS AND DIAGNOSTIC STUDIES]
The presence of white blood cell casts [choice D] in the urine indicate either infection of upper GU tract due to Pyelonephritis or inflammation involving the renal interstitium (Acute interstitial nephritis).
As the white blood cells from upper urinary tract infection or inflammation enter the collecting duct, they take the shape of the tubules, forming cellular casts (white cell casts).

All of the other choices can be seen in both Acute cystitis and Pyelonephritis.

33. PSYCHIATRY/BEHAVIORAL – GRIEF REACTION [HEALTH MAINTENANCE]
<u>Abnormal grief</u> **should be suspected if**
- **symptoms >1 year [choice E]**
- **severe symptoms**
- **positive suicidal ideation**
- **psychosis**
- **illusions, or hallucinations that the patient perceives are real.**

Normal grief:
- usually resolves within 6 months to 1 year.
- peaks usually within the first couple of months after the loss.
- usually characterized by intense emotions, appetite or sleep disturbances, guilt, weight loss
- symptoms may include illusions or simple hallucinations of the deceased that the patient understands is not real.

Patients are usually able to function.

34. EENT – ACUTE OTITIS EXTERNA (APPLYING FOUNDATIONAL CONCEPTS]

The most common pathogenic organisms responsible for external otitis are:
- **Pseudomonas aeruginosa (41%) [choice E], the most common cause, and**
- **Staphylococcus aureus (15%).**

Other gram-positive and -negative bacteria can also cause external otitis.
Anaerobic pathogens make up 17% of cases especially Bacteroides [choice C] and peptostreptococci.
Candidal infection [choice B] occurs more commonly in patients who use hearing aids. Fungal infection [choice B] make up 2-10% of cases of external otitis and usually are associated with occurring after treatment of bacterial infection.

35. PULMONARY – LUNG ABSCESS [APPLYING FOUNDATIONAL CONCEPTS]

Impaired swallowing [choice C] and enteral feeding while supine are risk factors for the development of Lung abscess and aspiration Pneumonia.
Neurological conditions increase the risk of Aspiration (this patient has ALS).

Lung abscess are most commonly a complication of aspiration of oropharyngeal secretions especially in patients with recurrent aspiration who have dental, gingival, or periodontal infection or paranasal sinusitis.
Therefore, these infections are often polymicrobial with oral flora, including microaerophilic streptococci and anaerobes (*Peptostreptococcus, Prevotella, Bacteroides* [usually not *B. fragilis*]), and *Fusobacterium* spp.

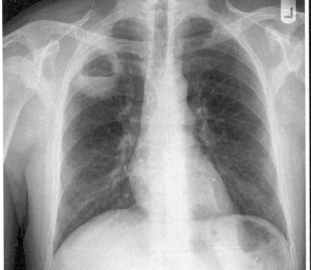 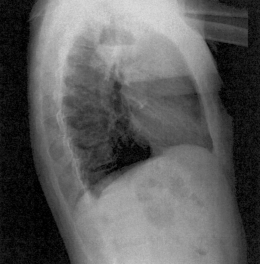

Chest radiograph typically shows a thick-walled cavity with an air-fluid level, with or without a surrounding opacity (in this case a thick-walled right upper lobe cavitary lesion with an air fluid level).

36. GENITOURINARY – ORCHITIS [CLINICAL INTERVENTION]

Patients with Viral orchitis (in this case Mumps orchitis) are treated symptomatically with bed rest, nonsteroidal anti-inflammatory agents (NSAIDs), support of the inflamed testis, and application of cold packs to the scrotum [choice B].

Clinical manifestations may include scrotal swelling, pain, and tenderness with erythema and shininess of the overlying skin.

Choice A [Perform testicular ultrasound to rule out a testicular mass] may be indicated if a mass was palpated suggestive of Testicular cancer.

Choice C [Surgical referral for Orchiopexy] is recommended in young children >4-6 months of age with Cryptorchidism.

Choice D [Initiate Trimethoprim-sulfamethoxazole] is not needed in Viral orchitis.

Choice E [Refer to urology for urological workup] is not indicated in this patient with uncomplicated Viral orchitis.

37. HEMATOLOGY – VON WILLEBRAND DISEASE (MOST LIKELY)

Von Willebrand disease (VWD) [choice D], the most common inherited bleeding disorder, should be suspected in patients who present with:
- **Bruising, mucocutaneous bleeding, heavy menstrual bleeding, and postpartum bleeding.**
- **Normal or increased activated partial thromboplastin time (aPTT)**
- **Normal platelets** (except for the rare form VWD type 2B, which may be associated with thrombocytopenia).

Choice A [Hemophilia A] is also associated with a prolonged aPTT but with deep tissue bleeding.

Choice B [Factor V Leiden mutation] is the most common inherited thrombophilic disorder, presenting with Deep vein thrombosis (DVT) and Pulmonary emboli (PE).

Choice C [Antiphospholipid syndrome] is associated with increased risk of venous thrombosis (DVT and PE).

Choice E [Hemophilia B] is also associated with a prolonged aPTT but with deep tissue bleeding.

38. EENT – ACUTE RHINOSINUSITIS [CLINICAL INTERVENTION]

Amoxicillin-clavulanic acid [choice E] is often the antibiotic of choice for Acute sinusitis in patients with symptoms present for an extended period of ≥10-14 days with worsening of symptoms or earlier if severe.

Second line antibiotics include Doxycycline (can be used first-line if Penicillin allergy). Third-generation oral Cephalosporin (eg, Cefixime, Cefpodoxime) with or without Clindamycin are other options.

Respiratory fluoroquinolones (Levofloxacin, Moxifloxacin) usually reserved to prevent resistance.

Choice A [Ibuprofen, intranasal sterile saline spray, and reassess in 48-72 hours] can be used in patients who present within the first 10 days of symptoms.

Choice D [Water's view radiographs] would not change the management of this patient and expose them to unnecessary radiation.

39. GASTROINTESTINAL/NUTRITIONAL – ACUTE COLONIC PSEUDO-OBSTRUCTION [LABS AND DIAGNOSTIC STUDIES]

Elevated serum lactate [choice B] is sensitive but not specific for mesenteric ischemia and increases the possibility of bowel ischemia and possible bowel infarction.

When peritonitis is suggested (guarding, rigidity, &/or rebound tenderness), an elevated blood lactate level requires an emergent surgical consult and is considered a contraindication for conservative management of Acute colonic pseudo-obstruction (Ogilvie syndrome).

Although most cases of Acute colonic pseudo-obstruction are managed conservatively, surgical management is indicated for patients with colonic ischemia, perforation, peritonitis, and those that are refractory to medical and conservative management.

Choice A [White blood cell count] is often elevated due to inflammation of the postoperative state; it is a nonspecific finding, and in most cases would not significantly change management when assessed solely.

Choice C [Urinalysis] may be abnormal if there is a postoperative urinary tract infection but would not significantly alter the management of acute colonic pseudo-obstruction.

Choice D [Amylase and lipase] elevations, indicative of Acute pancreatitis, is not a contraindication to conservative management of Acute colonic pseudo-obstruction.

Choice E [AST and ALT] elevations, indicative of Acute hepatitis, is not a contraindication to conservative management of Acute colonic pseudo-obstruction.

40. INFECTIOUS DISEASE – VACCINES DURING PREGNANCY [HEALTH MAINTENANCE]

Live attenuated vaccines are contraindicated during pregnancy, including:
- **Varicella (Chickenpox) [choice E]**
- Measles, Mumps, Rubella (MMR)
- Polio
- BCG

Other contraindicated vaccines include:
- Inactivated: HPV vaccine
- Intranasal influenza
- Yellow fever (in most)
- Smallpox

41. ENDOCRINE – CENTRAL ADRENAL INSUFFICIENCY [MOST LIKELY]

The most common cause of central (secondary and tertiary) adrenal insufficiency is long-term therapy with pharmacologic doses of glucocorticoids [choice D].

Long-term steroid use at high doses of glucocorticoids decrease both hypothalamic CRH synthesis and secretion as well as anterior pituitary ACTH synthesis and secretion via negative feedback.

This results in the hallmark laboratory finding of both decreased cortisol and inappropriately low ACTH levels in central (secondary and tertiary) adrenal insufficiency.

Choice A [Waterhouse-Friderichsen syndrome] results from adrenal hemorrhage and subsequent infarction associated with meningococcemia. It is a cause of Primary adrenal insufficiency, so it is associated with increased baseline ACTH and decreased serum cortisol.

Choice B [Tuberculosis] can destroy the adrenal glands due to calcification and spread of the infection to the adrenal glands. Infectious adrenalitis is a cause of Primary adrenal insufficiency, so it is associated with increased baseline ACTH and decreased serum cortisol.

Choice C [Autoimmune adrenalitis] is the most common cause of Primary adrenal insufficiency; therefore, it is associated with increased baseline ACTH and decreased serum cortisol.

Choice D [Cushing disease] is due to ACTH-secreting pituitary adenoma or hyperplasia, resulting in increases in both serum ACTH and cortisol.

42. NEUROLOGY – MIGRAINE HEADACHE [PHARMACOLOGY]

5-hydroxytryptamine–1 (5-HT 1b/1D) receptor agonists — (Triptans, Sumatriptan-Naproxen, Ergotamines) either alone or in combination with Dopamine receptor antagonists (eg, Metoclopramide, Prochlorperazine, Chlorpromazine) [choice B] are Migraine-specific agents used for moderate to severe Migraine attacks.

Other options for abortive therapy include:
- CGRP antagonists (eg, Ubrogepant)
- 5-HT1F receptor agonists (Lasmiditan).

Migraine headaches are characterized by:
- Headache: [1] episodic lateralized (unilateral), throbbing (pulsatile) headache localized in the frontotemporal & ocular area, moderate to severe in intensity,
- [2] usually 4-72 hours in duration
- [3] Often associated with nausea, vomiting, photophobia, &/or phonophobia.
- Worsened with routine physical activity (eg, walking climbing stairs), stress, lack or excessive sleep, alcohol, specific foods, hormonal (eg, oral contraception, menstruation), odors, skipped meals.

Choice A [Verapamil and Ubrogepant] combination can be used for prevention of Migraines.

Choice C [100% oxygen via nonrebreather and Ibuprofen] is the management of a Cluster headache.

Choice D [Carbamazepine] is the management of Trigeminal neuralgia.

Choice E [Ethosuximide] is the management of an Absence seizure.

43. GENITOURINARY – CHRONIC PROSTATITIS [MOST LIKELY]

The classic findings of Chronic prostatitis [choice E] on digital rectal examination include an edematous (boggy), nontender or minimally tender, prostate.

Chronic bacterial prostatitis is associated with chronic or recurrent urogenital symptoms in the setting of documented bacterial infection of the prostate.

Choice A [Prostate cancer] is associated with a hard, asymmetric prostate, often with nodularity on digital rectal examination.

Choice B [Acute cystitis] and Prostatitis can present with irritative symptoms, but Acute cystitis has no examination findings on prostate examination.

Choice C [Acute prostatitis] is associated with an edematous (boggy), warm ("hot'), and exquisitely tender prostate on digital examination.

Choice D [Benign prostatic hyperplasia] is associated with a firm, rubbery, symmetrically enlarged prostate without tenderness or edema.

44. RENAL – GLOMERULONEPHRITIS [MOST LIKELY]

Immune complex-mediated Membranoproliferative (MPGN) [choice A] is most commonly secondary to hepatitis C and B viral infections.

Other causes of MPGN include autoimmunity (eg, SLE, and, less often, Sjögren's disease or Rheumatoid arthritis).

The hallmark findings of MPGN on biopsy include:
- **[1] <u>thickened basement membrane</u>:** the capillary basement membranes are thickened by interposition of mesangial cells and matrix into the capillary wall. This gives rise to the tram-track or double-contoured appearance of the capillary wall.
- **[2] <u>proliferation</u>: hypercellularity** (due to glomerular inflammation).

Choice B [Postinfectious glomerulonephritis] is characterized by electron-dense, glomerular dome-shaped subepithelial immune complex deposits ("humps") of IgG, IgM, & C3.

Choice C [IgA Glomerulonephritis] IgA mesangial deposits on immunofluorescence microscopy.

Choice D [Minimal change disease] is a type of Nephrotic syndrome associated with a normal appearing glomerulus and fatty casts; it is not associated with red cell casts or hypercellularity (nephritic syndrome).

Choice E [Focal segmental glomerulosclerosis] is associated with focal areas of narrowing. FSGS is commonly seen with HIV, Heroin use, and Hypertension.

45. GENITOURINARY – NEPHROLITHIASIS [CLINICAL INTERVENTION]

Emergency intervention for urgent decompression of the collecting system [choice C] is usually recommended for:
- **Struvite stones (as in this patient) – surgery is usually required to successfully manage struvite stones.**
- **obstructing stones**
- **<u>complicated Nephrolithiasis</u>: eg, urinary tract infection (UTI), Acute kidney injury.**

Medical therapy alone is **not** preferred and should be reserved for patients who are too ill to tolerate, or who refuse, stone removal surgery.

Large stones ≥10-mm often require urology referral for stone removal.

Struvite (magnesium ammonium phosphate) stones are strongly associated with urinary tract infections (UTIs) with urea-splitting organisms (eg, *Proteus mirabilis*).

Struvite stone should be suspected in patients with:
- recurrent or persistent UTIs
- persistently alkaline urine pH (>8)
- magnesium ammonium phosphate crystals present in the urine sediment, or
- a staghorn calculus identified by abdominal imaging (see photo below)

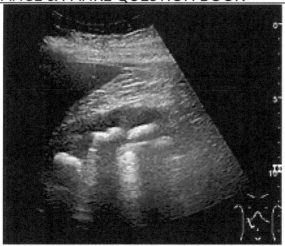

Staghorn calculi filling the entire collecting system and creating pronounced shadowing.

Choice A [Percutaneous nephrostomy tube insertion] can be used in patients who are not surgical candidates.

Choice B [Extracorporeal shock wave lithotripsy] alone would be insufficient as this struvite stone is filling the entire renal calyx.

Choice D [Discharge home with Ibuprofen, increased fluid intake, and Tamsulosin to facilitate stone passage] is used in the management of small stones <5 mm as they have >80% chance of spontaneous passage.

Choice E [Perform a CT scan of the abdomen and pelvis with intravenous contrast] is often the preferred initial imaging for Nephrolithiasis but is not necessary as the Ultrasound clearly outlines the stone and the involvement of the calyx.

46. ENDOCRINE – PHEOCHROMOCYTOMA [APPLYING FOUNDATIONAL CONCEPTS]

Pheochromocytoma is a catecholamine-secreting tumor that arises from chromaffin cells of the adrenal medulla [choice B].

Because the tumor can secrete catecholamines (eg, epinephrine, norepinephrine, and dopamine), the classic triad of symptoms in patients with a Pheochromocytoma include "PHE"

- **P**alpitations and tachycardia (B1 receptor activation); **P**allor (alpha-1 mediated vasoconstriction)
- **H**eadache (episodic) due to Hypertension (alpha-1 mediated vasoconstriction)
- **E**xcessive sweating

Choice A (Disease of the adrenal cortex) is one of the causes of Cushing syndrome, which presents with abdominal striae, buffalo hump, supraclavicular fat pad, moon faces, and centripetal obesity.

Choice C [Narrowing of the renal artery] associated with Renovascular disease is often associated with an abdominal bruit.

Choice D [Aldosterone-producing adenoma] results in Primary hyperaldosteronism, which classically presents with the triad of hypokalemia, metabolic alkalosis, and Hypertension.

Choice E (Coarctation of the aorta) classically presents with brachiofemoral delay, hypertension, decreased femoral pulses, and a systolic murmur.

47. CARDIOLOGY – SECOND-DEGREE ATRIOVENTRICULAR BLOCK (COMPLETE HEART BLOCK) [CLINICAL INTERVENTION]

Treatment for a Mobitz type II involves initiating temporary cardiac pacing [choice D] as soon as this rhythm is identified.

If no identifiable reversible cause is found, permanent pacemaker is definitive management.

Unlike Mobitz type I (Wenckebach), patients that are bradycardic and hypotensive with a Mobitz type II rhythm often do not respond to Atropine as the block is usually infranodal.

Patients with Mobitz type II second-degree AV block who are symptomatic or hemodynamically unstable should be urgently treated with:
- beta-adrenergic agonist (eg, Isoproterenol, Dopamine, or Epinephrine) if myocardial ischemia is not likely, and in most,
- temporary cardiac pacing (either with transcutaneous or, if immediately available, transvenous pacing)

Choice A [IV Dopamine] can be used as third-line therapy in patients with Complete heart block if the patient remains unstable despite treatment with [1] Atropine followed by [2] transcutaneous pacing in the setting of a low blood pressure.

Choice C [IV Dobutamine] can be used as third-line therapy in patients with Complete heart block if the patient remains unstable despite treatment with [1] Atropine followed by [2] transcutaneous pacing in the setting of Heart failure.

Choice E [Observation and reassurance it is self-limiting] can be used for asymptomatic bradycardia excluding Mobitz II and Third-degree AV blocks.

48. CARDIOLOGY – ACUTE DECOMPENSATED HEART FAILURE/CONGESTIVE HEART FAILURE (CHF) [PHARMACOLOGY]

Initial therapy of Acute decompensated Heart failure includes supplemental oxygen to treat hypoxemia (SpO$_2$ <90%), assisted ventilation if needed, and a loop diuretic, such as IV Furosemide [choice C] for volume overload.

Early initiation of an effective IV loop diuretic regimen reduces symptoms due to overload (eg, dyspnea), and has been shown to reduce in-hospital mortality.

Loop diuretics remove excess volume, relieving the pulmonary and peripheral edema.

Choice A [Nitroglycerin] is a vasodilator that can be used as an adjunct to diuretic therapy for patients with ADHF/CHF without adequate response to diuretics.

Choice B [Digoxin] can be used in the long-term management of Heart failure in patients who have maximized initial pharmacotherapy.

Choice D [Sacubitril-Valsartan] is a first-line long-term agent in the management of Compensated Heart failure.

Choice E [Carvedilol] can be used in the long-term management of Compensated Heart failure, but dosage is usually reduced or temporarily discontinued in patients with Decompensated heart failure.

49. NEUROLOGY – BASILAR SKULL FRACTURE [HISTORY AND PHYSICAL EXAMINATION]

Hallmark features of a Basilar skull fracture include:

- **Hemotympanum (blood behind the tympanic membrane) [choice D]** and generally appears within hours of injury. Hemotympanum is detected by otoscopy, which reveals the blue to purple hue taken on by the tympanic membrane.
- **Retroauricular or mastoid ecchymosis (eg, Battle sign)** typically appears one to three days after the fracture
- "**Raccoon eyes" (periorbital ecchymosis)**, which suggests a basilar skull fracture or anterior or middle fossa facial trauma, often 1-3 days after the injury.
- **Clear rhinorrhea or otorrhea** is found in up to 20 percent of temporal bone fractures. Such leaks may be detected within hours or up to several days after trauma.

Choice A [Diplopia with upward gaze] is indicative of an Orbital floor fracture.
Choice C [Upward Babinski] indicated an upper motor neuron finding.
Choice C [Irregular tear-shaped pupil] suggests an Open globe injury.
Choice E [Papilledema] suggests Intracranial hemorrhage.

50. REPRODUCTIVE – ENDOMETRIAL CANCER [HEALTH MAINTENANCE]

Because Raloxifene [choice E] is an estrogen antagonist in the uterus, it is not linked with an increased risk of Endometrial cancer (think Raloxifene "relaxes" the uterus, so there is no risk). Raloxifene is an estrogen antagonist in the uterus and breast, which is why it can be used as Prophylaxis for Breast cancer. It is an estrogen agonist in the bone and liver.

Increased number of menstrual cycles and chronically increased estrogen levels/activity can increase the risk of Endometrial cancer:

- chronically increased estrogen levels/activity:
  - Tamoxifen use: Tamoxifen is an estrogen agonist in the breast, bone, liver, and uterus, increasing the risk of Endometrial hyperplasia and cancer (think "Tamoxifen is toxic to the uterus; unlike Raloxifene, which relaxes the uterus")
  - Obesity
  - Chronic anovulation: eg, PCOS
  - Unopposed estrogen therapy
- increased number of cycles:
  - early menarche
  - nulliparity
  - late menopause

51. PULMONARY – SILICOSIS [HISTORY AND PHYSICAL EXAMINATION]

Occupations that involves processing, crushing, grinding, or using silica-containing rock [choice E] or ores increase the risk for Silicosis, such as:

- **stone cutting**, foundry work, and ceramics.
- mining, quarrying, sandblasting, masonry

The hallmark findings of Silicosis are:

- PFTs: restrictive pattern [normal or increased FEV1/FVC; decreased lung volumes (RV, TLC, RV/TLC)]

- Chest radiographs: small (<1 cm) nodules predominantly in the mid to upper lung zones, eggshell calcifications, nodules.

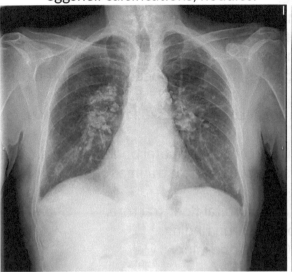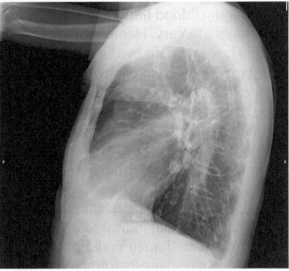

SILICOSIS
- **Frontal**: Ill-defined bilateral hila with multiple calcified adenopathies in it and in the retrocardiac space. Right costophrenic angle blunting. Aortic arch elongated and calcified.
- **Lateral:** The "eggshell" calcification of multiple adenopathies along the mediastinum and bilateral pulmonary hila.

Choice A [30 pack-year smoking history] increased the risk for Chronic obstructive pulmonary disease, which has an obstructive pattern on PFTs.

Choice B [Cystic fibrosis] is often associated with Bronchiectasis, both of which are classically associated with an obstructive pattern on PFTs.

Choice C [Occupation as a plumber and pipefitter] is hallmark of Asbestosis, which classically presents with lower lobe predominance and pleural plaques.

Choice D [Working in a fluorescent light bulb and electronics manufacturing plant] is a risk for the development of Berylliosis, which classically presents with bilateral hilar lymphadenopathy on chest imaging, similar to Sarcoidosis.

52. NEUROLOGY – MOTOR NEURON DEFECTS [HISTORY AND PHYSICAL EXAMINATION]
Classic findings of an upper motor neuron lesion include:
- **Hypertonicity: increased deep tendon reflexes (hyperreflexia) [choice C] and clonus**
- Spastic paralysis
- Upward Babinski
- Little to no muscle atrophy or fasciculations.

Classic findings of a lower motor neuron lesion include:
- Hypotonicity: decreased deep tendon reflexes (hyporeflexia)
- Flaccid paralysis
- Downward Babinski
- Muscle atrophy
- Fasciculations.

Depending on the spinal cord injury, it can present as either an upper motor neuron lesion or lower motor neuron lesion with varying loss of motor, sensory and autonomic function, either temporary or permanent depending on the level and type of injury to the Spinal Cord or Cauda Equina.

53. PROFESSIONAL PRACTICE – INFORMED CONSENT
Informed consent is not needed in an emergency when delayed treatment would be dangerous for the patient [choice E].
Delaying defibrillation for ≥2 minutes decreases survival rate compared to patients receive immediate defibrillation.
Unless the patient has a Do not resuscitate order documented, he should undergo treatment for pulseless VT.

Informed consent is required in all the other choices listed.

54. REPRODUCTIVE – MENOPAUSE [PHARMACOLOGY]
In patients with moderate to severe Menopause without contraindications to estrogen and an intact uterus, combined estrogen-progestin [choice B] are the first line therapy for the symptoms of Menopause.
Estrogen relieves the symptoms and progestin prevents endometrial hyperplasia as a result of unopposed estrogen.

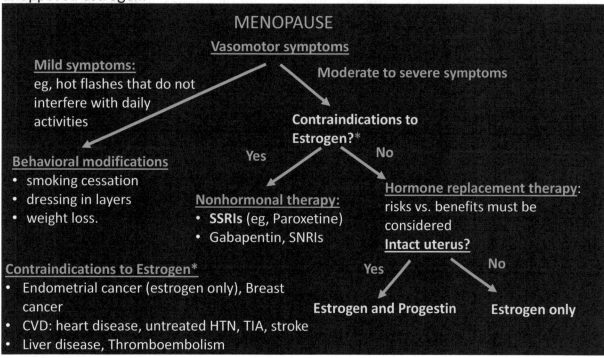

Choice E [Oral Estrogen] can be used in patients with moderate to severe Menopause without contraindications to estrogen without an intact uterus.

Choice A [Gabapentin] and choice E [Oral Sertraline] are alternatives for moderate to severe symptoms of Menopause when estrogen is contraindicated (eg, Endometrial cancer, Breast cancer, CVD: heart disease, untreated HTN, TIA, stroke; Liver disease, Thromboembolism).
Choice C [Oral Tamoxifen] is not used in the management of Menopause.

55. INFECTIOUS DISEASE – MENINGITIS (MENINGOCOCCAL PROPHYLAXIS) – [HEALTH MAINTENANCE]

Meningococcal prophylaxis should be administered to all close contacts and consists of either:
- **<u>Rifampin</u> 600 mg every 12 hours 2 days (4 doses) of oral therapy [choice D], or**
- **<u>Ceftriaxone</u> 250 mg single IM dose, or**
- **<u>Ciprofloxacin</u> 500 mg single dose (if there is no suspicion for increased resistance)**

Antimicrobial chemoprophylaxis should be administered for close contacts as early as possible (ideally <24 hours after identification of the index patient and not >14 days after exposure) as per the United States Centers for Disease Control and Prevention (CDC).

Choice B [Azithromycin 500 mg single dose] is an alternative agent for prophylaxis if one of the preferred agents cannot be used.

56. GASTROINTESTINAL/NUTRITIONAL – APPENDICITIS [HISTORY AND PHYSICAL EXAMINATION]

In patients with suspected Appendicitis, the Rovsing sign [choice B] refers to pain in the right lower quadrant with palpation of the left lower quadrant. It has a sensitivity 22-68%; specificity 58-96%.

Other signs for Appendicitis include:
- <u>McBurney</u> [choice D] point tenderness is described as maximal tenderness at 1.5 to 2 inches from the anterior superior iliac spine (ASIS) on a straight line from the ASIS to the umbilicus.
- <u>Psoas sign</u> [choice E] is positive is when passive extension of the iliopsoas muscle with hip extension causes right lower quadrant pain. The psoas sign is associated with a retrocecal appendix.
- <u>Obturator sign</u> [choice C] is right lower quadrant pain elicited by flexing the patient's right hip and knee, followed by internal rotation of the right hip.

Choice A [Murphy] sign is positive if right upper quadrant pain occurs on inspiration, when the inflamed gallbladder comes into contact with the examiner's hand in patients with Acute cholecystitis.

57. REPRODUCTIVE – CERVICAL CANCER SCREENING [HEALTH MAINTENANCE]

In women ≥ 35 years with Atypical glandular cells of undetermined significance (AGC), Colposcopy AND endocervical sampling (curettage) and endometrial biopsy [choice B] should be performed.
AGC can represent either [1] Cervical cancer &/or [2] Endometrial cancer (although 90% of Endometrial cancer is Adenocarcinoma, 10% are Squamous cell carcinoma).
The presence of AGC on cervical cytology is a significant marker for premalignant disease of the cervix or endometrium; therefore, evaluation includes testing of both sites.

Choice A [Serum CA-125] is a tumor marker for Ovarian cancer
Choice C [Loop electrosurgical excision procedure] is a therapeutic procedure if biopsy reveals Cervical cancer.

Choice D [Return to routine Pap screening] is not recommended at this time because the presence of AGC on cervical cytology is a significant marker for premalignant disease.

Choice E [Colposcopy alone] isn't usually recommended because the presence of AGC on cervical cytology is a significant marker for premalignant disease of the cervix or endometrium; therefore, evaluation includes testing of both sites.

58. PULMONARY – MYCOPLASMA PNEUMONIA [PHARMACOLOGY]

The empiric treatment for Community-acquired pneumonia treated as an outpatient include:
- **Macrolide: Azithromycin [choice C],**
- **Doxycycline, or**
- **Respiratory Fluoroquinolone (eg, Levofloxacin or Moxifloxacin).**

There 3 empiric regimens are active against both "typical" pathogens (eg, *Streptococcus pneumoniae*) as well as atypical pathogens, such as *M. pneumoniae.*

Factors suggestive of pneumonia due to *Mycoplasma pneumoniae* include:
- concurrent URI symptoms (eg, rhinorrhea, pharyngitis, earache)
- non-respiratory tract manifestations (eg, Cold agglutinin disease).

Because *M. pneumoniae* is spread via respiratory droplets, outbreaks frequently occur among persons living in close quarters (eg, universities, schools, military).

Choice A [Amoxicillin and supportive care] is an alternative treatment for Community acquired pneumonia treated as an outpatient but because *M. pneumoniae* lacks a cell wall, cell wall synthesis inhibitors, such as Penicillins, lack coverage for *M. pneumoniae.*

Choice B [Supportive care only] does not consider he has an active bacterial infection.

Choice D [Piperacillin-tazobactam] and other cell wall synthesis inhibitors lack coverage for *M. pneumoniae* because *M. pneumoniae* lacks a cell wall,

Choice E [Doxycycline and Ceftriaxone] is a treatment option for CAP treated as an inpatient. There are no indications for admission in this young, healthy patient.

59. ENDOCRINE – SHEEHAN SYNDROME [MOST LIKELY]

Sheehan syndrome [choice D] (post-partum pituitary necrosis) refers to the necrosis of the anterior pituitary gland due to hypotension, following significant post-partum bleeding, hypovolemia, and shock.

The acute presenting condition of Sheehan syndrome is usually evident when the mother of the newborn has difficulty with breastfeeding or cannot produce milk (agalactorrhea).

Lab values may reflect hypoglycemia, hyponatremia, and/or anemia.

Endocrine studies often show a secondary pattern (any combination of decreased FSH, LH, ACTH, prolactin, &/or TSH).

Choice A [Waterhouse-Friderichsen syndrome] results from adrenal hemorrhage and subsequent infarction associated with meningococcemia. It is a cause of Primary adrenal insufficiency. The patient's central pattern of hypothyroidism (decreased TSH and free T4) suggests a secondary (pituitary cause).

Choice B [Prolactinoma] would more likely present with galactorrhea as opposed to reduced milk production.

Choice C [Postpartum thyroiditis] is a primary cause of Hypothyroidism, reflected by increased serum TSH and decreased T4. The patient's central pattern of hypothyroidism (decreased TSH and free T4) suggests a secondary (pituitary cause).

Choice E [Addison disease] is Primary adrenal insufficiency. The patient's central pattern of hypothyroidism (decreased TSH and free T4) suggests a secondary (pituitary cause).

60. NEUROLOGY - HUNTINGTON DISEASE [MOST LIKELY]

Huntington disease [choice C] is a neurodegenerative disorder affecting mood, movement, and memory (psychiatric issues, choreiform movements, and dementia).

Huntington disease should be suspected in patients with "ABCD"

- **Atrophy of the caudate (striatum)** on neuroimaging, resulting in "boxcar" shape of the ventricles.
- **Behavioral changes**: eg, irritability, depression, dysphoria, agitation, apathy, anxiety, paranoia, delusions, and hallucinations.
- **Chorea**: involuntary movements,
- **Dementia**: cognitive decline and executive dysfunction (often in the later stages of the disease).

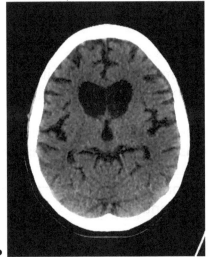

-
- Significant brain atrophy compared to patient age; frontal horns exhibit the classic box-shaped appearance.

The diagnosis of HD is confirmatory with genetic testing for the disease-causing trinucleotide (cytosine-adenine-guanine [CAG]) repeat expansion in the huntingtin (*HTT*) gene.

Although there is often a family history of HD, up to 8% of patients with genetically proven HD have no family history.

Choice A [Parkinson disease] is associated with the triad of bradykinesia, rigidity, and tremor. Dementia is a late feature of PD.

Choice B [Wilson disease] can also present with Chorea, but is more associated with liver dysfunction, Kayser-Fleischer rings, drooling, and other neurological findings.

Choice D [Tourette syndrome] can present with motor tics but is not associated with personality changes or atrophy on neuroimaging.

Choice E [Alzheimer dementia] can present with dementia in older patients and is not associated with chorea or tic-like findings.

61. PSYCHIATRY/BEHAVIORAL MEDICINE - SCHIZOPHRENIFORM DISORDER [MOST LIKELY]

Schizophreniform disorder [choice A] is characterized by psychotic symptoms lasting from 1 month to 6 months [eg, delusions, hallucinations, disorganized speech (formal thought disorder), disorganized or catatonic behavior, or negative symptoms.

Schizophreniform disorder is categorized under "schizophrenia spectrum disorders and other psychotic disorders" due to its classic presentation with psychotic symptoms.

Choice B [Schizophrenia] is characterized by persistent psychotic symptoms lasting for ≥6 months.

Choice C [Schizoaffective] is the presence of psychotic symptoms that meet the criteria for Schizophrenia in the setting of a mood disorder.

Choice D [Schizotypal disorder] is associated with bizarre thinking.

Choice E [Brief psychotic disorder] is characterized by brief psychotic symptoms lasting for <1 month.

62. MUSCULOSKELETAL – PATELLAR TENDON RUPTURE [MOST LIKELY]

A high-riding patella (patella alta) [choice A] is most consistent with a patellar tendon rupture.

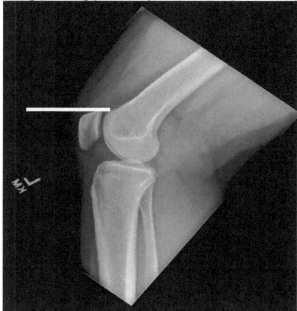

Normal knee radiograph

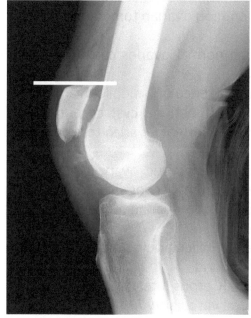

Patellar tendon rupture
The patella is high-riding with avulsion fracture fragments from its inferior pole.

Physical examination findings may include
- swelling, tenderness localized to the tendon insertion,
- a palpable defect at the inferior pole of the patella at the tendon site, and
- inability to perform a straight leg raise due rupture of the extensor mechanism.

The most common mechanism of injury for patellar and quadriceps tendon ruptures is forceful quadriceps contraction (eg, fall on a flexed knee, walking up or down stairs, or if the patient falls backward with a planted foot).

Patellar rupture usually occurs in patients <40 years. Quadriceps rupture usually occurs >40 years of age.

Choice B [Patella dislocation] is usually associated with lateral or medial displacement of the patella.

Choice C [Quadriceps tendon rupture] has a similar mechanism of injury to Patellar tendon rupture and is also associated with inability to perform straight leg raise but is associated with a low-riding patellar and a palpable defect above the patella.

Choice D [ACL injury] is usually associated with normal radiographs or a Segond fracture. Patients are usually able to perform the straight leg raise.

Choice E [Knee dislocation] is associated with anterior or posterior displacement of the tibia from the femur on radiographs.

63. REPRODUCTIVE – OVARIAN TORSION/CYSTIC (DERMOID) TERATOMA [MOST LIKELY]

The presence of a markedly hyperechoic nodule within the mass, especially if the hyperechoic nodule has distal acoustic shadowing, is a strong indicator for the presence of a Teratoma [choice D].

Mature cystic teratomas account for more than 95 percent of all ovarian teratomas are the most common ovarian tumor in females in the second and third decade of life

Although normal ovaries can undergo torsion, the primary risk factors for Ovarian torsion include

- the presence of a mobile ovarian mass (especially if >5-cm), seen in >85% [eg, physiologic cyst (functional cyst, corpus luteum) or benign neoplasm], PCOS and
- prior history of Ovarian torsion (although normal ovaries can undergo torsion).

Choice A [Polycystic ovary syndrome] appears as multiple small fluid-filled follicles with increased stromal echogenicity with a "sting of pearls" appearance.

Choice B [Tubo-ovarian abscess] appears as a multiloculated complex solid or cystic mass on Ultrasound.

Choice C [Follicular cyst] that are simple appear as anechoic fluid filled cysts with a thin wall on Ultrasound.

Choice E [Corpus luteal cyst] appears as a thick-walled cyst with a characteristic "ring of fire" peripheral vascularity.

64. PULMONARY – HEMOTHORAX [MOST LIKELY]

Classic physical examination findings of a Hemothorax (collection of blood in the pleural space) [choice C] reflect blood in the pleural space, manifesting as dyspnea, tachypnea, decreased or absent breath sounds, dullness to percussion, decreased fremitus.

In severe cases, hypovolemic shock can occur (eg, hypotension, narrow pulse pressure, chest wall asymmetry, flat neck veins, and contralateral tracheal deviation).

Tube thoracostomy is the first line management of Hemothoraces, with immediate bloody drainage of >20 mL/kg (~1,500 mL) being an indication for emergent surgical thoracotomy.

Blunt thoracic trauma is a common cause of a Hemothorax.

In the setting of trauma (eg, MVA), hypovolemic shock is attributed to hemorrhage until proven otherwise.

Choice A [Pleural effusion] is also associated with decreased breath sounds and dullness to percussion but usually accumulates slowly. In the setting of an MVA and hypovolemic shock and signs of trauma, Hemothorax is a more likely diagnosis. Analysis of the pleural fluid can more reliably distinguish between the two.

Choice B [Tension pneumothorax] presents with obstructive shock (distended neck veins instead of flat neck veins) and would show a large air collection in the pleural space on chest imaging.

Choice D [Pulmonary contusion] can also occur with blunt trauma. Opacification of the pulmonary parenchyma are classic radiograph findings of a pulmonary contusion and is often not evident until up to 24 hours after the injury.

Choice E [Cardiac tamponade] can also present with obstructive shock (distended neck veins instead of flat neck veins seen with hypovolemic shock), muffled (distant) heart sounds, and clear lungs. Chest radiographs may show a pericardial effusion or enlargement of the heart.

65. INFECTIOUS DISEASE – COCCIDIOIDOMYCOSIS [APPLYING FOUNDATIONAL CONCEPTS]

Coccidioidomycosis [choice C] should be suspected in individuals living in or having traveled to an endemic area (SW United States) with any of the following:
- **Valley fever: diffuse symmetrical arthralgias and rash (especially erythema nodosum or erythema multiforme).**
- **Flu-like symptoms:** night sweats, fatigue, weight loss.
- A respiratory illness with an infiltrate on chest radiograph, **especially if there is upper lobe involvement or hilar or mediastinal adenopathy.**

Choice B [Pneumocystis jirovecii] is associated diffuse infiltrates in patients with an immunocompromised state.

Hilar and mediastinal adenopathy do not occur in bacterial pneumonia (choices A, D, and E) and should alert the practitioner to the possibility of Coccidioidomycosis.

66. PSYCHIATRY/BEHAVIORAL MEDICINE MAJOR DEPRESSIVE DISORDER [PHARMACOLOGY]

Selective serotonin reuptake inhibitors (SSRIs), such as Sertraline [choice B], are the first line pharmacological therapy for Major depressive disorder because of their efficacy, selectivity [they have little or no effect on other receptors (dopamine, norepinephrine, histamine, or acetylcholine (except for Paroxetine)], and there are less complications in cases of overdose. Selective norepinephrine reuptake inhibitors (SNRIs), based upon their efficacy and tolerability in randomized trials.

67. CARDIOLOGY – ST ELEVATION MYOCARDIAL INFARCTION [CLINICAL INTERVENTION]

In patients with Cardiogenic shock due to Myocardial infarction, early successful revascularization via Coronary angiography [choice E] improves outcomes compared with medical treatment.

Some patients will require only percutaneous coronary intervention (PCI) of the infarct-related artery; others may require immediate coronary artery bypass graft surgery (CABG).

Acute ST-Elevation Myocardial Infarction (STEMI) Anterolateral

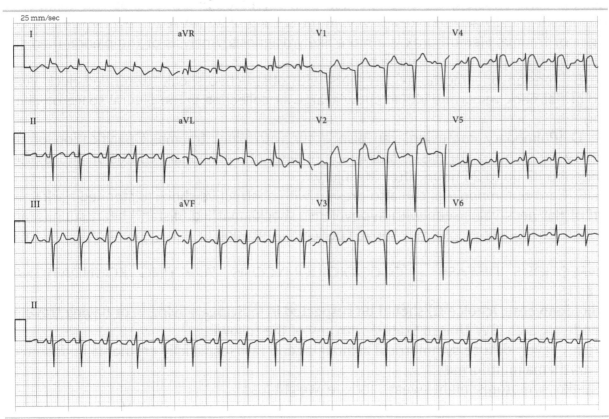

Choice A [IV Nitroglycerin] is contraindicated in patients with Hypotension.

Choice B [IV Metoprolol] is contraindicated in patients with Hypotension.

Choice C [IV Furosemide] is not indicated because it is contraindicated in patients with Hypotension and the patient is in Cardiogenic shock due to STEMI.

Choice D [Emergent pericardiocentesis] is the treatment of Obstructive shock due to Cardiac tamponade.

68. ENDOCRINE – DIABETIC NEUROPATHY [PHARMACOLOGY]
In addition to strict glucose control, first-line pharmacotherapy for Diabetic neuropathy include either:
- <u>Serotonin-norepinephrine reuptake inhibitors</u>: Duloxetine [choice C], Venlafaxine or
- <u>Tricyclic antidepressants</u> Amitriptyline, Nortriptyline, Desipramine or
- <u>Gabapentinoid</u>: Pregabalin, Gabapentin.

Although not fully understood, Duloxetine blocks the uptake of serotonin and norepinephrine, neurotransmitters thought to play a role in the experience of pain (mediates synaptic norepinephrine and effects on central perception of pain).

Options for patient who do not tolerate any of the first line pharmacotherapy either alone or in combination include:
- Capsaicin cream [choice B]
- Lidocaine patch [choice D]

- Transcutaneous electrical nerve stimulation [choice E]
- Spinal cord stimulation

Choice A [Tramadol 50 mg] is a potential second line agent.

69. CARDIOLOGY – PERIPHERAL ARTERIAL DISEASE [HISTORY AND PHYSICAL]
Claudication pain in the upper two thirds of the calf is usually due to the narrowing of the artery in the mid-thigh (the superficial femoral artery) [choice C].
Claudication pain occurs due an imbalance of increased demand (ambulation) + decreased blood supply to the lower extremities (due to peripheral arterial narrowing).
Calf claudication is the most common complaint and is most usually associated with superficial femoral and popliteal artery disease.

Choice A [Popliteal] artery narrowing results in pain in the lower third of the calf due to disease in the artery behind the knee (the popliteal artery).
Choice B [Common femoral] often results in thigh claudication due to narrowing of the artery in the groin (the common femoral artery) or mid-thigh (the superficial femoral artery) but can also be caused by blockage of the vessels above the groin (the aorta and iliac arteries).
Choice D [Tibial] and choice E [Peroneal] often results in foot pain due to narrowing of an artery in the lower part of the leg below the knee (the tibial or peroneal artery).

70. PULMONARY – MESOTHELIOMA [MOST LIKELY]
Clinical suspicion for Malignant pulmonary Mesothelioma (MPM) [choice E] should be increased in patients with respiratory symptoms in the context of unilateral pleural thickening or calcification, or an effusion on chest imaging and a history of asbestos exposure.
Although these features increase the suspicion of MPM, a biopsy is required to confirm the diagnosis of MPM.
Occupational exposure to Asbestosis, the primary risk factor for the development of Mesothelioma, including shipbuilding and shipyard work.
In addition to insulation, asbestosis is used on ships to insulate boilers, incinerators, and for gaskets.

Choice A [Caplan syndrome] is the combination of Rheumatoid arthritis and Pneumoconiosis that is associated with well-defined homogenous intrapulmonary nodules on chest imaging.
Choice B [Loffler syndrome] is a transient pneumonitis that occurs in certain parasitic infections (eg, Ascariasis), and is reflected by transient pulmonary infiltrates.
Choice C [Large cell carcinoma] usually presents as a large peripheral mass with prominent necrosis. It is extremely rare and often a diagnosis of exclusion.
Choice E [Bronchial carcinoid tumor] presents as a pulmonary nodule with or without symptoms of carcinoid syndrome (cutaneous flushing, wheezing, diarrhea).

71. PULMONARY – EMPHYSEMA [HISTORY AND PHYSICAL]
Classic findings of Emphysema include:
- **Air trapping: distant (decreased) breath sounds [choice D], hyperresonance to percussion, wheezes, crackles at the lung bases, and/or distant heart sounds are heard on auscultation.**

- **"pink puffers,"** meaning they are often cachectic and non-cyanotic. Expiration through pursed lips raises airway pressure and prevents airway collapse during respiration, and the use of accessory muscles of respiration indicates advanced disease.

It is important to note that many individuals with Chronic obstructive pulmonary disease (COPD) have elements of both Emphysema and Chronic bronchitis, with one being more dominant.

Classic findings of Chronic Bronchitis include
- Noisy lungs: rales, rhonchi
- "Blue bloaters": obese habitus, cyanosis, and peripheral edema due to severe chronic hypoxemia
- Cor pulmonale: (signs of right-sided Heart failure due to pulmonary Hypertension from chronic hypoxemia): peripheral edema, distended neck veins.

72. NEUROLOGY – TENSION-TYPE HEADACHES [HISTORY AND PHYSICAL EXAMINATION]
Increased pericranial muscle tenderness [choice A] is the most common abnormal finding on examination in patients with Tension type headache (TTH).
Muscle tenderness may be noted head, neck, or shoulders and is often worse with the headache episode.

Classic features of Tension-type headache (TTH) include:
- mild to moderate bilateral headaches describe as "dull," "pressure," "head fullness," "head feels large," "like a tight cap," "band-like,".
- nonpulsating: pressing or tightening
- not aggravated by routine physical activity such as walking or climbing stairs
- Both of the following: No nausea or vomiting; no more than one of photophobia or phonophobia.

Choice B [Conjunctival erythema] is a feature of Cluster headache.
Choice C [Papilledema] is a feature of Idiopathic intracranial hypertension.
Choice D [Nausea and vomiting] is a feature of Migraine headache.
Choice E [Pain reproduced with stroking the face and chin] is a feature of Trigeminal neuralgia.

73. INFECTIOUS DISEASE – CHANCROID [APPLYING FOUNDATIONAL CONCEPTS]
The causative agent of Chancroid is *Haemophilus ducreyi* [choice A].
Patients with Chancroid classically present with
- **painful genital ulcer (often deep and well demarcated); multiple ulcers may develop.**
- **painful (tender) regional lymphadenopathy.**
Chancroid is very rare in the United States and most other developed countries.

The management of choice for Chancroid is either:
- Azithromycin (single dose) 1 gram orally OR
- Ceftriaxone 250 mg intramuscularly.

Choice B [*Klebsiella granulomatis*], also known as Donovanosis, classically presents as a painless, progressive ulcerative lesion without regional lymphadenopathy. The ulcerative lesions are highly vascular and beefy red in appearance.

Choice C [Herpes simplex virus 2] is classically associated with multiple grouped vesicles on an erythematous base; multiple, shallow, tender ulcers that may be vesicular are often present.

Choice D [*Chlamydia trachomatis* serovars] may result in Lymphogranuloma venereum (LGV). LGV classically presents as a small, shallow, painless ulcer or vesicle with tender inguinal or femoral lymphadenopathy (buboes).

Choice E [*Treponema pallidum*] is associated with a chancre (nontender ulcer) and nontender regional lymphadenopathy.

74. REPRODUCTIVE – BREAST MASS [LABS AND DIAGNOSTIC STUDIES]

Mammography [choice D] is the initial modality to evaluate breast masses in women >40 years of age.

Mammography is a most useful tool in the initial imaging of a breast mass in older women as early as 40 years of age due to less glandular breast tissue.

Grouped microcalcifications & spiculated high-density masses (most specific feature) are highly suspicious for malignancy.

Choice A [Ultrasound of the breast] is the recommended initial modality to evaluate breast masses in women <40 years of age due to high density of breast tissue. Ultrasound may also be used to guide FNA with biopsy or determine if a mass seen on mammogram is cystic or solid.

Choice B [Core needle biopsy] is the most commonly used diagnostic modality for histological evaluation of a suspicious mass seen on imaging (eg, MRI or US).

Choice C [Fine needle aspiration] can be used after imaging if deemed necessary.

Choice E [MRI of the breast] may be used to screen some women at high risk for Breast cancer.

75. GASTROINTESTINAL/NUTRITION – CELIAC DISEASE [LABS AND DIAGNOSTIC STUDIES]

Tissue transglutaminase IgA antibody [choice C] is the single preferred initial test for detection of Celiac disease in adults.

Evaluation is initiated with serologic testing.

Patients with positive serologic testing should undergo an upper endoscopy with small bowel biopsy to confirm the diagnose Celiac disease (criterion standard).

Dermatitis herpetiformis is common rash in patients with Celiac disease.

Dermatitis herpetiformis is characterized by multiple intensely pruritic papules and vesicles that occur in grouped ("herpetiform") configurations.

Upper endoscopy with small bowel biopsy [choice A] is the definitive diagnostic test to establish the diagnosis in patients with suspected Celiac disease after serological testing.

Choice B [Sweat chloride testing] is used in the diagnosis of Cystic fibrosis.

Choice D [Hydrogen breath testing] is used to establish the diagnosis of Lactose intolerance.

Choice E [Skin scraping with KOH preparation] may be used to diagnose fungal dermatological infections.

76. GASTROINTESTINAL/NUTRITIONAL – HEPATOCELLULAR CARCINOMA [HEALTH MAINTENANCE]

For most at-risk individuals, Abdominal ultrasound [choice C] every 6 months is recommended for Hepatocellular carcinoma surveillance, with or without serum Alpha-fetoprotein.

Alpha-fetoprotein is an oncofetal protein normally produced by the fetal liver and yolk sac and becomes undetectable shortly after birth.

Elevated levels of alpha-fetoprotein can be seen associated with Hepatocellular carcinoma and Nonseminomatous germ cell testicular cancer.

Because elevated levels of alpha-fetoprotein can also be seen in cirrhosis and viral hepatitis, it not used alone (without Ultrasound) for surveillance for HCC.

Choice A [Colonoscopy] screening is initiated at age 50 (class A recommendation) or age 45 (Class B recommendation) for patients with average risk.

Choice B [CT scan of the abdomen and pelvis] is not used as the primary imaging for surveillance for HCC. The primary role of CT is for further workup of any suspicious lesions seen on screening Ultrasound (eg, lesions ≥1 cm identified during surveillance).

Choice D [Cancer antigen 19-9] is a more useful tumor marker for Pancreatic and biliary duct malignancies.

Choice E [Carcinoembryonic antigen] is a more useful tumor marker for Colorectal cancer.

77. CARDIOLOGY – ACUTE ARTERIAL OCCLUSION [CLINICAL INTERVENTION]

In an immediately threatened limb, anticoagulation with IV unfractionated Heparin [choice E] should be initiated following a clinical diagnosis of embolism prior to proceeding with imaging to minimize thrombus propagation and preserve microcirculation, along with fluid resuscitation, & pain control.

In patients with suspected arterial embolization, a Heparin drip should be initiated and vascular surgery consult, immediately followed by imaging (CT angiography typically often preferred imaging) [choice C], followed by a possible endovascular procedure to save the limb.

Atrial fibrillation is a common predisposing factor for Acute arterial occlusion.
The classic presentation of Acute arterial occlusion are the 6 P's [eg, paresthesias, pain, pallor, poikilothermia (cold), pulselessness, and paralysis.

Revascularization for reperfusion is the mainstay of treatment — surgical procedures include surgical or catheter-based thrombectomy [choice B] with a balloon catheter (Fogarty), bypass surgery and adjuncts such as endarterectomy, patch angioplasty, and intra-operative thrombolysis depending on the duration of the ischemia and the extent of occlusion.

CT angiography of the right lower extremity [choice C] is the imaging of choice to confirm the presence and site of the thrombus or embolism, but anticoagulation should not be delayed waiting on completion of CT angiography reduce the risk of thrombus propagation.

78. RENAL – HYPERNATREMIA [PHARMACOLOGY]

In patients with Hypernatremia who are concurrently volume depleted, priority should be to restore euvolemia using isotonic fluids (eg, 0.9% normal saline) [choice B], followed by Hypotonic fluids to correct any remaining free water deficit.

If urine sodium is <20 mEq/L, that often indicates Hypovolemia, reflecting the kidney is actively retaining as much sodium as possible to help improve the volume status.

This patient has signs of Hypovolemia (eg, flat neck veins, sunken fontanelles, and delayed capillary refill, urine sodium <20 mEq/L) most likely due to GI volume loss from vomiting due to Infantile hypertrophic Pyloric stenosis.

Choice A [Dextrose 5% in water] is the first line for most patients with Hypernatremia to replace free water deficit; the notable exception is volume depleted patients (as seen in this patient).

Choice C [0.45% sodium chloride solution] is an alternative hypotonic fluid that can be used after repleting this patient's volume with Normal saline.

Choice D [3% sodium chloride solution] is used in the management of severe Hyponatremia.

Choice E [Fluid restriction] is used in the management of Isovolemic hypotonic hyponatremia. This patient is already at a fluid deficit so fluid restriction would worsen his Hyponatremia.

79. DERMATOLOGY – NONBULLOUS IMPETIGO [PHARMACOLOGY]

Topical therapy with Mupirocin [choice D] or Retapamulin are the first line options for limited Nonbullous impetigo.

Patients should be treated for a 5-day course.

In patients with more extensive lesions, systemic antibiotic therapy with coverage of both *S. aureus* and streptococcal species is recommended [eg, Dicloxacillin (choice C) and Cephalexin (choice A)] for 7 days.

Choice B (Oral Valacyclovir) can be used for Varicella zoster and Herpes simplex infections.

Choice E [Topical Neomycin] is not recommended because it has gram-negative coverage and doesn't reliably cover *S. aureus* and streptococcal species.

80. MUSCULOSKELETAL – FROZEN SHOULDER (ADHESIVE CAPSULITIS) [HISTORY AND PHYSICAL EXAMINATION]

Patients with Diabetes mellitus [choice D] are at greater risk of developing Frozen shoulder [FS (Adhesive capsulitis)].

Overall, FS affects ~11%-30% of people with Diabetes as compared to 2%-10% people without diabetes.

Although Frozen shoulder (Adhesive capsulitis) can be primary (idiopathic) it is often associated with other diseases and conditions including:
- Diabetes mellitus
- Thyroid disease
- Trauma
- Dupuytren contracture
- Systemic sclerosis (Scleroderma).

FS classically presents as pain-stiffness syndrome with significantly reduced passive and active ranges of motion.

81. EENT – HERPANGINA [MOST LIKELY]
Classic features of Herpangina [choice B] include:
- **abrupt onset with high fever**
- **sore throat: oral lesions in the posterior pharynx** (discrete vesicles and ulcers surrounded by an erythematous ring) on the anterior fauces, tonsils, and soft palate that may interfere with oral intake
- associated symptoms include vomiting, anorexia, irritability, or fussiness.

The diagnosis is usually made clinically, and supportive therapy is the mainstay of treatment.

Choice A [Herpetic gingivostomatitis] is associated with a prodrome of fever, anorexia, irritability, malaise, and headache precedes the appearance of oral changes. Oral changes initially consist of erythema and edema of the gingiva with clusters of vesicles. The gums are friable and bleed easily.

Choice C [Aphthous ulcers] are characterized by painful. Shallow circumscribed ulcers with a greyish base. Aphthous ulcers are not associated with skin lesions.

Choice D [Hand, foot, and mouth disease] are associated with painful oral lesions in the anterior pharynx and a rash on the palms and soles. Both HFMD and Herpangina are caused by the same virus.

Choice E [Varicella] is associated with pruritic crops of lesions that rapidly progress to papules followed by vesicles and, ultimately, crusts all seen (rash in different stages at the same time).

82. RENAL – RHABDOMYOLYSIS [LABS AND DIAGNOSTIC STUDIES]
The diagnosis of Rhabdomyolysis is met with a marked acute elevation in serum Creatine kinase (CK) [choice C] and any of the following criteria:
- **Classic symptoms &/or signs: muscle weakness, muscle tenderness, and/or dark-colored urine**
- **Urinalysis consistent with myoglobinuria: heme positive by dipstick but with <5 RBCs per high-powered field on microscopic examination** (minimal RBCs)
- **One or more causative or inciting factors,** eg, trauma, crush injury, compartment syndrome, extreme exertion, severe heat exposure/hyperthermia, prolonged immobilization, or intoxication.

Although there is no absolute cut-off value for CK elevation, the CK is usually at least five times the upper limit of normal and is usually greater than 5,000 units/L.

Choice A [Serum myoglobin] is useful in the early presentation of rhabdomyolysis, but the level returns to normal within 24 hours

Choice B [Anti-Jo-1 and anti-signal recognition peptide antibodies]

Choice D [Serum potassium] and Acute kidney injury can occur as complications of Rhabdomyolysis, but they are not diagnostic.

Choice E [Electromyography] is not part of the diagnostic criteria for Rhabdomyolysis.

83. GENITOURINARY – BLADDER CANCER [LABS AND DIAGNOSTIC STUDIES]
After a Urinalysis is performed, the next best step in diagnosing Bladder cancer is a Cystoscopy with biopsy [choice D], which is the criterion standard for the initial diagnosis and staging of Bladder cancer.
Cystoscopy allows for biopsy of any suspicious lesions.

Transitional cell carcinoma is the most common type of Bladder cancer.

The most common presentation of Bladder cancer is painless microscopic or gross hematuria. Irritative symptoms may also occur.
Risk factors for Bladder cancer includes smoking cigarettes and occupational exposure (eg, industrial dyes, leather, and rubber).

Choice A [Urine cytology] is an adjunctive to Cystoscopy for the diagnosis of Bladder cancer. By itself, Urine cytology has a high specificity but low sensitivity.
Choice B [Intravenous pyelogram] is rarely used now as CT has replaced IVP for staging and evaluation of the urinary tract.
Abdominal CT scan [choice E], Ultrasound [choice C], or MRI may later be necessary for staging.

84. CARDIOLOGY – PROLONGED QT [PHARMACOLOGY]
Medications associated with causing a prolonged QT interval include:
- **Antibiotics: eg, Fluoroquinolones [choice A], Macrolides**
- **Antiarrhythmic agents**
- **Antidepressants**

Propranolol [choice B] or Nadolol are Beta blockers that can be used in the long-term management of Congenital QT syndrome.
These patients may need a cardiology referral and genetic counseling to assess if implantation of a cardiac defibrillator would be necessary for individuals with increased risk of sudden cardiac death.

85. EENT – CORNEAL ABRASION [CLINICAL INTERVENTION]
Patients with corneal abrasions but no corneal infiltrate and a history of recent contact lens wear should be treated with topical antibiotics effective against *Pseudomonas* species with either:
- **Topical Fluoroquinolones: eg, Ciprofloxacin, Ofloxacin [choice B],**
- **Topical Aminoglycosides: eg, Tobramycin or Gentamicin.**
Early referral to an ophthalmologist or optometrist for daily follow-up care is important.

Treatments that should be avoided in Corneal abrasions, especially in contact lens wearers include:
- **Topical corticosteroids** [choice A] due to increased potential for secondary infection or exacerbation of missed herpes simplex virus or microbial keratitis.
- **Black fabric patches** [choice C] because they do not keep the lid down as a properly applied pressure patch does and increase the risk of further abrading the cornea.

Choice D [Topical Erythromycin ointment 0.5%] does not have adequate coverage of Pseudomonas.
Choice E [Topical Proparacaine 0.5%] may be used initially for analgesia but to prevent overuse (<24 hours), they should not be prescribed to patients.

86. PULMONARY – ASTHMA [PHARMACOLOGY]

In patients with mild persistent Asthma not fully controlled on low-dose inhaled glucocorticoids, the options include
- **Add a long-acting beta agonist (LABA), such as Formoterol [choice A] often preferred or**
- **Increased the ICS to medium dose.**

Formoterol has advantages over other LABAs with long duration in that it has a faster onset of action.

The management of Mild persistent Asthma include:
- GINA guidelines: Low-dose ICS-Formoterol as needed (preferred). Alternative: Low-dose ICS.
- NAEPP guidelines: Low-dose ICS daily and SABA as needed. Alternative option(s): Daily LTRA and SABA as needed.

Definition of Mild persistent Asthma:
- daytime symptoms >2 but <7 days/week
- Nocturnal awakenings 3-4 nights/month
- minor interference with activities
- FEV1 within the normal range
- Exacerbations ≥2/year.

Choice B [Discontinue Fluticasone and switch to Salmeterol] is incorrect because LABAs should not be used as monotherapy in persistent Asthma.
Choice C [Add Omalizumab] is an alternative for severe or refractory Asthma.
Choice D [Add oral Prednisone] is used for Acute Asthma exacerbations.
Choice E [Add Cromolyn sodium] is not the best next step as per both guidelines.

87. REPRODUCTIVE – POSTPARTUM HEMORRHAGE [APPLYING FOUNDATIONAL CONCEPTS]

Uterine atony [choice E] is diagnosed as the cause of Postpartum hemorrhage (PPH) when the uterus does not become firm to palpation (eg, flaccid, boggy, dilated uterus) after expulsion of the placenta.
Prolonged labor (as seen in this patient) and prior PPH are strong risk factors for atony-related PPH. Magnesium sulfate administration (as seen in this patient), also increases the risk.

The 4 main causes of PPH include:
- Tone: uterine atony — flaccid, boggy, dilated uterus.
- Trauma: laceration (visible lacerations), rupture (usually abrupt onset of pain)
- Tissue: retained tissue, blood clots, or placenta accreta spectrum (PAS) — may be seen on examination &/or ultrasound
- Thrombin: coagulopathy.

Choice A [Uterine rupture] due to Uterine trauma [choice C] is usually painful and evident on physical examination.
Choice B [Retained placenta] is unlikely with an Ultrasound showing no placental products.
Choice D [Uterine inversion] is unlikely with a normal ultrasound.

88. GASTROINTESTINAL/NUTRITIONAL – PYRIDOXINE (VITAMIN B6) DEFICIENCY [HEALTH MAINTENANCE]

Taking supplemental Pyridoxine (Vitamin B6) [choice E] concurrently with Isoniazid can prevent Pyridoxine deficiency and therefore prevent Isoniazid-induced neuropathy.

The US CDC recommends that 10-50 mg of Pyridoxine be given daily to anyone taking Isoniazid or if symptoms of peripheral neuropathy develop on Isoniazid therapy.

Symptoms of Pyridoxine (Vitamin B6) deficiency includes nonspecific stomatitis, glossitis, cheilosis, irritability, confusion, and depression, and peripheral neuropathy.

Choice A [B1] deficiency can also present with symmetric peripheral neuropathy as well as dilated cardiomyopathy, Wernicke's encephalopathy, and Korsakoff dementia.

Choice B [Vitamin B12] deficiency can also present with gait abnormalities but is also associated with a macrocytic anemia.

Choice A [Vitamin A] deficiency presents with night blindness and Bitot spots on the conjunctiva.

Choice D [Vitamin C] deficiency presents with perifollicular bleeding and easy bruising.

89. PULMONARY – SOLITARY PULMONARY NODULE [HEALTH MAINTENANCE]

Solid nodules 6-8 mm can be followed with CT scan for surveillance with monitoring for changes [choice B].

Nodules 5-9 mm have a 2-6% probability of cancer.

Nodules <6 mm do not require routine follow-up in the patient without risk factors for lung cancer [choice A] because nodules <5 mm have a <1% risk.

Follow-up CT at 12 months is optional for the patient with risk factors.

Choice C [Bronchoscopy] is used for centrally located nodules with intermediate probability for cancer.

Choice D [Transthoracic needle aspiration] is used for peripherally located nodules with intermediate probability for cancer.

Choice E [Resection with biopsy] is used for lesions with a high probability for cancer.

90. DERMATOLOGY – SEBORRHEIC DERMATITIS [MOST LIKELY]

Seborrheic dermatitis [choice D] is a chronic papulosquamous dermatitis due to increased production of sebaceous and hypersensitivity to *Malassezia* species, a fungus that is part of the skin flora.

Seborrheic dermatitis is characterized by erythematous plaques or papules with yellow greasy scales on areas with increased sebum production (eg, central face, scalp, eyebrows, chest, and groin).

Management includes topical antifungals (eg, Ketoconazole 2%, Ciclopirox 1%, Selenium sulfide, or Zinc pyrithione).

Topical corticosteroids may be added in severe or refractory cases.

In patients with HIV infection, SD may be more extensive or more severe.

Choice A [Psoriasis] also presents with erythema and scaling; however, the lesions are sharply demarcated and associated with thick silver-white scales and involves the extremities.

Choice B [Rosacea] also affects the face but is more associated with telangiectasias, and papulopustular with minimal to no scaliness.

Choice C [Systemic lupus erythematosus] can present with an erythematous malar rash or discoid lesions. Greasy scales are not a common finding.

Choice E [Tinea versicolor] can also present with a scaly rash but lack the erythema seen with SD.

91. MUSCULOSKELETAL – REACTIVE ARTHRITIS [PHARMACOLOGY]

Treatment of Reactive arthritis involves relieving the pain and decreasing the inflammation with Nonsteroidal anti-inflammatory drugs, such as Naproxen [choice A], Diclofenac, or Indomethacin.

C. trachomatis-triggered reactive arthritis improves faster with antibiotics.

Reactive arthritis often occurs 2-6 weeks after an episode of urethritis or GI infection (as in this patient), which triggers active inflammation in the joint without infection in the joint.

It classically presents with the triad of ("can't pee, can't see, can't climb a tree"):
  • Urethritis, which can occur even when the arthritis is induced by Enterobacteriaceae
  • Conjunctivitis
  • Oligoarthritis.

Enthesitis (Achilles tendon, plantar fascia) may also occur, as seen in this patient).

Synovial fluid analysis will show increased white cell count but no organisms (the inflammation and arthritis is reactive not septic).

Choice B [Colchicine] can be used in the management of Gout and Pseudogout.

Choice C [Ceftriaxone] and other antibiotics can be used if thought to be due to a GU infection (this patient had a recent GI infection, which probably triggered his symptoms). In general, antibiotics are not indicated for uncomplicated enteric infections, especially if the GI symptoms have resolved.

Choice D [Acetaminophen] is an analgesic, but it lacks anti-inflammatory properties, making it not as useful for Reactive arthritis.

Choice E [Intraarticular Triamcinolone acetonide] or other intraarticular glucocorticoid may be used in patients with persistent symptoms of Reactive arthritis despite treatment with NSAIDs. If not responsive to intraarticular glucocorticoids, systemic glucocorticoids may be used.

92. EENT – ORAL LEUKOPLAKIA [HISTORY AND PHYSICAL EXAMINATION]

Oral leukoplakia is a potentially malignant white patch or plaque in the oral cavity that cannot be scraped off and is strongly associated with tobacco use [choice A].

Risk factors for Oral leukoplakia are similar to those for Squamous cell carcinoma (SCC), including
  • tobacco use (smoked and smokeless)
  • alcohol drinking
  • human papillomavirus (HPV) infection
  • dental malocclusion.

Biopsy is used to make a definitive diagnosis and to rule out malignancy.

Choice B [Uncontrolled Diabetes mellitus] can be associated with Oral Candidiasis (Thrush).

Choice C [Herpes simplex virus 1] is not a risk factor for Oral leukoplakia.

Choice D [Epstein-Barr virus] is a risk factor Oral hairy leukoplakia.
Choice E [Inhaled glucocorticoids] can be associated with Oral Candidiasis (Thrush).

93. PSYCHIATRY/BEHAVIORAL MEDICINE - SCHIZOTYPAL PERSONALITY DISORDER [MOST LIKELY]

Schizotypal personality disorder [choice E] is a pervasive pattern of social and interpersonal deficits marked by acute discomfort with, and reduced capacity for, close relationships as well as by cognitive or perceptual distortions and eccentricities of behavior.

Features include:
- [1] Ideas of reference (excluding delusions of reference).
- [2] Odd beliefs or magical thinking that influences behavior and is inconsistent with subcultural norms (eg, superstitiousness, belief in clairvoyance, telepathy, or "sixth sense")
- [3] Odd thinking and speech (eg, vague, circumstantial, metaphorical, overelaborate, or stereotyped).
- [4] Suspiciousness or paranoid ideation.
- [5] Inappropriate or constricted affect.
- [6] Behavior or appearance that is odd, eccentric, or peculiar.
- [7] Lack of close friends or confidants other than first-degree relatives.

Choice A [Schizophreniform disorder] is characterized by psychotic symptoms lasting for 1-6 months.
Choice B [Schizophrenia] is characterized by persistent psychotic symptoms lasting for ≥6 months.
Choice D [Schizoid personality disorder] is characterized by social isolation and preference for solo activities.
Choice E [Paranoid personality disorder] is characterized by a pervasive pattern or paranoia. Magical thinking is not a classic component.

94. MUSCULOSKELETAL – OSTEOPOROSIS [HEALTH MAINTENANCE]

Bisphosphonate therapy, such as oral Alendronate [choice C] is the first line pharmacotherapy for Osteoporosis based on T-score (T-score ≤-2.5) or fragility fracture.
Oral bisphosphonates are contraindicated in those with esophageal disorders (eg, esophageal stricture) or known malabsorption (eg, Roux-en-Y gastric bypass.

Choice A [Teriparatide] or Romosozumab are anabolic agents used in patients with severe high fracture risk: eg, T-score of ≤-2.5 plus a fragility fracture, T-score of ≤-3.0 in the absence of fragility fracture[s], history of severe or multiple fractures.
Choice B [Raloxifene] is the selective estrogen receptor modulator (SERM) of choice for Osteoporosis when there is an independent need for Breast cancer prophylaxis because it reduces the risk of fracture, has eight-year safety and efficacy data; However, in general Bisphosphonates are preferred over SERMs for Osteoporosis.
Choice D [Denosumab] can be used in patients with severe high fracture risk who cannot tolerate anabolic agents or if they are contraindicated.

95. CARDIOLOGY – DEEP VEIN THROMBOSIS [HISTORY AND PHYSICAL]

Unilateral edema or swelling with a difference in calf or thigh circumferences [choice D] is the most useful finding for suspected Deep vein thrombosis (DVT).

Patients with a difference in calf circumference >3 cm are twice as likely to have DVT as unilateral edema is the most specific symptom.

Other findings of DVT include:
- Leg pain occurs in 50% of patients but is nonspecific
- Tenderness occurs in 75% of patients but is nonspecific.
- Warmth or erythema of the skin over the area of thrombosis (also nonspecific)

Homans' sign (calf pain on passive dorsiflexion of the foot) [choice E] is unreliable for the presence of DVT.

96. INFECTIOUS DISEASE – VACCINATIONS/HERPES ZOSTER VACCINATION [HEALTH MAINTENANCE]

Zoster vaccine recombinant, adjuvanted [choice A] is an FDA-approved vaccine for the prevention of Herpes zoster (Shingles) in adults 50 years and older.

In addition to reducing the risk of Shingles it also reduces the risk of Postherpetic neuralgia.

Choice B [Tetanus-diphtheria-pertussis toxoid booster] would be recommended 10 years after the last booster or if the patient has a deep &/or dirty laceration with a last booster ≥5 years.

Choice C [20-valent pneumococcal conjugate vaccine] is indicated in adults ≥65 years or <65 years with risk factors.

Choice D [Pneumococcal polysaccharide vaccine (*PPSV23*] is given 1 year after PCV 15 as an alternative to the PCV20 in adults ≥65 years or <65 years with risk factors.

Choice E [Meningococcal B vaccine] is a childhood vaccination given at 2, 4, and 12 months.

97. MUSCULOSKELETAL – SYSTEMIC LUPUS ERYTHEMATOSUS [LABS AND DIAGNOSTIC STUDIES]

The 2 autoantibodies that are specific for Systemic lupus erythematosus are:
- **Anti-Smith (anti-Sm) [choice C] — think "Smith most Specific**
- **Anti-double-stranded DNA (anti-dsDNA) — also useful for monitoring flares and treatment of flares (levels increase during flares); thinks anti-<u>ds</u>DNA <u>d</u>isease <u>s</u>oars.**

This patient has classic symptoms and signs of Systemic lupus erythematosus [eg, young patient with fatigue, arthralgia, pleuritic chest pain, a pleural friction rub, arthritis, and renal involvement (hematuria, proteinuria)].

Choice A [Anti-topoisomerase I antibodies], also known as Anti Scl-70 antibodies, are hallmark of diffuse Systemic sclerosis (Scleroderma).

Choice B [Antinuclear antibodies] are sensitive for SLE, but they are not specific as positive ANA can be seen in many inflammatory autoimmune conditions.

Choice D [Anti-Ro antibody], or anti-SSA antibodies, are commonly seen in Sjögren's disease.

Choice E [Anti cyclic citrullinated peptide antibody] are specific for Rheumatoid arthritis.

98. INFECTIOUS DISEASE – STAPHYLOCOCCAL TOXIC SHOCK SYNDROME [HISTORY AND PHYSICAL]

Rapid onset of hypotension (systolic blood pressure ≤90 mmHg) [choice B] is hallmark of Staphylococcal toxic shock syndrome (TSS), often resulting in tissue ischemia and organ failure.

The hypotension is caused by toxin-induced cytokine release which decreases systemic vascular resistance and causes leakage of fluid from the intravascular to the interstitial space.

Staphylococcal TSS should be suspected in patients with rapid onset of fever, rash, hypotension, and multiorgan system involvement.

Use of tampons are associated with 50% of cases of TSS;

Nonmenstrual causes include surgical and postpartum wound infections, mastitis, sinusitis, osteomyelitis, arthritis, and burns.

Choice A [Raised target lesions] is hallmark of Erythema multiforme.

Choice C [Pulse rate <60 beats per minute] is a nonspecific finding. Patients with TSS are often tachycardic to compensate for the hypotension to maintain cardiac output.

Choice D [Splinter hemorrhages on the nailbeds] may be seen with Infective endocarditis.

Choice E [Diffuse petechiae] can be seen with Rocky Mountain spotted fever or thrombocytopenia.

99. DERMATOLOGY - ALOPECIA AREATA [CLINICAL INTERVENTION]

Intralesional corticosteroids [choice D] is the first line treatment for limited, patchy hair loss in adults with Alopecia areata (eg, <25% scalp hair loss).

The goals of treatment are to promote regrowth and limit hair loss.

Alopecia areata is usually self-limiting, with complete regrowth of hair in 80% of patients, but some mild cases are resistant.

Alopecia areata should be suspected if there are:
- smooth, circular, discrete areas of complete hair loss that develop over a period of a few weeks.
- exclamation point hairs: short broken hairs for which the proximal end of the hair is narrower than the distal end may also be seen.

Choice A [Topical Minoxidil] can be used in the management of Androgenetic alopecia.

Choice B [Refer for psychiatric counseling] is used for Trichotillomania, which appears as a round patch of alopecia on the vertex with a tonsure pattern ("Friar tuck sign") and broken hairs of different lengths.

Choice C [Oral Baricitinib] can be used for extensive hair loss.

Choice E [Topical Diphenylcyclopropenone (DPCP)] can be used for refractory Alopecia areata.

100. PROFESSIONAL PRACTICE – PATIENT AND PROVIDER RELATIONSHIPS

Only with the patient's expressed permission should family members be informed of medical information as the patient's wishes should be honored [choice A].

It is the patient's right to share whatever to whomever they choose to.

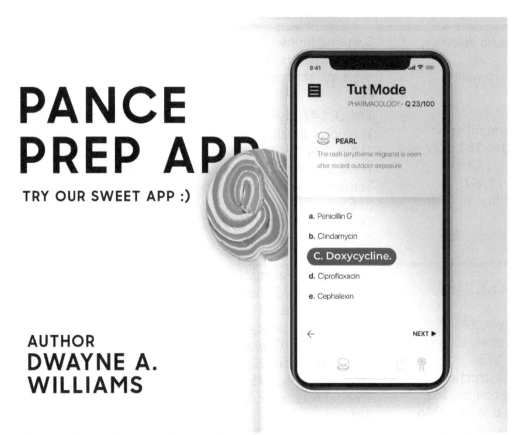

PANCE PREP APP

TRY OUR SWEET APP :)

AUTHOR
DWAYNE A. WILLIAMS

Over 15,000 clinically-based practice examination questions specifically formulated to enhance clinical skills and improve performance on examinations, such as the PANCE, PANRE, OSCES, USMLE, end of rotation examinations and comprehensive medical examinations.

Special clinical pearls, disease review, explanation of the answers, test taking strategies and much more.

3 modes,
Timed mode to simulate the exams
Tutor mode that allows you to review the disease states in addition to the questions and **improve mode** to enhance your weak areas.

For every question in tutor mode, there is a feature for a hint to see if you are going in the right direction, answer explanation, a clinical pearl, and a bonus questions. Create your own examination based on organ systems or task areas. The ultimate study and exam preparation app!

PANCE PREP QUESTION APP

EARN 20 CATEGORY 1 SELF-ASSESSMENT CME CREDITS

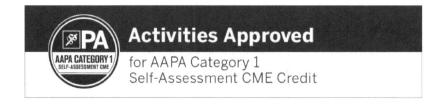

Activities Approved
for AAPA Category 1
Self-Assessment CME Credit

ALSO AVAILABLE

CYTOCHROME P450 INDUCERS

John was **wort**hy when referred & <u>**inducted**</u> into sainthood for giving up **chronic alcohol** use & placing him**self on a real** fast, **fend**ing off **greasy carbs**, leading to **less warfare** with **theo**logians.

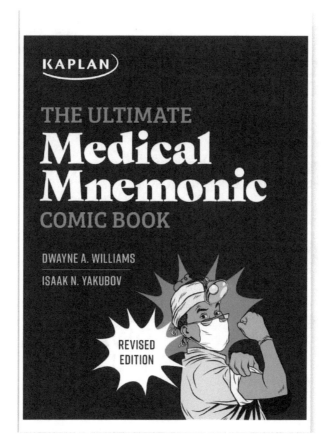

drugs that induce CP450 system can lead to decreased levels of certain drugs ex. warfarin (less warfare), theophylline (theologians) and phenytoin

INDUCERS OF THE P450

- **St. Johns Wort**
- **rifampin** (referred)
- **chronic alcohol use**
- **sulfonylureas**
     (self on a real)
- **Phenytoin**
- **Phenobarbital** (fend)
- **Griseofulvin** (greasy)
- **Carbamazepine**
     (carbs)

KAPLAN

THE ULTIMATE
Medical
Mnemonic
COMIC BOOK

DWAYNE A. WILLIAMS

ISAAK N. YAKUBOV

REVISED EDITION

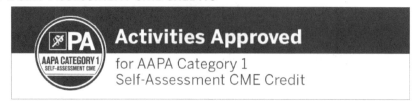

Activities Approved
for AAPA Category 1
Self-Assessment CME Credit

B

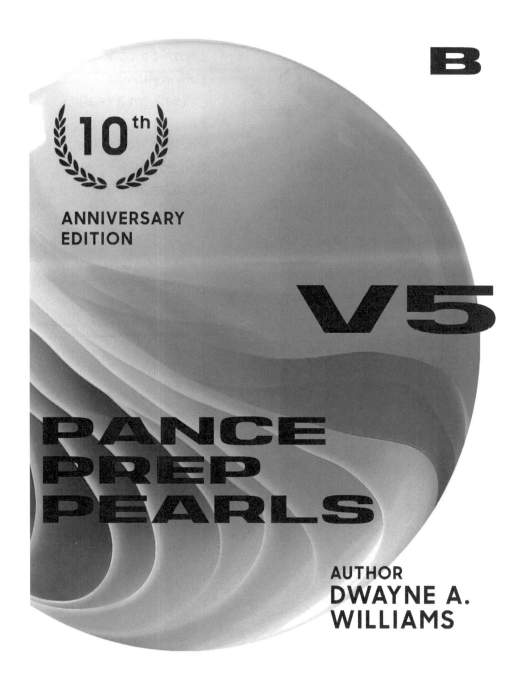

10th

ANNIVERSARY EDITION

V5

PANCE PREP PEARLS

AUTHOR
DWAYNE A. WILLIAMS

Made in United States
Troutdale, OR
10/04/2024

23433342R00257